INFECTION PREVENTION AND CONTROL

2ND EDITION

Infection Prevention and Control

Applied microbiology for healthcare

Dinah Gould

and

Chris Brooker

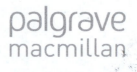

First published 2000
Reprinted twice
Second edition 2008

Published by
PALGRAVE MACMILLAN
Houndmills, Basingstoke, Hampshire RG21 6XS and
175 Fifth Avenue, New York, N.Y. 10010
Companies and representatives throughout the world

PALGRAVE MACMILLAN is the global academic imprint of the Palgrave Macmillan division of St. Martin's Press, LLC and of Palgrave Macmillan Ltd. Macmillan® is a registered trademark in the United States, United Kingdom and other countries. Palgrave is a registered trademark in the European Union and other countries.

ISBN-13: 978–0–230–50753–1
ISBN-10: 0–230–50753–0

This book is printed on paper suitable for recycling and made from fully managed and sustained forest sources. Logging, pulping and manufacturing processes are expected to conform to the environmental regulations of the country of origin.

A catalogue record for this book is available from the British Library.

10 9 8 7 6 5 4 3 2 1

17 16 15 14 13 12 11 10 09 08

Printed and bound in China

Contents

8   Wound infections   165

9   Respiratory infections   190

10   Infections associated with intravascular devices   208

11 Enteric infection 221

12 Infection risks from blood and body fluids 244

List of Figures

List of Tables

Preface

All staff working in health and social care settings encounter patients or residents who are at risk of infection or already have an established infection. One in every 10–12 patients admitted to acute hospitals will develop a healthcare-associated infection (HCAI), and people in a variety of community settings, including their own homes, will have infections. In addition to problems of infection that have existed for decades, and the resurgence of others such as tuberculosis, many 'new' conditions of major concern such as severe acute respiratory syndrome (SARS) and human immunodeficiency virus (HIV) are caused by infective agents.

Knowledge of how infection occurs, the precautions required to contain it and methods of preventing infection occurring in the first place are essential information for everybody who works in health and social care settings. Experienced practitioners and infection prevention and control specialist nurses have access to a wide range of advanced texts and specialist resources, but the needs of students and non-specialist practitioners have tended to be overlooked.

This second edition is aimed at exactly this group of readers and has been expanded to cater for the needs of staff employed in social care because they work collaboratively with the healthcare team. The book introduces the important concept of applied microbiology with the aid of information boxes and new practice application boxes with suggested activities to enhance clinical application and understanding. The text has been fully updated with new reference material, including many new web-based sources, although we have been careful to refer readers to important seminal works where relevant. (Please note that all websites cited have been accessed by us in 2007 and the early part of 2008.)

The book has been reorganized into three sections to improve clarity. Part I, Microbiology, covers fundamental information about microbiology with emphasis on clinical application, drawing on a wide range of practical examples. Part II, Principles of Infection Prevention and Control, presents the principles of infection prevention, control and treatment. Part III, Applying Knowledge to Practice, has specific chapters that deal with particular aspects such as urinary and wound infections and the risks posed by blood and body fluids. The concluding chapter looks at the epidemiology of selected communicable diseases, both old and new. Numerous cross-references between chapters help to link microbiological theory with what health and social care workers do and see in practice.

Each chapter is extensively referenced and where appropriate readers are offered suggestions for further reading and other sources of information. Many informative illustrations help readers to 'make sense' of new material. Chapter outcomes at the beginning of each chapter inform the reader about what they should know after reading the chapter, and provide a framework for learning. Self-assessment questions for each chapter (with answers provided in Appendix I) enable readers to check their knowledge and identify topics needing further work. A comprehensive glossary of the 'language' of microbiology and infection prevention is provided in Appendix II.

This book will help readers to develop their evidence-based practice and, most importantly, will assist in the continual efforts required to improve the quality of health and social care.

DINAH GOULD, *London*
CHRIS BROOKER, *Norfolk*

Acknowledgements

Special thanks to Elspeth Hardy, infection prevention and control specialist nurse, The Queen Elizabeth Hospital, King's Lynn, Norfolk.

Note

This book should not be used as a primary source for prescribing, dispensing or administering drugs. While all reasonable care has been undertaken to ensure accuracy, the authors and publishers are not responsible for any damage caused to any person, which may occur if a reader prescribes, dispenses or administers drugs on the basis of information given here. Readers are responsible for checking the manufacturer's product information and a national formulary before calculating doses or administering any drug.

Readers should also be aware that the publication of new research findings and guidelines concerning infection prevention and control will continue to affect their evidence-based practice.

Every effort has been made to trace all the copyright holders but if any have been inadvertently overlooked the publishers will be pleased to make the necessary arrangements at the first opportunity.

Website

This book is also supported by an engaging companion website, available at www.palgrave.com/nursing/GouldBrooker. A useful resource containing self-test sections, hotlinks and critical thinking questions, it is designed to help the reader monitor and enhance their understanding of the subject matter.

Foreword

Second editions of books are not published by accident; they are published because, in the eyes of the publisher, they have been successful and they have been purchased and found useful by readers. It is, therefore, a pleasure and an honour to be asked again to write the foreword of this book: *Infection Prevention and Control: Applied Microbiology for Healthcare*.

Since the theory of spontaneous generation was disproved by Louis Pasteur and antibiotics were discovered by Alexander Fleming, we know, respectively, what causes infection and how to kill bacteria. Other simple principles, such as the root mean square law, which dictates that you keep as far away from a source of infection as possible unless you are taking barrier precautions, have meant we know just about everything that we need about infection control. The euphoria when penicillin was discovered and produced in commercially viable amounts must have been immense, and many subsequent antibiotics have been invented to deal with a wider spectrum of infections. Similarly, until recently, we believed we knew how to keep infections at bay and possibly even thought that hospital acquired infections would soon become a historical curiosity. However, in the UK and the USA, the phenomenon of MRSA has emerged and it is only part of a growing catalogue of bacteria that greet the immunologically compromised (the old, the very young and the injured) in hospitals. Of course, the existence of some of these 'superbugs' is a direct consequence of the continued indiscriminate use of antibiotics. Family doctors, in particular, are faced daily with the consequences of either treating the person in front of them or taking decisions for the greater good that may mean, on occasion, restricting their prescription of antibiotics.

It is clear, therefore, that the necessity for infection control is as high as ever and the existence of this book is quickly justified. It is hard to say, professionally, who is at the 'front line' in infection control: the doctor, the nurse or the cleaner; but, regardless of who is there in a working capacity, the patient is always on the front line, and the nurse/carer is part of a team that can make infection prevention and control the difference between life and death. In addition, health professionals increasingly are being allowed to prescribe a wider range of drugs and, to use antibiotics wisely, they need to be aware of the possibility of any adverse consequences of their actions.

The subject of infection prevention and control is in very safe hands with the authors of this book who have done a superb job of revising and updating the text. It is practical throughout, beginning with a very cogent overview of microbiology: What are microorganisms? How does the body react? How do we know? How can we treat infection? Part II of the book covers infection control: policies and practice. However, the largest section is Part III in which knowledge is applied to practice and this covers a wide range of topics from wound infections to sexually transmitted diseases. Each chapter is meticulously referenced and up to date.

It is likely that, like the poor, infections will always be with us, but, as a result, we have this superb second edition of *Infection Prevention and Control* to help prepare and refresh health and social care students, registered nurses and other health professionals in one of the most essential features of their job – doing the patient or client no harm.

ROGER WATSON
Professor of Nursing
University of Sheffield

PART I

Microbiology

CHAPTER 1

Microorganisms and disease

CHAPTER OUTCOMES

After reading this chapter, you should be able to:

➤ List the main groups of microorganism causing infection

➤ Explain the terms 'infection', 'colonization', 'commensal', 'pathogen', 'opportunist' and 'virulence'

➤ List the possible signs and symptoms of infection

➤ Give examples of bacteria of the following morphological types: bacilli, cocci, spirochaetes and vibrios

➤ Give an example of each of the following: Gram-negative bacterium, Gram-positive bacterium, acid-fast bacillus, a spore-forming bacterium, an aerobe and an anaerobe

➤ State the ways in which microorganisms gain access to the internal tissues of the host, and give an example for each mechanism suggested

➤ List the ways in which bacteria multiply, and point out their clinical significance

➤ List the main mechanisms by which microorganisms are disseminated, and give an example for each route suggested

➤ Explain how viruses cause disease and give an example

➤ Give one example of a human disease caused by a fungus, a protozoon, a *Chlamydia* and a helminthic (worm) infestation

Introduction to medical microbiology and microorganisms causing disease

Microbiology is the study of microorganisms – living organisms that are too small to be examined without a microscope. Organisms with a diameter of 0.1 mm are just visible to the naked eye, but magnification is required to study them in detail. Medical microbiology is the study of microorganisms that play a role in human infection.

Infection is caused by bacteria, viruses, fungi, protozoa and a few minor groups (mycoplasmas, rickettsiae and chlamydiae). Parasitic worms are multicellular and often clearly visible to the naked eye, but their eggs and larvae are microscopic, so the presence of infection is frequently detected in specimens sent to the microbiology department. In recent years, minute virus-like protein particles called 'prions' have also been implicated in causing infection. An example is the agent causing Creutzfeldt–Jakob disease (CJD) (Chapter 14).

Bacteria

Bacteria live everywhere. Most are saprophytes (organisms that live on dead organic material) present in soil and water. They play a vital role degrading complex organic molecules from dead animals and plants into simple organic ones. These molecules are recycled during metabolism by living organisms.

Pathogenic activity

Approximately 50 species of bacteria are 'pathogenic' (able to cause disease). Virulence – the ability to generate infection – is a complex phenomenon related to the physiology of both pathogen and host. Some bacteria are always highly virulent. For example, exposure to *Yersinia pestis* (bacterium causing plague) will almost certainly result in infection. However, some bacteria, particularly those causing infections in hospital, are of low pathogenicity. They cause infection only in people whose immune status is compromised by illness, drugs or the invasive procedures they have undergone (for example surgery, intubation or the insertion of an intravenous line). They do not attack healthy tissues. These bacteria are called 'opportunists'. *Pseudomonas, Klebsiella* and *Proteus* are typical opportunists.

Other bacteria live harmlessly in or on one particular part of the body. These make up the normal flora and are called 'commensals' (Table 1.1). They receive shelter and benefit the host by keeping potentially dangerous microorganisms at bay. If they gain access to a different anatomical location, however, they can generate infection. *Escherichia coli* (*E. coli*), normally present in the bowel, can cause urinary tract infection if it gains access to the bladder. This is an example of endogenous (self-) infection, occurring when the organisms responsible originate from the same individual. Exogenous (cross-) infection occurs when microorganisms originate from another source: patients, residents, staff or the environment.

Table 1.1 The normal human flora

Anatomical location	Organisms
Skin	*Staphylococcus epidermidis*, micrococci, diphtheroids
Upper respiratory tract	*Streptococcus viridans*, diphtheroids, *Moraxella catarrhalis* (*Neisseria catarrhalis*)
Large intestine/bowel	*Bacteroides* spp., *Escherichia coli*, *Streptococcus faecalis*, *Proteus*, clostridia, lactobacilli
Vagina	Lactobacilli, *Staphylococcus epidermidis*

Infection and colonization

Infection occurs when pathogens gain access to host tissues and elicit a response. Infection in a wound is indicated by the appearance of inflammation and pus. The patient may become pyrexial, and a wound swab will indicate the presence of large numbers of the causative organism.

The response to the pathogens may, however, be slight or absent, a situation described as 'colonization'. A colonized wound is free from inflammation, a swab indicating scanty bacterial growth. When colonization occurs, several species of bacteria may be present, often referred to as 'mixed bacterial growth' on laboratory reports. Colonization is of clinical significance because the organism may multiply in large numbers to form a reservoir. Colonization is usually the precursor to infection when outbreaks occur (Muder et al., 1991), and even if the original patient escapes the clinical signs and symptoms of disease, cross-infection may still occur.

There are many situations in which infection may be difficult to diagnose: the very young, older adults, people with communication difficulties and people with some mental health problems or a learning disability (see below).

▬ PRACTICE APPLICATION 1.1 ▬

Being Alert to the Possibility of Infection

The expected signs of infection may not be present, for example an elevated temperature may not always be present in older people. Health and social care practitioners need to be alert to other signs, symptoms and changes in behaviour that may indicate an infection.

For example:

➤ Complaints of feeling generally unwell

➤ A rash characteristic of the infection

➤ Chills and shivering

➤ Changes in vital signs other than temperature, such as an increase in respiratory rate

➤ General aches and pains in the muscles and joints

➤ A dry mouth with a furred tongue

➤ Loss of appetite

➤ Nausea and vomiting

➤ Diarrhoea

➤ Headache

➤ Loss of continence in adults

➤ 'Accidents' in previously continent toddlers and children

➤ Behavioural changes in children, becoming fretful and miserable

➤ Increasing confusion and disorientation in older adults

➤ Enlarged and tender lymph nodes

NB The knowledge that a particular infection, for example chickenpox or gastroenteritis, is present in the population at the time should alert health and social care practitioners to the possibility of infection.

Activity

Think about a patient, client or resident in your care who had an infection without the usual signs being present.

➤   What first alerted you to the possibility of an infection?

➤   Which of the features listed above were present?

Describing bacteria

Bacteria can be described in terms of their:

- Morphology (shape)
- Ultrastructure (fine detail)
- Response to dyes used on microscope specimens, for example the Gram stain reaction
- Spore formation
- Oxygen requirement.

Morphology

Four morphological forms exist (Figure 1.1):

- **Cocci** are round. When they are arranged in pairs, they are known as 'diplococci'. Examples include *Streptococcus pneumoniae* (which causes pneumonia) and *Neisseria gonorrhoeae* (leading to gonorrhoea). Clusters of cocci are termed 'staphylococci'. Examples include *Staphylococcus aureus*, a constituent of the normal skin flora, which in some members of the population is also able to operate as a wound pathogen, and *Staphylococcus epidermidis*, an opportunist able to cause infection in very sick people, although not in the healthy. 'Streptococci' are round bacteria attached to one another in chains. They cause sore throats and a wide range of other infections encountered in hospital and the community.

- **Bacilli** (for example *Pseudomonas*, *Klebsiella*, *Proteus* and *E. coli*) are rod shaped, occurring singly or in chains. They are notorious for their ability to cause serious infection in hospital. An extended-spectrum beta-lactamase (ESBL)-producing *E. coli*, which is resistant to several antibiotics, can cause urinary infection and is responsible for around 2,000 cases of blood poisoning each year in England and Wales (Health Protection Agency, 2007) (see Chapter 4 for beta-lactamase-producing bacteria). Several bacteria which cause food poisoning, including *Shigella* and *Salmonella*, also belong to this group.

- **Vibrios** are curved bacteria. Examples include *Vibrio cholerae* (resulting in cholera) and *Campylobacter* (responsible for food poisoning).

■ **Spirochaetes** are very small, flexible, spirally shaped bacteria. Typical members of the group include *Treponema pallidum* (which causes syphilis), *Leptospira interrogans* (serotype *icterohaemorrhagiae*) (Weil's disease, which is transmitted to human hosts from infected rats) and *Borrelia burgdorferi* (Lyme disease).

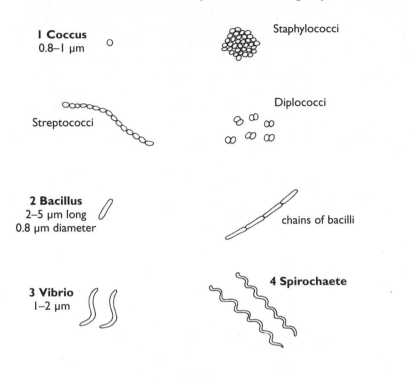

Figure 1.1 Bacterial morphology I

All bacteria are unicellular, but their size and shape vary widely (Figure 1.1). Specimens must be 'fixed' (killed) and stained before they can be examined with the light microscope. Advances in electron microscopy have made it possible to study the ultrastructure of cells. The cells are, however, still dead because examination must be performed with the specimens in a vacuum. The image that appears does not represent the dynamic, living state.

Ultrastructure

The bacterial cell ultrastructure differs from that of multicellular organisms. The cells of multicellular organisms are 'eukaryotic' (that is, they have a true nucleus). Their genetic material is enclosed in a membrane to form this nucleus. Numerous cytoplasmic organelles (minute, subcellular structures in the cytoplasm that perform specific functions in a cell) are also present, a few exceptions being membrane bound. In contrast, bacteria are 'prokaryotic' (lacking a true nucleus and nuclear membrane). The chromosome containing the genetic material (nucleic acid) lies directly in the cytoplasm, as do all the organelles, including the ribosomes (sites of protein synthesis) and storage granules. The mesosome, an infold of the outer membrane, is the site of respiration, analogous to the eukaryotic mitochondria.

Figure 1.2 depicts a 'typical' bacterial cell, although few species display all the possible features shown. Some species (for example *N. gonorrhoeae*) possess hair-like processes called 'pili' used to attach the bacterium to a potential host, while other, highly motile forms (for example *Salmonella* and *Proteus*) have one or more flagella (Figure 1.3). However, all bacterial species are surrounded by a rigid cell wall, giving the cell support and protecting its contents. This is absent in eukaryotic cells. Some bacteria have a mucous capsule around the cell wall, reducing the risk of desiccation in dry conditions. Strains of *Klebsiella* equipped with a mucous capsule are particularly likely to contribute to cross-infection and to result in outbreaks of disease because they survive well on dry skin (Casewell and Desai, 1983).

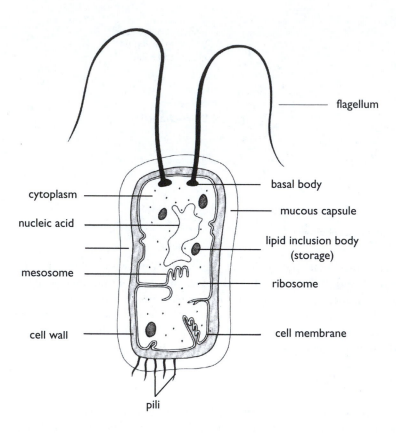

Figure 1.2 The 'typical' bacterial cell

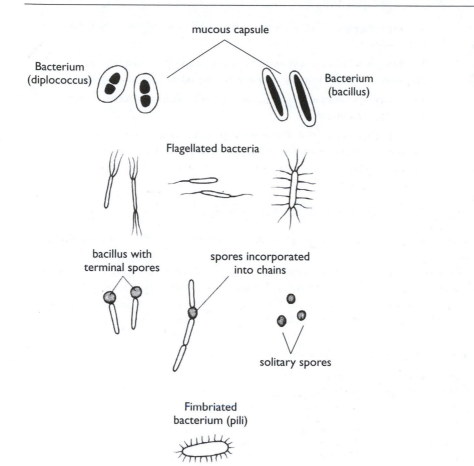

Figure 1.3 Bacterial morphology II

The Gram stain reaction

In the natural condition, bacteria are colourless. The Gram staining reaction is used in the first step of laboratory identification (see below).

The Gram stain reaction

➤ A thin film of the specimen is smeared onto the surface of a glass microscope slide

➤ The slide is passed through the flame of a Bunsen burner 3–4 times to 'fix' (kill) the microorganisms

➤ The slide is covered with purple dye (methyl or crystal violet) for 15 seconds, the excess fluid then being poured away

> ➤ The slide is flooded with Gram's iodine for up to 1 minute, after which the iodine is drained

> ➤ The slide is flooded with acetone for 2–5 seconds before being washed with water or ethanol to rinse away any dye not taken up by the bacteria

> ➤ The bacteria are counterstained by pouring a red dye (carbol fuchsin) onto the slide for 20 seconds

> ➤ The slide is blotted dry and is then ready for examination. Gram-positive organisms retain the violet dye and appear deep purple. Gram-negative bacteria stain pink because they lose the violet stain, taking up the red counterstain instead

Examples of typical Gram-positive and Gram-negative bacteria are shown in Table 1.2.

Mycobacterium does not respond well to Gram staining because the thick, waxy cell wall is impermeable to the dyes. It can be identified by the acid-fast (Ziehl–Neelsen) staining technique. *Mycobacterium tuberculosis* (tuberculosis) is thus described as being 'acid fast' or as the 'acid-fast bacillus' (AFB).

Table 1.2 Typical Gram-positive and Gram-negative bacteria

Gram-positive bacteria	Gram-negative bacteria	
Bacillus	Acinetobacter	Neisseria
Clostridium	Bacteroides	Proteus
Corynebacterium	Escherichia coli	Salmonella
Staphylococcus	Haemophilus	Vibrio
Streptococcus	Klebsiella	Yersinia

The Gram stain reaction is valuable because it distinguishes structural differences between Gram-positive and Gram-negative bacteria and provides an indication of their behaviour. Much of the difference between the two groups is explained by a variation in the chemical composition of the cell wall (see Chapter 4). Gram-positive bacteria tend to be more resistant to desiccation (dehydration) and tolerate dry conditions. Gram-negative species thrive in damp situations and are generally more resistant to antibiotics. Few species of Gram-positive bacteria are flagellated, so they lack motility.

Spore formation

Clostridium and *Bacillus* form spores under adverse conditions. A thick, protective capsule surrounds the cell, and its metabolism slows. In favourable conditions, the spore germinates, releasing the bacterium. Spores are very resistant to heat and desiccation, remaining viable over long periods. The ability to form spores that will survive in adverse environmental circumstances is restricted to the Gram-positive species. The spores of *Bacillus anthracis* (causes anthrax) and *Clostridium tetani* (causes tetanus) survive dormant for years, able to withstand extremes of temperature and exposure to disinfectants that would destroy vegetative cells. Germination occurs when conditions become favourable for growth and reproduction.

Oxygen requirement

Bacteria display a variety of oxygen requirements (Table 1.3):

- Obligate aerobes – their growth demands an environmental oxygen supply
- Obligate anaerobes – those unable to tolerate the presence of oxygen
- Facultative aerobes – can grow whether or not oxygen is available.

Table 1.3 Oxygen requirements of some medically important bacteria

Oxygen requirement	Example
Aerobic/facultatively aerobic	Campylobacter Escherichia coli Klebsiella Neisseria gonorrhoeae Neisseria meningitidis Proteus Salmonella Shigella
Anaerobic	Bacteroides Clostridium Treponema pallidum

Establishing infection

Before infection is possible, a susceptible host must encounter a virulent microorganism. The pathogen must complete the following stages:

- Gain access to the host tissues
- Move to a favourable site
- Multiply successfully in spite of the defence mechanisms mustered by the host
- Reproduce so that new pathogens can escape to be disseminated, thus completing the life cycle.

Invasion: portals of entry

Invasion occurs by inhalation or ingestion, via the urogenital (urinary and genital) tracts, by inoculation and by vertical transmission:

- **Inhalation** occurs via the respiratory tract, the nose or mouth being the route taken by colds and influenza viruses and organisms causing tuberculosis, diphtheria and the infections of childhood (measles and mumps). Infectious airborne particles are released as aerosols. Droplet transmission only occurs when an individual with an infectious respiratory condition exhales forcefully, sneezes or coughs. Only the smallest particles (1–5 μm) can reach the lower airways. The length of contact between the source and the potential new case increases the risk of transmission. This is because the longer the period of exposure, the greater the risk of inhalation.

- **Ingestion** via the mouth into the gastrointestinal tract occurs when food or water is contaminated. *Salmonella, Shigella, Campylobacter, Vibrio* and the virus causing poliomyelitis enter by being ingested.

- The **urogenital tract** is the route taken by pathogens causing sexually transmitted infections *(N. gonorrhoeae, T. pallidum* and *Trichomonas vaginalis)*. Urinary pathogens, principally Gram-negative bacilli, gain access via the urethra.

- The **inoculation** of pathogens via the skin or mucous membranes can occur during surgical incision, accidental injury or injection with a needle (hepatitis B, hepatitis C and human immunodeficiency virus – HIV), or via the mouthparts of an insect (*Plasmodium* following a mosquito bite).

- **Vertical transmission** occurs via the placenta from the maternal to the fetal circulation (for example rubella virus and *T. pallidum*) or by contamination as the fetus travels down the birth canal at parturition. *N. gonorrhoeae* and other microorganisms can be transferred to the eyes of the infant from an infected mother in this way, resulting in ophthalmia neonatorum (pus discharging from the eyes of an infant commencing within 21 days of birth). *Chlamydia trachomatis* can cause serious respiratory and eye infections in babies exposed to the organism during birth. Women infected with HIV may transmit the infection to the fetus via the placenta, in breast milk or at parturition when the infant is exposed to contaminated blood and cervical secretions. A baby may develop shingles if its mother had varicella (chickenpox) during pregnancy (Enders et al., 1994).

Virulence

The ability to establish an infection depends on virulence. Several factors contribute, including the size of the inoculating dose and the ability to invade host tissues and damage them.

Size of the inoculating dose

Except in the case of very virulent pathogens, a large number of microorganisms is more likely to overwhelm the host defences, and there is a greater chance that at least some will reach a site suitable for growth and multiplication. Most pathogens invade specific sites. *N. gonorrhoeae* invades the delicate cervical and urethral epithelia but not the tough squamous epithelial cells lining the mouth or vagina. Viruses responsible for colds invade the nasal epithelium and conjunctivae but not the oral mucosa.

Ability to invade host tissues

This depends on the bacterium's morphological characteristics and its production of enzymes and toxins.

Morphological characteristics

Pili on the surface of *N. gonorrhoeae* allow it to attach to epithelial cells on the cervix uteri and urethra. Mutant strains without pili lack virulence. The presence of a protective mucous capsule surrounding the cell wall reduces the risk of desiccation in particular strains of Gram-negative bacteria, so they survive longer on the hands and are more likely to cause cross-infection (Cooke et al., 1981).

Enzyme production

Enzyme production is a property of many bacteria. Staphylococci, streptococci and *Clostridium perfringens* release haemolytic enzymes, which destroy erythrocytes (red blood cells). *Staphylococcus aureus* releases an enzyme called 'coagulase', which clots plasma, thus protecting the bacteria from phagocytosis (Chapter 2).

Toxins

Toxins are of two types, depending on the mechanism of synthesis and secretion:

1. **Exotoxins** are secreted by Gram-positive bacteria and released outside the cell into the surrounding extracellular fluid, dissolving and being carried throughout the tissues. Exotoxins destroy host cells or inhibit specific metabolic functions. They include some of the most lethal chemicals known. The exotoxin secreted by *Clostridium botulinum* (which causes botulism) interrupts the transmission of nervous impulses, paralysing the victim. *Clostridium tetani* releases an exotoxin that excites neurones in the central nervous system. The muscular spasms of 'lockjaw' result. Exotoxins released by *Staphylococcus aureus* and *Bacillus cereus* result in food poisoning.
2. **Endotoxins** develop as part of the cell wall of Gram-negative bacteria. They include *Salmonella enterica* serovar Typhi (which causes typhoid), *Neisseria meningitidis* (meningococcal meningitis) and *Shigella sonnei* (dysentery). The release of endotoxins corresponds with the symptoms of fever and malaise experienced by the host.

Ability to damage host tissues

The ability to damage host tissues is closely related to the ability to invade. Damage may be structural (the tissues being physically destroyed) or physiological (normal function becoming disturbed). In most cases, both types occur. *Staphylococcus aureus* destroys tissue because the infection causes abscess formation. Pyrexia occurs simultaneously with this.

Bacterial growth requirements

Knowledge of bacterial growth requirements is essential when attempts are made to grow and identify organisms in the laboratory. Bacteria are unicellular and therefore more susceptible to environmental fluctuations than larger, more complex multicellular organisms. As with higher forms of life, their growth requirements include:

- Water
- An energy source
- A suitable pH
- A suitable temperature
- Protection from ultraviolet rays.

Water

Water accounts for more than 80 per cent of the bacterial cell volume and is essential for the growth and survival of vegetative bacterial cells. Some Gram-positive species (for example *Bacillus* and *Clostridium*) avoid desiccation by forming resistant spores under adverse conditions.

Energy source

Nourishment is derived from substances available within the environment. Bacteria vary enormously in their ability to utilize different sources of nourishment:

- Phototrophs use carbon dioxide as their sole source of carbon to synthesize all the complex organic molecules they need. Like plants, they obtain their energy from sunlight.
- Chemotrophs obtain energy by oxidizing inorganic material.
- Heterotrophs require a supply of nutrients such as carbohydrates or amino acids produced by other organisms. Most pathogens are heterotrophs. Generally speaking, the more adapted the organism is to a strictly pathogenic existence, the more demanding its growth requirements (for example *Pseudomonas*, *E. coli* and *Klebsiella*). In contrast, *N. gonorrhoeae* has complex growth requirements and cannot survive long outside the human host. *T. pallidum*, which is even more fastidious, has never been cultured outside living tissues.

Bacteria also vary in their ability to use sources of energy during respiration (see Oxygen requirement, above):

- Obligate aerobes (for example *M. tuberculosis*) are unable to grow in the absence of oxygen.
- Facultative aerobes are tolerant of the presence of free atmospheric oxygen in their environment and will grow whether or not it is available. Most human pathogens belong to this group.
- Obligate anaerobes cannot grow unless all traces of oxygen are removed from their environment. They tend to cause infections deep within the tissues. *Clostridium* spp. cause gangrene and tetanus, infections originating when the bacteria gain access to the deep tissues.
- Microaerophilic bacteria grow more rapidly in the presence of only traces of free oxygen.

A suitable pH

Bacteria vary widely in their tolerance of acidic or alkaline conditions, ranging from pH 4 to 9. Human pathogens generally prefer a pH within the range 7.2–7.6, but there are exceptions. Cholera vibrios, for example, thrive best at pH 8. They affect the small intestine, which receives pancreatic fluid at the same pH. Lactobacilli (part of the normal flora) inhabiting the vagina grow best at a pH of about 4.

A suitable temperature

All species have a preferred temperature range, but within this there is an optimum temperature at which they grow best:

- Mesophilic bacteria thrive within the 25–40 °C range. Human pathogens fall into this group, thriving optimally at 37 °C.
- Psychrophilic bacteria grow best at approximately 20 °C and slowly at 4 °C. They influence health not by causing infection, but by their ability to spoil food that has not been properly refrigerated.
- Thermophilic bacteria, growing at temperatures of 55–90 °C do not operate as human pathogens.

Protection from ultraviolet rays

Most pathogenic bacteria grow best in darkness and are rapidly destroyed by ultra-violet light, whether it is natural, in sunlight or arising from an artificial source. This is the rationale behind 'airing' clothing in the sun as it dries.

Bacterial reproduction and genetics

Bacteria reproduce asexually by simple binary fission, or by sexual reproduction in which there is transfer of genetic material.

Binary fission

Binary fission is a simple, asexual process involving the division of a bacterial cell into two genetically identical daughters. The rate of binary fission depends on the particular species and the environmental circumstances. In ideal conditions (for example a warm, damp hospital ward), a typical Gram-negative bacillus such as *E. coli* will divide about once every 20 minutes. Others, for example *M. tuberculosis*, divide very slowly. The results of laboratory tests for *E. coli* are available within 24 hours, but a diagnosis of tuberculosis may not become available for weeks. Treatment for tuberculosis is, however, started on the basis of clinical findings and other tests, for example skin tests, radiography and the presence of AFBs in a sputum specimen.

Asexual reproduction does not involve the exchange of genetic material so there can be no provision for genetic variation, a disadvantage as the organisms are thus limited in their ability to respond and adapt to environmental pressures.

Sexual reproduction

Sexual reproduction is, however, possible in particular bacteria containing a small amount of extrachromosomal deoxyribonucleic acid (DNA) lying within the cytoplasm. This is called a 'plasmid'. It accounts for approximately 1 per cent of the total amount of genetic material present in those cells which contain it. A transfer of genetic material between bacteria is possible according to three mechanisms: conjugation, transduction and transformation (Figure 1.4).

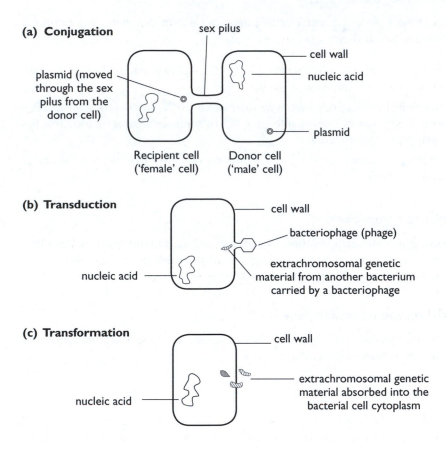

Figure 1.4 Sexual reproduction in bacteria (diagrammatic)

Conjugation

Conjugation (Figure 1.4a) is an important means of genetic exchange, particularly among Gram-negative bacilli. Sex pili coded by the DNA of a donor or 'male' cell attach to the recipient or 'female' cell. Plasmid replication follows, one copy passing to the recipient, the other remaining within the cytoplasm of the donor.

Transduction

Transduction (Figure 1.4b) occurs when a bacteriophage (a viral parasite of bacteria) invades a bacterial cell. Bacteriophages (or phages) operate in a manner similar to that of conventional viruses, entering the bacterium and replicating to release a large number of new infective agents, which in turn attack more bacteria. Transduction results when new phages carry extrachromosomal genetic material from the old host to a new one that previously lacked a plasmid.

Transformation

Transformation (Figure 1.4c) takes place when a strand of extrachromosomal DNA is absorbed via the cell wall into the cytoplasm of a bacterium.

Sexual reproduction in bacteria is of great clinical significance as genes conferring antibiotic resistance can be exchanged, resulting in the emergence of antibiotic-resistant strains (see below). The widespread, indiscriminate use of antibiotics encourages the survival of bacteria carrying plasmids conferring antibiotic resistance on their hosts (Chapter 4).

PRACTICE APPLICATION 1.2

Plasmid-mediated Antibiotic Resistance

Plasmid-mediated antibiotic resistance occurs between enterococci. Plasmids carrying the genes for vancomycin resistance can also spread between enterococci and other more virulent bacteria, including *Staphylococcus aureus* (Tenover et al., 2004).

Commonly, resistance to glycopeptide antibiotics (vancomycin and teicoplanin) occurs in the bowel commensals *Enterococcus faecium* and *Enterococcus faecalis*. These enterococci are known as glycopeptide-resistant enterococci (GRE) or vancomycin-resistant enterococci (VRE).

Activity

➤ Consider the implications of a vancomycin-resistant gene transferring from enterococci to meticillin*-resistant *Staphylococcus aureus* (MRSA). For example, how it will influence the choice of antibiotic therapy for infections caused by *Staphylococcus aureus*.

*The new British Approved Name (BAN) for methicillin.

Escape and dissemination

In many cases, bacteria leave the body via the entry route, but there are exceptions. Those causing gastroenteritis gain access via the mouth and leave in the faeces, thus being said to be disseminated by the faecal-oral route.

Microorganisms are spread from one individual to the next by direct and indirect contact. Dissemination is also possible via the airborne route, in contaminated food and water, and by insects.

Contact

Contact is the major route of spread in hospital and probably in the community too (Gould, 1991).

In hospital, bacteria are spread chiefly on the hands of staff because patients and equipment are handled so frequently, increasing the number of opportunities for cross-infection. Ignaz Semmelweiss first demonstrated the relationship between handwashing and a reduction in infection rate in a series of epidemiological studies in the 1840s. Since this time, controlled trials in hospital have been notable by their absence because withholding hand decontamination would be ethically and aesthetically undesirable (Larson, 1988). There is, however, a wealth of indirect evidence to implicate hands as vectors of cross-infection.

Persuasive evidence is provided by Casewell and Phillips (1977), who demonstrated that the hands of staff in an intensive care unit were contaminated with *Klebsiella* of the same strain as those colonizing and infecting the patients. Laboratory studies indicated that the bacteria could remain viable for up to 150 minutes following artificial inoculation onto the hands of volunteers – ample time for cross-infection to occur during normal nursing activities. Clothing, air and ward dust were seldom contaminated with the same strains, confirming earlier views that Gram-negative bacteria are not readily disseminated by the airborne route (Noble et al., 1976). In later studies within the same unit, the rate of cross-infection declined following the introduction of a strict regimen of hand decontamination (Casewell and Phillips, 1977).

In the community, there is evidence that many pathogens traditionally thought to rely on droplet spread are in fact disseminated by contact (Worsley et al., 1994). Laboratory simulations demonstrate that individuals are more likely to develop upper respiratory tract infection after contact with hands and objects (fomites) contaminated with the virus than after exposure to virus-laden aerosols (Gwaltney et al., 1978). It has been suggested that coughing and sneezing release infected droplets that settle onto surfaces, including clothes, in the immediate environment. Hands then transfer them to other objects (crockery, door handles and so on), reaching new victims after their hands have in turn become contaminated. The virus reaches the nose and conjunctivae when the face is touched. Hand hygiene can reduce the incidence of upper respiratory tract infection.

Similarly, rotavirus, responsible for vomiting and diarrhoea, although released in droplets, appears to be spread by hand contact. In an experimental incidence study conducted in a day nursery, a reduction in the rate of infection was demonstrated when handwashing was promoted among children and the staff attending them (Black et al., 1981). It is worth remembering that handwashing is a simple and cost-effective way to reduce infection (Gould, 1997) (see below).

PRACTICE APPLICATION 1.3

Handwashing

Handwashing is the most effective infection control measure, but it is performed too seldom by hospital staff, often because they are too busy. Hands should be washed even when gloves are worn because virus particles can leak through and contamination can occur as the gloves are removed (Gould, 1994).

Hand hygiene is equally important in the community, where it can be more difficult to achieve. For example, difficulties arise when a large number of people are seen quickly in clinics and health centres (Gould, 1997).

Activity

➤ Reflect on the frequency of your own handwashing when dealing with patients, clients or residents.

➤ Have there been occasions when it was difficult to wash your hands?

Airborne spread

Airborne spread occurs only over short distances for Gram-positive pathogens and for viral infections such as chickenpox. An extensive review of the literature confirms that cross-infection by this route is unusual outside high-risk environments such as operating theatres and burns units (Ayliffe and Lowbury, 1982). In theatre, skin scales laden with staphylococci gain access to open tissues, often by landing on the drapes from the air. They may originate from either the patient or the attendants. The airborne route is also important in burns units. The skin is the body's chief defence against bacteria, and when it is no longer intact, patients become extremely susceptible to infection.

Contaminated food and water

Contaminated food readily operates as a vehicle for bacteria. Such infection is the result of poor hygiene in homes, restaurants, fast-food outlets, shops and factories (North, 1989). In most cases, contamination occurs via the hands. *Salmonella* contaminating the fingers from infected food sources can survive handwashing. Spread is therefore by the faecal-oral route.

Waterborne spread occurs in areas where sanitation is poor. Cholera is endemic throughout much of the developing world, including Asia, but outbreaks rarely occur in the UK. Typhoid is also transmitted via contaminated water. Legionnaires' disease (caused by the bacterium *Legionella pneumophila*) is disseminated in contaminated aerosols (Woo et al., 1986); outbreaks of this have occurred in the UK.

Insect vectors

Insect vectors disseminate infection by mechanical and biological transmission. Mechanical transmission occurs when pathogens are transferred from one locality to another via the surface of the insect, often on its feet. Houseflies operate as mechanical vectors for *Shigella* (Cohen et al., 1991). In hospital, flies, Pharaoh's ants and other arthropods may carry pathogenic bacteria present within the clinical environment (Fotedar et al., 1992).

Biological transmission involves a complex interaction between pathogen and vector. *Plasmodium*, the agent responsible for malaria, multiplies within the gut of the mosquito, increasing the number of protozoa available to contribute to an infective dose. Transmission occurs when the insect bites a human host.

Reservoirs of infection

Reservoirs of infection develop when favourable conditions promote the growth and reproduction of a large number of bacteria. Reservoirs may develop on the skin of staff, patients or residents, leading to cross-infection. The contribution of environmental reservoirs to cross-infection depends on their situation. A large reservoir of bacteria in a drain is unlikely to contribute to healthcare-associated infection (HCAI) because there are few opportunities for transfer to susceptible individuals, but if the reservoir involves objects that have the potential for contact with patients, residents or staff, the risks are considerable.

Viruses

Viruses are the smallest microorganisms known to be infective agents. They vary in size between 10 and 300 nm, being visible only under the electron microscope. Each virus particle consists of a core of nucleic acid – either DNA or ribonucleic acid (RNA) but never both (Table 1.4). The nucleic acid is surrounded by a protein coat (or capsid) to protect it from adverse environmental conditions (Figure 1.5). Prions (see above) are less complex structures that consist of proteins but no nucleic acids. 'Enveloped' viruses are surrounded by a lipid and protein capsule with structures permitting them to attach to their hosts. Attachment is always at specific sites on the cell surface for which the virus has particular affinity. For example, the influenza virus attaches itself to mucoprotein receptors. Viruses lacking a capsule are described as 'naked'. Viruses are classified by their shape and by the type of nucleic acid they contain – DNA or RNA.

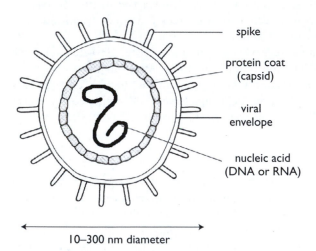

spike

protein coat (capsid)

viral envelope

nucleic acid (DNA or RNA)

10–300 nm diameter

Figure 1.5 The structure of a typical virus

Table 1.4 Examples of some medically significant viruses

Viruses	Diseases/conditions
DNA viruses	
Adenoviruses	Sore throat, conjunctivitis
Herpes viruses Herpes simplex types 1 and 2 (HSV-1, HSV-2) Varicella zoster virus (VZV) Epstein–Barr virus (EBV) Cytomegalovirus (CMV)	Cold sores, genital infections Chickenpox (varicella), shingles (herpes zoster) Glandular fever (infectious mononucleosis), Burkitt's lymphoma Cytomegalovirus infection
Hepadnavirus Hepatitis B virus (HBV)	Hepatitis B
Papovaviruses Human papilloma virus (HPV)	Warts, tumours (for example cervix)
Poxvirus Smallpox virus	Smallpox (variola)
RNA viruses	
Picornaviruses Enteroviruses, poliovirus, echoviruses, coxsackie viruses Rhinovirus Hepatitis A virus (HAV)	Poliomyelitis, respiratory infection Common cold (coryza) Hepatitis A
Togaviruses Flaviviruses Rubella virus	Yellow fever, dengue, West Nile fever, hepatitis C German measles (rubella)
Reoviruses Reovirus Rotavirus	Respiratory tract infection, gastroenteritis Gastroenteritis
Calicivirus Norovirus	Gastroenteritis
Rhabdovirus Rabies virus	Rabies
Arenavirus Lassa virus	Lassa fever
Orthomyxovirus Influenza viruses	Influenza
Paramyxoviruses Parainfluenza virus Respiratory syncytial virus (RSV) Mumps virus Measles virus	Parainfluenza Respiratory infection Mumps (infectious parotitis) Measles (morbilli)
Retrovirus Human immunodeficiency virus (HIV-1, HIV-2) Human T cell lymphotropic viruses (HTLV-I, HTLV-II)	HIV disease Leukaemia
Filoviruses Ebola virus Marburg virus	Ebola fever Marburg fever

Viruses are responsible for a wide range of human, animal and plant infections. Some, called 'bacteriophages' (phages), attack bacteria. Viruses depend on living organisms to provide a host; they are not capable of growth or reproduction outside living cells. Lacking cellular structure and the characteristics of living organisms, they may occupy the 'grey' zone between animate and inanimate organisms, perhaps resembling life as it first appeared on earth. It is, however, more likely that they represent degeneration into highly successful and sophisticated parasites. Their existence as the earliest form of 'life' in the absence of potential victims is hard to explain.

Life cycle

The virus gains entry by 'endocytosis' (a bulk transport process that transfers material into cells) and is carried into the cytoplasm in a vacuole via the cell membrane (plasma membrane), leaving its protein capsule redundant on the cell's surface (Figure 1.6). Viral nucleic acid is then released to take over the genetic

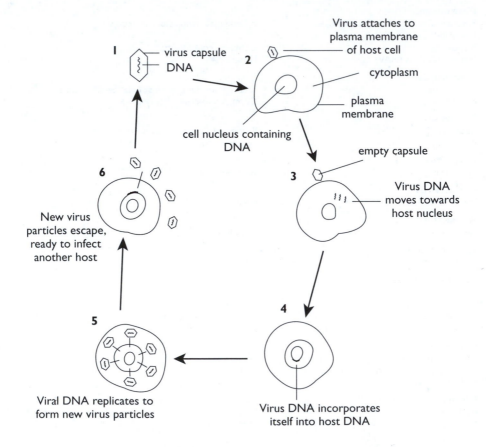

Figure 1.6 The life cycle of a typical virus

machinery of the host cell. Viral DNA becomes incorporated into the DNA of the host, assuming command of genetic control. The host synthesizes viral proteins rather than its proteins, so that new virus particles are generated and eventually released, completing the life cycle. RNA viruses use the enzyme 'reverse transcriptase' to manufacture DNA templates of their own RNA for incorporation into the genome of the host. Some viruses lie dormant within the host cell for long periods of time but can become activated to produce active infections, a good example being herpes zoster (shingles).

Viruses and malignancy

The earliest relationship between viruses and malignancy was demonstrated in 1908 when it was established that, in poultry, a certain type of leukaemia could be transmitted to previously healthy birds from those with the disease. It is now known that viruses are responsible for malignancies in many animals, and they appear to play a role in the development of some human cancers. There is an established association between the human papilloma virus (HPV) and cervical cancer, the Epstein–Barr virus and Burkitt's lymphoma, and the hepatitis viruses and hepatocellular cancer (Campbell, 2006). A vaccine against HPV types 6, 11, 16 and 18 has been licensed for use for females aged 9–26 years. In the UK, the vaccine against the HPV is to be added to the routine NHS immunization programme (Department of Health, 2007). It will be routinely offered to girls aged 12–13 years from the autumn of 2008, with a later catch-up programme for girls aged up to 18 years.

Fungi

Fungi are classified independently of plants and animals. Over 300,000 species are known but like bacteria, most are harmless saprophytes. Approximately 200 species cause human disease. In common with other microorganisms, some fungi (for example *Candida albicans*) can cause opportunistic infections in people who are immunocompromised (Arkell, 2003), especially those with a malignant disease (Krcmery and Barnes, 2002). *Aspergillus* species can cause severe, frequently fatal infections in people who are already immunocompromised (Kibbler, 2003). All fungi are eukaryotic, and because of the similarities between fungal and mammalian cells, it has never been easy to develop antifungal agents. The drugs used to treat fungal infections are often highly toxic, and few are available without a prescription. Some fungi, for example yeasts, assume a simple structure and exist as single cells, but complex forms exist with filamentous hyphae branching to form an extensive interwoven mesh called a 'mycelium' (Figure 1.7). These forms are visible to the naked eye, but as microscopic examination is necessary for identification, the diagnosis of fungal infection (mycosis) is made in the microbiology laboratory.

There are three types of mycosis:

1. **Superficial mycoses** occur when infection is superficial or restricted to the skin and its appendages (hair and nails), for example athlete's foot (*Trichophyton interdigitale*), or mucous membranes, as in the case of vaginal thrush (*Candida albicans*).

2. **Subcutaneous mycoses** (for example mycetoma) affect the skin, subcutaneous tissues and bone. Slow, localized spread occurs.

3. **Systemic mycoses** (caused by, for example, *Cryptococcus*) develop, and then the hyphae penetrate the deeper tissues. In temperate climates, systemic mycoses are uncommon except in the immunocompromised patient.

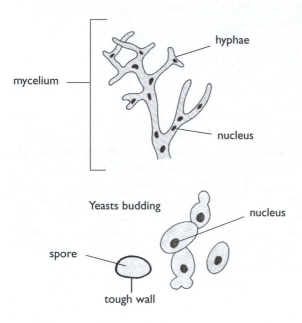

Figure 1.7 Fungal morphology

Table 1.5 gives examples of fungi that may cause human disease.

Table 1.5 Human mycoses

Fungus	Mycosis
Candida albicans	Thrush (candidiasis/candidosis)
Trichophyton interdigitale	Athlete's foot (tinea pedis)
Cryptococcus neoformans	Meningitis (immunocompromised patients)
Microsporum audouini	Ringworm (commonly affecting the scalp)
Aspergillus fumigatus	Respiratory infection (immunocompromised patients)

Protozoa

Protozoa are unicellular, microscopic animals (Figure 1.8). Most species are harmless, but some operate as human pathogens, especially in hot climates. Others are a threat to the immunocompromised host (Table 1.6). *Plasmodium*, the protozoan responsible for malaria, is discussed in Chapter 14.

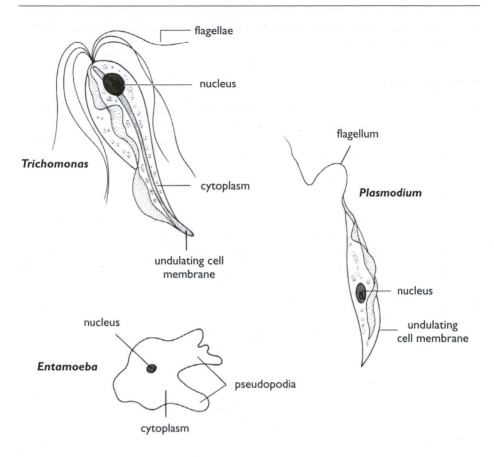

Figure I.8 Pathogenic protozoa

Table I.6 Pathogenic protozoa

Protozoan	Condition
Trichomonas vaginalis	Vaginal infection
Plasmodium spp.	Malaria
Trypanosoma rhodesiense, Trypanosoma brucei gambiense	Trypanosomiasis (some types known as 'sleeping sickness')
Leishmania donovani	Leishmaniasis – kala-azar (generalized visceral form)
Entamoeba histolytica	Amoebic dysentery
Toxoplasma gondii	Latent infection, damage to fetus in utero

Rickettsiae and chlamydiae

These microorganisms bridge the gap between viruses and bacteria. Like viruses, they are small and rely on their hosts to grow and reproduce, but they are suscepti-ble to antibiotics. Typhus, caused by *Rickettsia prowazeki*, is spread by human head and body lice. *Chlamydia trachomatis*, responsible for nonspecific urethritis (inflam-mation of the urethra), is discussed in Chapter 13. The microorganism also causes an eye condition known as trachoma or trachoma inclusion conjunctivitis (TRIC), which can lead to blindness.

Mycoplasmas

Mycoplasmas are similar to bacteria but lack cell walls. Without a rigidly supporting outer structure, they change shape readily during growth, often becoming filamentous. The most significant mycoplasma operating as a human pathogen is *Mycoplasma pneumoniae*, which infects the lungs.

Helminths

Numerous species of helminths (worms) give rise to human infestation. Some are large and multicellular, others microscopic (Figure 1.9). There are two main groups: round and flat (Table 1.7). It is impossible to cover all types and with that in mind only the threadworm will be discussed.

Table 1.7 Medically significant helminths

Helminth	Type
Enterobius vermicularis	Round (threadworm/pinworm)
Ascaris lumbricoides	Roundworm
Toxocara canis	Dog roundworm
Trichinella spiralis	Pork roundworm
Necator spp.	Roundworm (hookworm)
Strongyloides stercoralis	Roundworm
Taenia saginata	Beef tapeworm
Taenia solium	Pork tapeworm
Schistosoma haematobium	Fluke

Threadworms

Enterobius vermicularis, the threadworm, is probably the most common helminthic parasite in the Western world. Cats, dogs or any other domestic animals do not carry it; humans are the only hosts. The eggs are swallowed, hatch in the small intestine and migrate to the large intestine, where they live. Within two weeks, the worms reach maturity, mate and migrate to the rectum, emerging at night to lay their eggs on the perianal (around the anus) skin. The eggs adhere to the skin by a sticky fluid, which causes intense itching. When the victim scratches, large numbers of eggs are transferred to the hands and fingernails. These are thence transferred back to the mouth, recommencing the cycle of infection. People of any age can become infested with threadworms, but children are the most commonly affected (Blake, 2003). The entire family should be treated, however, as the eggs are easily transferred onto towels, soap and upholstery, and may be ingested with food if it is touched with inadequately washed hands (see Practice Application 1.4). The eggs can survive in the environment for several weeks. Threadworms are not dangerous but they can be a nuisance, causing discomfort, irritability and sleeplessness.

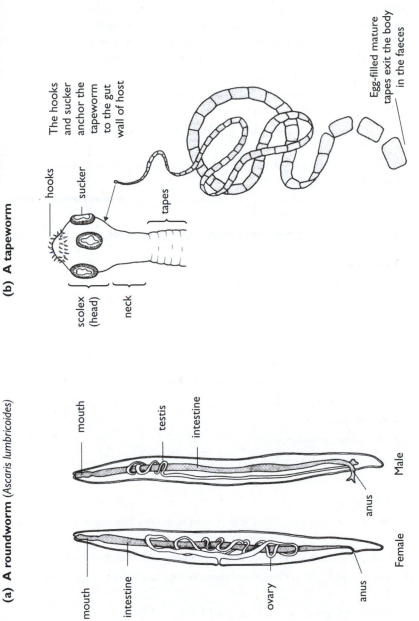

(a) A roundworm (*Ascaris lumbricoides*)

mouth

testis

intestine

anus

Male

mouth

intestine

ovary

anus

Female

(b) A tapeworm

The hooks
and sucker
anchor the
tapeworm
to the gut
wall of host

hooks

sucker

scolex
(head)

neck

tapes

Egg-filled mature
tapes exit the body
in the faeces

Figure 1.9 Helminthic infestation

PRACTICE APPLICATION 1.4

Controlling Threadworm Infestation

Control is achieved by:

➤ All household members taking one of the proprietary antihelminthic agents such as piperazine, which paralyses the worms, or mebendazole, which starves them by preventing sugar absorption. These preparations are available over the counter but instructions must be followed carefully.

➤ Good handwashing before eating and after using the lavatory and scrubbing of the nails, which should be kept short

➤ Vacuuming the house (carpets and upholstery) to remove eggs and avoid reinfestation

➤ Avoiding sharing towels and flannels. Towels, flannels and bed linen should be frequently laundered

SELF-ASSESSMENT

1. Most bacteria and fungi are pathogenic. True? or False?

2. Which of the following are typical opportunists?

    (a) *Staphylococcus aureus*

    (b) *Candida albicans*

    (c) *Legionella pneumophila*

    (d) None of these

3. Infection always causes an elevation in body temperature. True? or False?

4. Which of the following are bacilli?

    (a) *Pseudomonas*

    (b) *Staphylococcus epidermidis*

    (c) *Mycobacterium pneumoniae*

    (d) *Treponema pallidum*

5. What is virulence?

6. *Staphylococcus aureus* never forms spores, even under dry conditions. True? or False?

7. Most microorganisms are disseminated by the airborne route. True? or False?

8. Diseases caused by viruses include influenza, rubella and hepatitis A. True? or False?

9. Plasmodium is a protozoan. True? or False?

10. List the measures taken to control threadworm infestation.

REFERENCES

Arkell S (2003) Update on oral candidosis. *Nursing Times* **99**(48): 52–3.

Ayliffe GA and Lowbury EJ (1982) Airborne infection in hospital. *Journal of Hospital Infection* **3**: 217–40.

Black RE, Dykes AC, Kern EA et al. (1981) Handwashing to prevent diarrhoea in day centres. *American Journal of Epidemiology* **113**: 445–51.

Blake J (2003) An action plan to prevent and combat threadworms. *Nursing Times* **99**(42): 18–19.

Casewell M and Desai N (1983) Survival of multiply-resistant *Klebsiella aerogenes* and other Gram-negative bacteria on the finger tips. *Journal of Hospital Infection* **4**: 350–60.

Casewell M and Phillips I (1977) Hands as a route of transmission for *Klebsiella* colonisation and infection in an intensive care ward. *Journal of Hygiene* **80**: 295–300.

Campbell K (2006) Understanding how viruses can cause malignant disease. *Nursing Times* **102**(36): 30–1.

Cohen D, Green M and Block C (1991) Reduction of transmission of shigellosis by control of houseflies (*Musca domestica*). *Lancet* **337**: 993–7.

Cooke EM, Edmonson AS and Starkey W (1981) The ability of strains of *Klebsiella aerogenes* to survive on the hands. *Journal of Medical Microbiology* **14**: 443–50.

Department of Health (DH) (2007) *HPV Vaccine Recommended for NHS Immunisation Programme.* Available www.gnn.gov.uk/.

Enders G, Miller G, Craddock-Watson J et al. (1994) Consequences of varicella and herpes zoster in pregnancy: a prospective study of 1739 cases. *Lancet* **343**: 1548–51.

Fotedar R, Banerjee U, Singh S et al. (1992) The housefly (*Musca domestica*) as a carrier of pathogenic micro-organisms in a hospital environment. *Journal of Hospital Infection* **20**: 209–15.

Gould D (1991) Nurses' hands as vectors of hospital-acquired infection: a review. *Journal of Advanced Nursing* **16**: 1216–25.

Gould D (1994) Nurses' hand decontamination practice: results of a local study. *Journal of Hospital Infection* **28**: 15–30.

Gould D (1997) Giving infection control a big hand. *Community Nursing Notes* **15**: 3–6.

Gwaltney JM, Moskalski PB and Hendley JO (1978) Hand to hand transmission of rhinovirus colds. *Annals of Internal Medicine* **88**: 463–7.

Health Protection Agency (HPA) (2007) Press statement *Infections caused by ESBL-producing E. coli.* Available www.hpa.org.uk/.

Kibbler C (2003) Aspergillus: the invisible threat. *Nursing Times* **99**(48): 48–50.

Krcmery V and Barnes AJ (2002) Non-albicans Candida spp. Causing fungaemia: pathogenicity and antifungal resistance. *Journal of Hospital Infection* **50**: 243–60.

Larson E (1988) A causal link between handwashing and risk of infection? Examination of the evidence. *Infection Control and Hospital Epidemiology* **9**: 28–34.

Muder RR, Brennan C, Vickers RM et al. (1991) Methicillin resistant colonisation and infection in a long-term care facility. *Annals of Internal Medicine* **114**: 107–12.

Noble SW, Habbema JD, Van Furth R et al. (1976) Quantitative studies of the dispersal of skin bacteria into the air. *Journal of Microbiology* **9**: 53–61.

North N (1989) Food scares: the role of the Department of Health, in E Harrison and A Gretton (eds) *Health Care UK: An Economic, Social and Policy Audit.* Policy Journals, Newbury, pp. 65–77.

Tenover FC, Weigel LM, Appelbaum PC et al. (2004) Vancomycin-resistant *Staphylococcus aureus* isolate from a patient in Pennsylvania. *Antimicrobial Agents and Chemotherapy* **48**: 275–80.

Woo AH, Yu VL and Goetz A (1986) Potential in-hospital modes of transmission of *Legionella pneumophila. American Journal of Medicine* **80**: 567–73.

Worsley M, Ward K, Painer L et al. (1994) *Infection Control: A Community Perspective.* Daniels, Cambridge.

FURTHER READING AND INFORMATION SOURCES

Centers for Disease Control and Prevention (US agency) – www.cdc.gov/.

Greenwood D, Slack R, Peutherer J and Barer M (2007) *Medical Microbiology,* 17th edn. Churchill Livingstone, Edinburgh.

Health Protection Agency (UK agency) – www.hpa.org.uk/.

Peters W and Pasvol G (2006) *Atlas of Tropical Medicine and Parasitology,* 6th edn. Mosby, Edinburgh.

CHAPTER 2

Response of the body to infection

CHAPTER OUTCOMES

After reading this chapter, you should be able to:

➤ Name the cells of the immune system and list their functions

➤ Distinguish between innate and acquired immunity, and describe their roles in defending the body against infection

➤ Explain the meaning of 'antigen' and 'antibody' (immunoglobulin) and give examples

➤ List the factors that may influence individual susceptibility to infection

➤ Discuss the concept of 'herd immunity' and the factors that may affect it

➤ Discuss the principles of immunization

➤ Outline a standard immunization schedule used during childhood

➤ Explain why hospital inpatients are at particular risk of developing infection

Introduction to the immune response, immunity and immunology

Immunity is a state of resistance to an infectious agent. It depends on the ability of the body to recognize and dispose of foreign microorganisms and other naturally occurring organic substances, including pollen, dust and cells from other organisms. Immunology is the study of the cells and molecules responsible for recognizing and destroying foreign substances. The immune response involves:

■ Detecting foreign substances or their toxins within the body
■ Communicating this information to the parts of the system responsible for their neutralization and destruction
■ Recruiting the immune attack
■ Suppressing the immune response once the harmful agent has been eliminated.

Types of immunity

There are two types of immunity that interact and are necessary for survival. These are innate (natural, nonspecific) immunity – the same in health for every member of the species – and adaptive (specific), or acquired, immunity, which is subject to individual variation.

Innate immunity: preventing invasion

Innate immunity helps the body to resist invasion. These defences include intact skin, anatomical adaptations, normal flora and antimicrobial substances that include hydrochloric acid and lysozyme. If its mechanisms fail, it attempts to contain the pathogens by limiting their access to the tissues.

Intact skin and mucous membranes

The anatomical arrangement of the tissues, the secretion of fluids that wash foreign materials from the body and the presence of normal flora covering the skin and lining the gut prevent invasion. Intact skin and mucous membranes are the body's chief defences against infection. The skin has a low pH because sebaceous secretion is acidic (the 'acid mantle'), supporting a population of commensal bacteria that keep pathogens at bay. Infection supervenes when the skin is broken or becomes excessively moist. Moisture beneath the breasts or between the toes frequently leads to infection, especially if hygiene is poor.

Gastrointestinal tract

The gastrointestinal tract's powerful acid and alkaline secretions protect the gastrointestinal system. The pH of gastric acid is too low for most bacteria to survive. Its effectiveness has been demonstrated by an epidemiological investigation revealing that, during an outbreak of dysentery, infection was confined to patients whose natural gastric secretions had been suppressed by taking antacids (Horan, 1984). In the small intestine, the high pH (8–9) destroys most pathogens, although the bacteria responsible for typhoid and cholera survive.

Respiratory tract

The coughing and sneezing reflexes protect the respiratory system. Inside the nose, the nasal conchae increase the surface area of the mucosal surface and cause air to eddy, thus trapping small particles as inspired air travels over them. Lymphoid tissue in the pharyngeal, palatine and lingual tonsils traps any remaining pathogens. The entire respiratory tree, except for the alveoli, is lined with specialized mucus-secreting epithelium. The mucus traps foreign substances and is then carried upwards to the pharynx by the action of the cilia. Smoking paralyses the action of the cilia, eventually destroying them altogether and thus contributing to the development of lower respiratory tract infections in heavy smokers.

Female genital tract

The vagina contains lactobacilli, bacteria that metabolize glycogen in cervical secretions, forming lactic acid. The pH of the healthy adult vagina is approximately 4.5, inhibiting the growth of other organisms. Before the menarche and after the menopause, the cervical secretions are scant because oestrogen production is low. The vaginal pH is correspondingly higher, and infection is more common in older women. Women taking antibiotics to treat recurrent infections are at risk of developing vaginal infections such as candidiasis (thrush) because the normal vaginal flora are suppressed (Sawyer et al., 1994).

Urinary tract

The bladder has little protection against pathogens, and urinary infections are common, especially during pregnancy. This is probably because the hormone progesterone has a relaxing effect on the tissues, including the urethral aperture, allowing bacteria to enter the bladder more easily. However, the regular and complete emptying of the bladder tends to militate against infection by flushing microorganisms out of the bladder and urethra.

Antimicrobial substances

Lysozyme, an enzyme secreted by macrophages (leucocytes – white blood cells), is present in many body fluids, including tears and saliva. It destroys bacteria by attacking their cell walls but is inactive against strains protected by a thick extracellular mucus coat (see Chapter 1).

Innate immunity: limiting spread

After invasion, inflammation and the activity of phagocytic leucocytes in the blood and tissues limit the spread of the infection. These form part of the innate immune response because they offer the same protection for everybody, operating in the same way. The origins and the basic types of leucocytes are shown in Figures 2.1 and 2.2.

Inflammation and phagocytosis

Inflammation is the response of tissues to trauma, whether injury involves cuts, chemical damage, extremes of temperature, or pathogenic invasion (Figure 2.3). The classic hallmarks of inflammation are:

- Erythema (redness)
- Swelling
- Heat
- Pain
- Loss of function (depending on the site and extent of the injury).

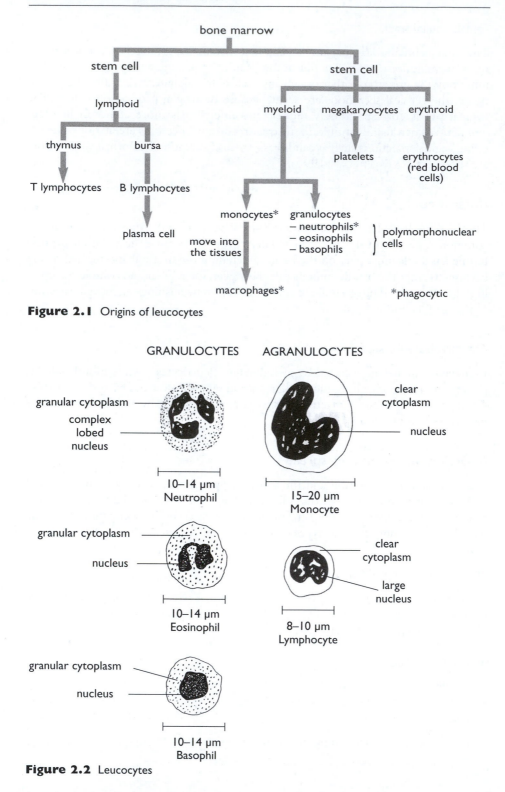

Figure 2.1 Origins of leucocytes

Figure 2.2 Leucocytes

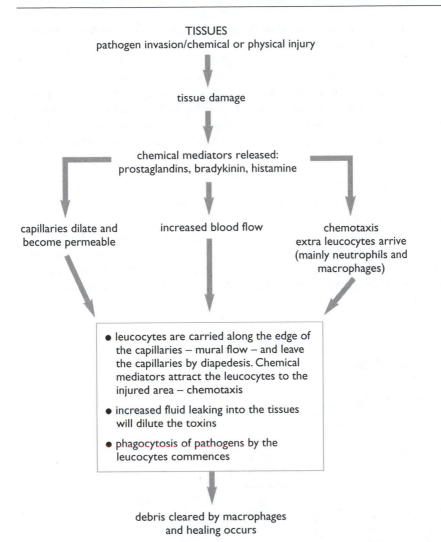

Figure 2.3 Events of inflammation: a summary

The walls of the capillaries dilate in an immediate response to injury, thus becoming more permeable. This action is triggered by the release of prostaglandins from platelets, and other locally acting hormones, particularly bradykinin and histamine. Bradykinin comes from the neutrophils and is responsible for the pain experienced during inflammation. Histamine is produced by the basophils.

Leakage of plasma through the capillary walls into the intercellular space accounts for the swelling (oedema) and contributes to the pain of inflammation by exerting pressure on adjacent nerve endings. Increased blood supply explains the erythema and sensation of heat. This increased blood supply is beneficial because it boosts the local availability of neutrophils (polymorphonuclear leucocytes) and macrophages (derived from monocytes, a type of white blood cell) to combat infection, while the greater volume of fluid helps to dilute the microbial toxins.

Neutrophils begin to appear within the damaged area about an hour after the initiation of inflammation, stimulated by the release of leucocyte-releasing factors, which increase the activity of leucopoietic (leucocyte-producing) tissue in the red bone marrow. Neutrophils entering the blood are carried along the edges of the capillaries to the site of injury (mural flow), escaping into the tissues via slits between the capillary cells (diapedesis). Migration to the injured area takes less than two minutes and is caused by chemical attraction (positive chemotaxis). As the inflammatory response progresses, macrophages begin to congregate within the damaged area, engulfing debris and spent neutrophils. The phagocytic and cytotoxic activity of both neutrophils and macrophages is similar.

Phagocytosis occurs when a neutrophil or macrophage engulfs a pathogen (Figure 2.4). The first step is opsonization, the attachment of a ligand (particle or group of molecules) to the surface of the phagocytic cell, stimulating the action of the contractile proteins myosin and actin that are present within the cytoplasm. Endocytosis follows: the pathogen is engulfed, entering a vacuole created by the phagocytic membrane. Lysosomes (enzyme-containing subcellular organelles) in the cytoplasm fuse with the vacuole, emptying strongly hydrolytic enzymes (catalase and myeloperoxidase) onto the pathogen and destroying it.

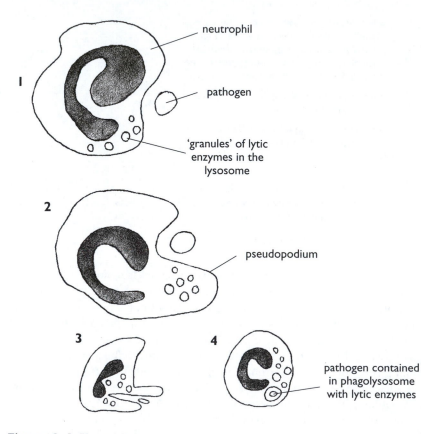

Figure 2.4 Phagocytosis

Opsonins are 'chemical tags' – antibodies and complement proteins with receptors enabling them to recognize and attach to receptors on the surface of foreign molecules, labelling them in order to enhance phagocytosis. Further receptors permit the opsonin to link itself in turn to a phagocyte so that it operates as a bridge between the pathogen and the cell that will engulf it.

Eosinophils (a type of white blood cell) are weakly phagocytic, strongly cytotoxic cells not dependent on opsonins for their action. Enzymes released from inclusions within their cytoplasm are poured onto the surface of the pathogen, destroying it by perforating the cell membrane. Their main activity appears to be the destruction of multicellular parasites too large for phagocytosis.

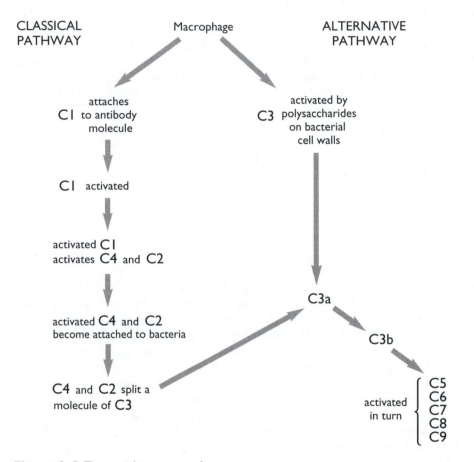

Figure 2.5 The complement cascade

Natural killer (NK) cells do not appear in Figure 2.1 (above), as their origin is obscure. They make up less than 1 per cent of the total leucocyte count, but are powerfully cytotoxic against the host cells that have become infected with viruses. NK cells attach to these cells and release enzymes that destroy the membrane. Their activity is promoted by lymphokines and interferon, and they may play a role in controlling the differentiation of cells in the immune system.

Basophils and mast cells (cells found in the tissues) initiate inflammation by degranulation – the release of histamine from granules in response to the attachment of a particular antibody (immunoglobulin E – IgE) to their membranes. Degranulation also requires a reaction between the antigen and the attached antibodies, and in some cases the action of complement proteins.

Interferons are proteins released by several types of leucocyte (white blood cell) during the immune response. They inhibit viral replication by disrupting the transcription of DNA into RNA.

Complement comprises a group of 20 or so proteins present in an inactive form in body fluids. Activation of the first complement in the sequence occurs on exposure to polysaccharides present in bacterial cell wall, parasites, and by the 'labelling' actions of opsonins and antibodies, an example of interaction between the body's innate and adaptive defence mechanisms. A cascade is triggered in which each active complement component activates the next one in the chain (Figure 2.5), as in the blood-clotting cascade. The final product is called a 'membrane attack complex'. It perforates the cell walls of bacteria, destroying them. The attachment of complement to an antigen–antibody complex results in its destruction (complement fixation).

Several complement proteins have additional functions important in the overall immune response, illustrating the highly complex and economic nature of immunity. For example, C3b is a potent opsonizer; C3a stimulates macrophages to release bactericidal agents and enhances mast cell degranulation; and C5b acts as a chemotactic attractor for neutrophils and macrophages.

Allergy (hypersensitivity)

Approximately 10 per cent of the population show an abnormal, hypersensitive reaction to otherwise harmless materials (pollen, dust, fur and a range of foods including nuts and shellfish, for example). This is the basis of allergy (Hendry and Farley, 2001). 'Anaphylaxis' describes a severe and potentially life-threatening allergic reaction (see below). Many allergic reactions involve the respiratory tract because potential allergens are so often inhaled and a large number of basophils and mast cells are present in the lungs. Immunoglobulin E (IgE) present on the surface of the mast cells and basophils binds to the allergen (foreign material), leading to the release of histamine and bradykinin. Allergic reactions to the latex in rubber examination gloves and other clinical and everyday items are a growing problem among health professionals, and patients who have regular contact with latex during repeated healthcare interventions. Protocols to reduce exposure to latex are required for NHS Trusts and other healthcare providers and these should include the identification of other products that contain latex, for example catheters and some mattresses.

▬ PRACTICE APPLICATION 2.1 ▬

Anaphylaxis

Anaphylaxis is defined as a severe allergic reaction that can lead to asphyxia, shock and cardiac arrest (Jevon, 2004). Its incidence is increasing in the UK and many other countries where it has been estimated that 0.3 per cent of the general population has an episode each year. Causes include allergies to nuts, shellfish, cows' milk, eggs, insect stings, latex and drugs (see Chapter 4). Signs and symptoms include:

➤ urticarial rash with weals

➤ swelling of lips, eyes and tongue

➤ respiratory distress

➤ stridor

➤ wheezing

➤ tachycardia

➤ hypotension

➤ a sensation of impending doom.

Accurate diagnosis can be difficult because reactions can vary in severity and rapid progression is not always the case. Consensus guidelines on the emergency medical treatment of anaphylaxis are available from the Resuscitation Council UK. If a patient or resident collapses and anaphylaxis is suspected, the emergency services must be alerted. It will necessary to maintain the airway and be ready to apply basic life support. Oxygen should be administered if it is available. Adrenaline (epinephrine) will be given as soon as possible to combat shock. It acts by reversing peripheral vasodilation, reducing oedema and encouraging bronchodilation.

Activity

➤ What protocols exist in your workplace/placement for the emergency treatment of anaphylaxis?

➤ What emergency equipment and drugs are available in the event of anaphylaxis?

Resource

Resuscitation Council UK – www.resus.org.uk/.

Pyrexia: in response to infection

Pyrexia is an innate response to infection. It occurs in all vertebrates and is thought to play some beneficial role, perhaps by increasing the metabolic rate so that bacteria and their toxins are more rapidly eliminated from the body. In addition, the rate of tissue repair is increased and the immune response is heightened (Mackowiak, 1994). Pyrexia, however, has its disadvantages. Fever is exhausting, draining the body of energy at a time when the individual is anorexic.

Complications include:

- **A negative nitrogen balance** – for every 1 °C rise in temperature above the norm, the adult pulse rises by approximately 10 beats per minute and the rate of breathing by seven respirations per minute. Glycogen stores become depleted, leading to nitrogen wastage, as protein is catabolized to provide energy.

- **Rigors** – uncontrollable attacks of violent shivering, often associated with the presence of bacterial toxins in the blood.

■ **Febrile seizures** (convulsions) – these typically occur in young children (six months to five years of age) and people with a history of epilepsy. Although transient, they are frightening and can be dangerous as they may lead to trauma, aspiration of secretions or asphyxia.

■ **Delirium** – this is most often seen in young children or older adults, or when pyrexia is marked. The person becomes confused and restless. This may add to the difficulties of isolating people with an infectious condition.

Temperature regulation and infection

Body temperature is controlled by the hypothalamus. An increase in body temperature is a systemic effect of the inflammatory response. Prostaglandins and proteins called 'pyrogens' released by the leucocytes induce fever.

The temperature-regulating centre is often compared to a thermostat. Human core temperature is fixed at about 37 °C in most people, deviations detected by receptor cells in the skin being relayed to the hypothalamus along afferent nerves (Figure 2.6). If the temperature falls below the set point of 37 °C, heat-conserving mechanisms are initiated, while a rise above the set point triggers heat loss (Table 2.1).

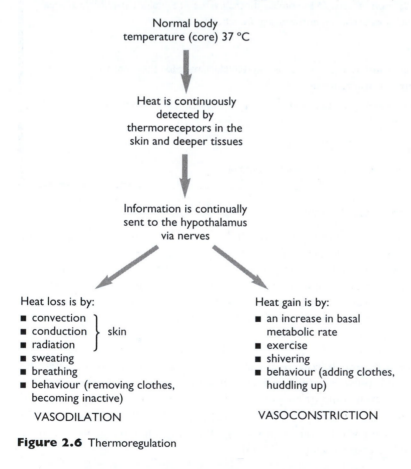

Figure 2.6 Thermoregulation

Table 2.1 Mechanisms of heat loss and conservation

Heat loss	Heat conservation
Skin capillaries dilate Increases heat loss by: ■ convection ■ conduction ■ evaporation (sweating)	Skin capillaries constrict Decreases heat loss by: ■ convection ■ conduction
	Shivering (involuntary muscular activity)
Behavioural activities: removing clothes, stretching out, reducing activity	Behavioural activities: huddling up, putting on extra clothes

When infection supervenes, surface antigens on the bacteria or viruses 'reset' the thermostat to a higher set point by stimulating neutrophils to release pyrogens. Temperature is maintained at this level until the foreign antigens have been neutralized and eliminated. Vasoconstriction and shivering are accompanied by an increase in metabolic rate. The patient feels cold and huddles up irrespective of the number of blankets provided. The magnitude of the fever depends on the infective organism. Mild infections may have little or no effect, but some pathogens (for example *Salmonella enterica* serovar Typhi) stimulate pyrexia of as much as 39–40 °C.

As the infection subsides, vasodilation and perspiration are stimulated. This promotes heat loss, and the patient feels hot and sticky (see below). Some infections are associated with characteristic changes in body temperature that aid diagnosis. In patients with brucellosis, the temperature gradually rises and then resolves over 10 days or so before the cycle repeats.

PRACTICE APPLICATION 2.2

Caring for People with Pyrexia

As fever develops, the patient feels cold and will suffer if attempts are made to reduce the temperature. Drugs that reduce temperature (antipyretics) may mask symptoms indicating the need for a change in treatment, for example a different antibiotic. The kindest and safest option is to allow extra bedclothes, and the appropriate action is to assist in identifying the infection by careful observation and obtaining specimens to aid laboratory diagnosis. Appropriate antibiotics can then be prescribed. Once the person's temperature begins to fall, they will appreciate the removal of any heavy blankets, as well as cold drinks and the use of a fan. Key points on a care plan will include:

➤ Regular monitoring of the temperature, pulse and respiratory rate

➤ Monitoring fluid intake and output

➤ Preventing dehydration

➤ Ensuring adequate nutrition (with sufficient energy, protein, vitamins and minerals)

➤ Ensuring adequate rest (both physical and mental)

➤ Help with hygiene, including mouth care and changing bedclothes and clothing if sweating is a problem

➤ Careful observation for signs of disorientation (febrile seizures in children under 5)

➤ The provision of bedclothes and equipment to ensure comfort at all times and heat loss when appropriate

Adaptive immunity

Adaptive immunity occurs through the coordinated functioning of lymphocytes and macrophages in response to antigens – foreign cells or molecules that have a structure incorporating a ligand able to bind them to the membranes of lymphocytes or the products of lymphocytes (antibodies). Traditionally, two types of adaptive immune response are described: humoral immunity, mediated by B lymphocytes (B cells) and cell-mediated immunity, regarded as the property of T lymphocytes (T cells) (see Figure 2.1 above). However, as research progresses, it is becoming increasingly obvious that the two interact closely, although for the sake of clarity they will be introduced separately here.

Humoral immunity

Humoral immunity refers to the activity of the B lymphocytes in body fluids (humors). They recognize and bind to antigens on the surface of pathogens, neutralizing them. Figure 2.7 shows that binding takes place between antigen-binding sites on the surface of the B lymphocyte and a small region of the pathogen called the 'epitope', which has a complementary shape. The antigen receptor sites on the B lymphocytes are the antibodies (immunoglobulins) with a complementary shape. Antigens are covered with numerous epitopes, and if the cell is large, more than one kind may be present.

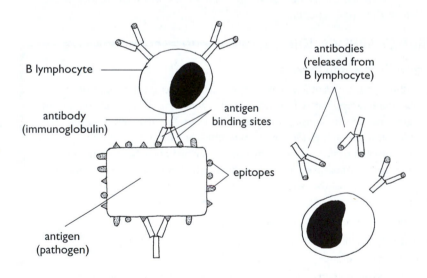

Figure 2.7 Simplified illustration of binding between B lymphocyte and antigen

Key features of adaptive humoral immunity include:

■ Antigen specificity
■ Clonal selection
■ Clonal expansion

- Clonal suppression and the formation of memory cells
- Antibodies (immunoglobulins).

Antigen specificity

B lymphocytes are able to recognize and respond to at least 10^8 different epitopes, so every different antigen encountered by the body is recognized independently of all the others. It is not possible for every single B lymphocyte to possess all the receptors necessary to recognize all the thousands of epitopes it could meet, because there would be insufficient physical space on the surface of the cell to hold them and insufficient DNA to code for them all. Instead, each B lymphocyte carries receptor molecules of unique structure and specificity to allow the recognition of just a few epitopes of a similar configuration (shape).

Clonal selection

All B lymphocytes appear the same during microscopic examination, but there are thousands of different types, each type responding to the same limited range of epitopes. B lymphocytes responding to the same epitopes form a clone. The body contains thousands of different clones that are 'selected' when the epitopes they match invade. A large bacterial cell carrying numerous different epitopes could select several different B lymphocyte clones.

Clonal expansion

This process involves the rapid replication of B lymphocytes in response to the arrival and binding of antigens. It results in the production of thousands of B lymphocytes able to react to the particular pathogen that is invading.

Clonal suppression

Clonal suppression occurs once the antigen has been eliminated. The immune response is 'switched off' once it becomes redundant, conserving metabolic resources and preventing an excessive response. The number of B lymphocytes belonging to the clone diminishes, although a few remain circulating in the plasma as memory cells. These allow a further rapid clonal expansion in response to a second invasion by the same pathogen, explaining why the immune response following re-exposure to the same organism is swift and will usually prevent reinfection (see also below).

Antibodies (immunoglobulins or Igs)

Antibodies are globular proteins carried on the surface of B lymphocytes, each B lymphocyte carrying about 10^5 immunoglobulins on its surface. Binding to the specific antigen takes place between the surface immunoglobulin molecule and a corresponding epitope (see Figure 2.7 above).

Immunoglobulin attachment is the signal for clonal expansion. Once a B lymphocyte binds to its epitope, it secretes additional immunoglobulins into the blood and body fluids rapidly – at a rate of thousands per second. Secreted immunoglobulins have numerous functions:

- They bind to their matching antigens. This does not destroy the antigen directly but results in clumping (agglutination) so that the resulting aggregates are more easily phagocytosed (see above).

- Once bound, immunoglobulins function as opsonins, labelling the antigen as a target for phagocytosis.

- Bound immunoglobulin enhances the cytotoxicity of NK cells and eosinophils (one example of the cooperation between innate and adaptive immunity).

- Binding between immunoglobulin and antigen operates as one of the triggers for the complement cascade (see above). This generates C3a and C3b, contributing to the inflammatory response, another example of the overlapping functions of the innate and adaptive responses.

If these activities were evoked without the binding signal, the immune response would take place wastefully and dangerously.

The primary and secondary immune responses and changes to antibody levels in the blood that occurs following immunization are illustrated below.

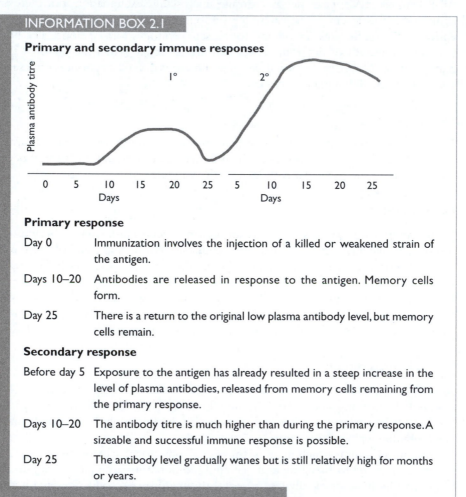

INFORMATION BOX 2.1

Primary and secondary immune responses

Primary response

Day 0	Immunization involves the injection of a killed or weakened strain of the antigen.
Days 10–20	Antibodies are released in response to the antigen. Memory cells form.
Day 25	There is a return to the original low plasma antibody level, but memory cells remain.

Secondary response

Before day 5	Exposure to the antigen has already resulted in a steep increase in the level of plasma antibodies, released from memory cells remaining from the primary response.
Days 10–20	The antibody titre is much higher than during the primary response. A sizeable and successful immune response is possible.
Day 25	The antibody level gradually wanes but is still relatively high for months or years.

There are several classes of immunoglobulins (IgG, IgA, IgM, IgD and IgE), which are found in different sites and perform a variety of functions, as shown below.

INFORMATION BOX 2.2

The immunoglobulins

IgG

Structurally the simplest immunoglobulin

The most abundant immunoglobulin

Has a major role in the secondary immune response

Neutralizes toxins and binds to antigens

Plasma levels provide an indication of recent exposure to antigens

Crosses the placenta in the last three months (third trimester) of pregnancy

IgA

Protects mucous membranes

Present in saliva, tears, breast milk and gut secretions

Particularly active against bacteria and fungi

IgM

Exclusively found in serum

Most abundant during the primary immune response

Has a major role in agglutination and complement activity

IgD

Present on B lymphocytes, where it functions as the antigen receptor for the B lymphocyte

May have other functions, but these are unclear

Maximum levels occur during childhood

IgE

Present on basophils in the lungs, skin and mucous membranes

Precipitates inflammation around parasites

Plays a role in hypersensitivity (allergic) reactions

Cell-mediated immunity

Cell-mediated immunity is a function of the T cells. They are released from the red bone marrow and migrate to the thymus gland, where they reach maturation. The functions of cell-mediated immunity include:

- Protection against viral and fungal infections and parasites

- Intracellular protection against bacteria with resistant cell walls able to survive phagocytosis; once inside the living cells of the host, they are sheltered from humoral defence mechanisms

- Maintaining the inflammatory response in cases of chronic infection (for example tuberculosis and leprosy)

- Surveillance against foreign cells, relevant in tumour detection and transplant rejection

- Regulation of the adaptive immune response.

Cell-mediated immunity is stimulated by the binding of an antigen to a receptor site on the surface of a T cell. The T cells respond by releasing chemical mediators called 'lymphokines'. These activate macrophages, enhancing phagocytosis, and stimulate the activity of many other cells vital for the immune response.

Types of T cell

T cells proliferate rapidly following exposure to an antigen, and undergo differentiation. Numerous subsets exist:

- **T cytotoxic cells** destroy specific target cells carrying surface antigens that they recognize. These include virally infected cells and cancer cells (as cells that have undergone neoplastic changes develop surface antigens different from those present in health).

- **T helper cells** initiate the immune response by promoting the maturation of B and other T lymphocytes once these have been triggered by antigens. This function is executed only after they have been stimulated by chemicals called 'interleukins' released from activated macrophages. It is thought that corticosteroids suppress fever by preventing the release of interleukins.

- **T suppressor cells** switch off the immune response by deactivating the T helper cells.

- **Delayed hypersensitivity T cells** are involved with other cells in chronic inflammation and cell-mediated delayed hypersensitivity.

In clinical settings, the T cells are generally classified according to the presence or otherwise of two surface molecules: CD4 and CD8. T helper cells are CD4+ or T4 cells, T cytotoxic and T suppressor cells being CD8 or T8 cells. The ratio of CD4+ to CD8+ cells is a useful guide to immune system function in viral infections or after transplantation; it is used to monitor progress of a person with HIV disease or established AIDS. Declining numbers of CD4+ helper T cells is a feature of HIV disease and AIDS.

Individual variation in the immune response and predisposition to infection

The activity of the immune system is depressed in some people and varies between individuals, reflecting the influence of genetic control. Some infections are species specific: distemper affects dogs, for example, but there are no recorded cases of transmission to a human host. Research on rhinoviruses, which cause the common cold, has never progressed well because so few laboratory species are susceptible to this illness. Some groups appear especially susceptible to certain infections, tuberculosis being particularly common among people of Asian extraction (Aditama, 1991). A genetic component appears to be operating in addition to environmental factors; if one twin of a monozygotic (identical) pair develops tuberculosis, the other is more likely to do so at some stage in his life than are other siblings who do not share all the same genes.

Some children are born with congenital or genetic deficiencies of the immune system and are highly susceptible to infection. Inherited lymphocytopenia (a low level of lymphocytes in the blood) and agammaglobulinaemia (the absence or deficiency of gammaglobulin in the blood) are X-linked disorders. Affected children (always males) rarely survive infancy. In chronic granulomatous disease, the affected subjects are highly susceptible to opportunistic infection because they have defective phagocytic enzymes and are unable to kill and digest bacteria.

Immunity throughout the lifespan

Immunity is also subject to variation throughout the lifespan and is influenced by a number of factors:

- **Age** – Infections occur less often between 20 and 40 years of age (Ayliffe et al., 1977), the young and the very old being most at risk. Infants acquire antibodies via the placenta and in breast milk, but the effects are short-lived (albeit valuable because they afford protection at a time when the adaptive system is still immature). At one time, antibody protection was thought to be impossible until the infant reached at least three months of age, but this is now disputed (Rudd, 1991). The ability to mount the inflammatory response and to form new antibodies declines with age.

- **Drugs** – Glucosteroids depress the inflammatory response and inhibit antibody formation. Antibiotics destroy the normal body flora, encouraging superinfection by extraneous strains of bacteria. The replacement of the normal flora in the bowel by pathogens may lead to diarrhoea and vomiting or more serious infections, superinfection with *Clostridium difficile*, for example, which is a serious complication of antibiotic treatment (Gammon, 1995).

- **Radiotherapy and chemotherapy** – These treatments depress the leucocyte count if the bone marrow or lymphatic tissues are involved. Patients with a depressed neutrophil count (neutropenia) are especially vulnerable to infection.

- **Metabolic disorders** – Such disorders reduce the immune response, but the mechanism by which they do this is unknown. Diabetes mellitus and malignant disease are both reported to have this effect. However, the mechanism increasing susceptibility to infection in patients with these two very different clinical conditions is unlikely to be the same.

- **Malnutrition** – Obesity reduces the ability to heal (Roberts and Bates, 1992). Undernutrition interferes with all aspects of the immune response, as shown by the devastating effects of measles in parts of the world where food supplies are poor. In malnourished patients, the capacity of the gastrointestinal mucosa to act as a barrier against pathogens is impaired (Reynolds et al., 1996).

- **Immobility** – Immobility contributes to susceptibility to infection because it inhibits the drainage of respiratory secretions, induces urinary stasis and increases the risk of pressure ulcers, which breach the normally intact cutaneous barrier and allow the entry of skin commensals that do not usually cause infection.

- **Psychological stress** – Stress appears to depress the immune response (Boore, 1978).

- **Specific and acquired immunity** – Immunity depends on the antigens to which an individual has been intentionally or accidentally exposed.

Immunity and community health

'Herd immunity' is the resistance to infectious disease exhibited by the population as a whole. High levels of herd immunity hinder transmission: epidemics are possible only when an infectious agent spreads throughout a susceptible population. The main source of herd immunity is exposure to naturally occurring infections. Before vaccination was introduced, outbreaks of measles and pertussis (whooping cough) occurred cyclically every few years, sporadic cases arising in between. A large number of infections occurring simultaneously was possible only when an entire cohort of children lacking immunity had built up through a lack of previous exposure, the number of infections waning once they had all been infected. In community health terms, sporadic infection is significant as epidemics are possible as long as individuals lacking immunity remain and are promoted by the geographical or social clustering of susceptible people (Bedford, 1993). The aim of immunization programmes is to induce acquired immunity in all susceptible people, preventing the development of outbreaks. It is generally believed that over 90 per cent of the population must be immune to a pathogen before a state of herd immunity can exist (Henderson, 1991).

The first vaccine was developed by Jenner in 1796 after his observation that milkmaids who had developed cowpox rarely contracted smallpox, a similar but much more serious infection. Jenner prepared a rudimentary vaccine from the cowpox virus that could induce immunity in people not previously exposed to cowpox or smallpox. This was a major scientific breakthrough as smallpox had claimed thousands of lives. The success of vaccination can be judged by the World Health Organization's declaration in 1980 that smallpox had been eradicated.

Childhood immunization programmes against infectious diseases starting with diphtheria were introduced in the UK from the 1940s onwards. Vaccines available in the UK include those against:

- Diphtheria
- Group C meningococcal disease (long-lasting vaccine)

- Hepatitis B
- *Haemophilus influenzae* type b (Hib)
- Human papilloma virus (HPV; types 6, 11, 16, 18)
- Influenza
- Measles, mumps and rubella (MMR)
- Pertussis (whooping cough)
- Pneumococcal disease
- Poliomyelitis
- Tetanus
- Tuberculosis.

There are also vaccines available for people at higher risk of a specific disease because of the nature of their work or condition. For example, vaccination against hepatitis A, an infection associated with poor hand hygiene after using the lavatory, can be offered to staff and residents considered to be at particular risk. People travelling to countries where other infectious diseases are endemic, for example yellow fever, typhoid fever and so on, can also be vaccinated. In the United States, varicella (chickenpox), hepatitis A and rotavirus vaccines are part of the childhood immunization schedule.

The terms 'vaccination' and 'immunization' are sometimes used interchangeably, although vaccination is strictly defined as the act of administering the vaccine, while immunization is the result of vaccination. The types of vaccine available are shown below.

INFORMATION BOX 2.3

Types of vaccines

> **Killed vaccine** – The active organism is destroyed, usually by heat. A primary dose followed by two boosters is needed to induce immunity, for example against pertussis. These organisms are not infectious, and are therefore harmless, but the period of protection is relatively short.

> **Live vaccines** – Viable organisms are attenuated (weakened) so that they are unable to harm the recipient but can still induce immunity, as, for example, with yellow fever. One dose will usually confer immunity, except for diseases such as poliomyelitis, for which three doses are required. A second advantage is that after a single dose, they can spread naturally within a population, helping to produce herd immunity. Care must be taken if these are required for immunocompromised patients.

> **Toxoids** – Inactivated toxins derived from the pathogen are injected.

> **Subunit vaccines** – These use part of the virus or bacterium to induce immunity.

> **Conjugate vaccines** – These combine antigenic parts of different organisms, thus inducing immunity to two or more infections in a single vaccine.

Throughout the 1980s, there was concern about the uptake of the vaccines, especially for measles and pertussis. Attention was drawn to the social costs and benefits of immunization and the dangers accruing to the population as a whole through a lack of compliance by a minority of parents refusing to present their children for vaccination either through ignorance or misplaced fears of side-effects associated with the vaccines. No vaccine can ever offer 100 per cent effectiveness, but the benefits of immunization are demonstrable (Bedford, 1993). Immunization against diphtheria and poliomyelitis has maintained a high degree of herd immunity within the population, and the side-effects of measles vaccine are slight, especially compared with the lasting damage that may accrue from the infection itself.

Standard immunization against infectious diseases

The routine immunization schedule for children and young people has been updated many times since the 1940s. For example, a vaccine against pneumococcal disease was introduced in 2006 and a vaccine against the human papilloma virus is to be introduced for girls aged 12–13 in the UK commencing autumn 2008 (Department of Health, 2007). Regular updating of the schedule and the provision of various one-off booster programmes occur, and for this reason a current schedule is not provided here. For up-to-date information, readers are always advised to check the contents of the current schedule by accessing the website www.immunisation.org.uk. An opportunity to reflect on uptake is provided below.

PRACTICE APPLICATION 2.3

Uptake of Immunization Schedule in Children and Young People

The uptake of immunization is critical in producing herd immunity. Since the publication in 1998 of unsubstantiated research that suggested a link between the MMR vaccine and the development of autistic disorders and Crohn's disease (an inflammatory bowel disease), many parents have not had their children vaccinated, or have opted for a course of single vaccines. This decline in the numbers of children vaccinated has caused serious concerns about the level of herd immunity. In August 2007, the Health Protection Agency (2007) reported that cases of measles were rising at a higher rate than expected for the time of year.

Activity

➤ Access the current schedule of immunization in your country. Find out what is offered and at what ages.

➤ How good is uptake in your local community?

➤ Reflect on the factors that influence the uptake of immunization.

Resources

NHS immunisation information – www.mmrthefacts.nhs.uk/library/.

World Health Organization – www.who.int/en/ and access Immunisation and Vaccines in Health topics.

Measles

Measles is caused by a paramyxovirus. It is endemic in many countries and globally it is estimated that one million children die from it each year, mostly in developing countries. Death is usually from complications such as encephalitis. It is highly contagious, with almost all non-immune children developing infection if exposed to the virus. The vaccine was introduced in 1968. Immunity is established in over 95 per cent of immunized subjects (Bedford, 2004). The extremely infectious nature of the virus means that a high level of immunity is needed in the population before herd immunity is reached. To reach this level, 90–95 per cent of preschool children must receive at least one dose of vaccine (Bedford, 2004). This level of coverage was attained in the UK in the mid-1990s. Since then, publicity regarding possible (unproven) side-effects and calls to separate vaccination for measles, rubella and mumps have increased parental concerns and reduced uptake (Jansen et al., 2003). Since 2000, measles outbreaks in England have been reported as a result of low uptake of the vaccine (Bedford, 2004). Outbreaks have also occurred in other European countries where uptake of the vaccine has declined. In 2006, there was an increase in the number of infections in the UK (Hainsworth, 2006).

Pertussis (whooping cough)

Pertussis may be accompanied by severe, occasionally fatal respiratory complications that are preventable by vaccination. Adverse publicity in 1975 led to a dramatic decrease in the uptake of vaccination, with epidemics occurring throughout England and Wales. There were suggestions that children had suffered brain damage after receiving the vaccine, eventually later refuted by case control studies (Alderslade et al., 1981). A similar association with sudden infant death syndrome (also known as sudden unexpected death in infancy) has never been proved, and there are now suggestions that undiagnosed pertussis may in fact be the cause of some unexplained infant mortalities (Bedford, 1993).

Rubella (German measles)

Rubella vaccination was introduced in the UK in 1970. The aim was initially to reduce the tragic consequences of infection during pregnancy rather than to eradicate the virus from the community, the vaccine being offered selectively to schoolgirls and susceptible women. Considerable success was achieved, so that by 1990 it was estimated that only 2–4 per cent of pregnant women were susceptible compared with 10–15 per cent before 1970. Congenital infections were, however, still reported to the Communicable Diseases Surveillance Centre, and as unvaccinated children were known to be operating as a reservoir of infection within the community, the immunization programme was extended so that the vaccine could be offered during routine childhood immunization. A major campaign to immunize schoolchildren in 1994 met with some opposition from certain groups objecting to the vaccine because the virus had been cultured on cells derived from fetal tissue.

Combined vaccines

The measles/mumps/rubella (MMR) vaccine for routine child immunization introduced in 1989 was intended to eliminate measles, mumps, rubella and congenital rubella syndrome from the UK. The uptake of MMR has recently declined because of a perceived risk that it may be linked to the development of autism, although a large study (Public Health Laboratory Service, 1999) has not shown a causal association between MMR and autism despite parental concern (Diggle, 2005). MMR is given at 13 months and a booster before starting school (between 3 years 4 months and 5 years).

Diphtheria, tetanus, poliomyelitis, Hib and pertussis vaccines are offered at 2, 3 and 4 months of age, replacing an earlier, more widely spaced, schedule. Preschool boosters are still recommended. This approach has been welcomed as it is likely to increase the uptake of vaccination at baby clinics: many mothers have returned to full-time employment by the time that their infants have reached 6 months of age, and attendance then becomes more difficult (Rudd, 1991).

Hib vaccine

The Hib vaccine, which acts against *Haemophilus influenzae* type b, was first developed in the early 1970s but was then only effective in children over 2 years of age. Most cases, however, occur during infancy, when the levels of maternal antibodies have waned but the baby has yet to develop its own natural immunity. *Haemophilus influenzae* is a Gram-negative organism often carried in the healthy throat. It has been associated with the development of respiratory infections and their associated side-effects of epiglottitis and otitis media. Infection is most damaging in young children and is the principal cause of bacterial meningitis in children under 5 years of age. It is a significant cause of mortality, and among survivors may cause neurological deficits including deafness, a learning disability and poor motor coordination. Its onset is insidious. Infection often follows a cold and the symptoms are nonspecific, so parents may not be aware that their child is becoming seriously ill. Currently, Hib vaccine is administered as part of the combined vaccine given at 2, 3 and 4 months (see above) with a booster combined with meningococcal group C around 12 months of age.

Group C meningococcal disease

A long-acting vaccine became available in 1999 for vulnerable groups. Group C *Neisseria meningitidis* causes meningitis and life-threatening septicaemia; most often affecting children and young adults. The vaccine is given at 3 and 4 months, and a booster combined with Hib around 12 months of age.

Pneumococcal disease

Pneumococcal disease is caused by *Streptococcus pneumoniae*, a bacterium that can cause otitis media, sinusitis, pneumonia, meningitis and septicaemia. It occurs most commonly in children under 5 years, with those under 2 years of age being most at risk. In addition, people over 65 years are at risk, as are those who have had a splenectomy (removal of the spleen), or with certain chronic conditions (Bedford and Lane, 2006). During childhood, the vaccine is given at 2 and 4 months, and a third dose at 13 months of age.

Hepatitis B

See Chapter 12.

Tuberculosis

See Chapter 14.

Health promotion

Health promotion and immunization form an important part of the work of health professionals employed in the community, especially health visitors (specialist community public health nurses), school nurses and practice nurses. Compliance can be increased by programmes to promote public awareness, especially in relation to side-effects and safety. There is, however, evidence that when failure occurs, it is more often caused by inadequate service provision or the misinterpretation of information than by a refusal to participate (Peckham et al., 1989).

Professionals clearly need to know the contraindications to vaccination but tend to be poorly informed and to emphasize harmful effects in a manner likely to result in a failure of uptake among eligible children (Walker, 1990).

Contradictions include:

- A history of anaphylaxis with a particular vaccine or its components
- Febrile illness
- Active infection
- Live vaccines should be avoided in pregnancy, immunosuppression and in people being treated for cancer with chemotherapy or radiotherapy
- People who are very sensitive to antibacterials present in some vaccines against viral diseases.

There is little doubt that parents seeking information from more than one source and receiving contradictory advice are less likely to present their children for immunization. One area in which there has been debate is the safety of vaccination in subjects for whom an allergy to egg has been reported, as the viruses are often cultured in eggs. Allergy is not, however, regarded as a contraindication (Aitken et al., 1994), but people with egg sensitivity and a history of anaphylaxis should not have certain vaccines, including that for influenza.

Storage of vaccines

INFORMATION BOX 2.4

Storage of vaccines

Storage of vaccines involves placing each new batch under the conditions stipulated in the national guidelines:

➤ The recommended temperature for polio vaccine is 0–4 °C, for all other vaccines it is 2–8 °C.

➤ A nominated, trained person should be responsible for storage, using the national guidelines, adapted as necessary to meet local needs.

➤ The temperature of the refrigerator should be monitored with a minimum and a maximum range thermometer, and should be recorded at regular intervals.

➤ Written procedures should be developed and followed if the refrigerator breaks down.

➤ The refrigerator should be defrosted regularly while the vaccines are placed in another refrigerator or cool box.

➤ Reconstituted vaccine should be used within the period recommended by the manufacturer, and partially used vials should be destroyed at the end of the clinic session.

➤ Stocks should be rotated so the oldest batch of numbered vaccines is available to be used first.

➤ Vaccines should be removed from the refrigerator and reconstituted only when they are about to be administered.

See Department of Health (DH) (2006, modified 2007) *Immunisation against Infectious Diseases (The Green Book)*, Chapter 3. TSO, Norwich.

Environmental factors, epidemics and vaccines

Environmental factors can play a major role in the promotion of epidemics in the human population:

- **Social factors** – overcrowding as people moved from rural areas to towns, for example during the Industrial Revolution, or are herded together in institutions.
- **The breakdown of previously successful control measures** – such as sanitation, resulting in epidemics of waterborne infection.
- **Altered behaviour** – human immunodeficiency virus (HIV) probably existed before the first reported cases in the late 1970s, but its incidence escalated in the early 1980s with an increase in high-risk activities such as unprotected intercourse with an infected person or the sharing of syringes and needles.

- **Geographical movement** – exposing people to pathogens that they have not encountered before. Travellers should seek expert advice about immunization and take sensible precautions before embarking on their journey.
- **Exposure to mutant strains of pathogens** – mutant strains of pathogens can possess new antigenic properties to which the population may not have had the opportunity to develop herd immunity. New vaccines are periodically developed for influenza, which demonstrates this phenomenon of 'antigenic drift'.

Development of new vaccines

Factors influencing the development of new vaccines and their introduction are promoted by:

- **Changing patterns of disease within the community** – As new pathogens are identified, the search for disease prevention inevitably commences, although it usually takes many years. There is currently no effective vaccine for HIV (a 'new' disease) or gonorrhoea (a significant community health problem that has been known since antiquity).
- **Perceptions about existing infectious diseases** – One of the consequences of an effective immunization programme is that a previously common disease becomes rare and the dangers of infection are forgotten (Bedford, 1993). Young health professionals and young parents, never having witnessed the effects of pertussis on a small baby, may be heavily influenced by media stories documenting complications associated with the vaccine.
- **Changes in the sectors of the population at risk** – Since the eradication of smallpox, routine vaccination is no longer required.

The need for vaccination is greatest in developing countries (Bird, 1996).

Risks in hospital

Hospital patients are at particular risk of infection because they:

- Experience high levels of physical and psychological stress, reducing their immune response
- Have close contact with a large number of different hospital staff, increasing the risks of cross-infection
- Are particularly likely to undergo invasive procedures and take drugs, both of which may depress the immune response
- Share facilities for personal hygiene to a much greater extent than at home
- Eat mass-produced food
- Are exposed to microorganisms not usually encountered.

Exposure to the above risk factors increases with the length of hospital stay and is greatest for those who are most sick. Immunization is not yet possible because effective vaccines still have to be developed. It may always remain impractical owing to the large number of different organisms capable of causing hospital-acquired infection.

SELF-ASSESSMENT

1. The bladder resists the invasion of pathogens by the presence of a resident population of lactobacilli. True? or False?

2. Name the five hallmarks of inflammation.

3. Briefly explain phagocytosis.

4. A care plan for a patient who is pyrexial should include monitoring vital signs and fluid intake and output. True? or False?

5. List four signs or symptoms of anaphylaxis.

6. Name five key features of humoral immunity.

7. Cell-mediated immunity involves T cells. True? or False?

8. Herd immunity is always a natural phenomenon. True or False?

9. *Haemophilus influenzae* is the most common cause of childhood:

   (a) viral meningitis
   (b) influenza
   (c) sore throats
   (d) none of these.

10. How many doses of the pneumococcal vaccine are given during the childhood immunization schedule?

    (a) 1
    (b) 2
    (c) 3
    (d) 4

REFERENCES

Aditama TY (1991) Prevalence of tuberculosis in Indonesia, Singapore and the Philippines. *Tubercle* **72**: 255–60.

Aitken R, Hill D and Kemp A (1994) Measles immunisation in children with allergy to egg. *British Medical Journal* **309**: 223–5.

Alderslade R, Bellman MH, Rawson N et al. (1981) The National Childhood Encephalopathy Study, in *Whooping Cough. Reports from the Committee on Safety of Medicines and the Joint Committee on Vaccination and Immunisation.* HMSO, London.

Ayliffe GA, Brightwell KM, Babb BJ et al. (1977) Surveys of hospital infection in the Birmingham region. *Journal of Hygiene* **79**: 299–313.

Bedford H (1993) Immunisation facts and fiction. *Health Visitor* **66**: 314–16.

Bedford H (2004) Measles and the importance of maintaining vaccination levels. *Nursing Times* **100**(26): 52–5.

Bedford H and Lane L (2006) Pneumococcal vaccination and the new child vaccination schedule. *Nursing Times* **102**(39) 44–5.

Bird C (1996) The battle continues. *Nursing Times* **92**(27): 66–8.

Boore J (1978) *Prescription for Recovery*. RCN, London.

Department of Health (DH) (2007) *HPV Vaccine Recommended for NHS Immunisation Programme*. Available www.gnn.gov.uk/.

Diggle I (2005) Understanding and dealing with parental vaccine concerns. *Nursing Times* **101**(46): 26–8.

Gammon J (1995) The difficult bug to beat. *Nursing Times* **91**(37): 57–8.

Hainsworth T (2006) Practice implications of the increase in measles infections. *Nursing Times* **102**(17): 19–20.

Health Protection Agency (HPA) (2007) Press statement *Book your back to school MMR jab*. Available www.hpa.org.uk/.

Henderson N (1991) Vaccination review. *Practice Nurse* October: 271–4.

Hendry C and Farley AH (2001) Understanding allergies and their treatment. *Nursing Standard* **15**(35): 47–52.

Horan MA (1984) Outbreak of *Shigella sonnei* dysentery on a geriatric assessment ward. *Journal of Hospital Infection* **5**: 210–12.

Jansen VA, Stollenwerk N and Jensen HJ (2003) Measles outbreaks in a population with declining vaccine uptake. *Science* **301**(5634): 804.

Jevon P (2004) An overview of managing anaphylaxis in the community. *Nursing Times* **102**(39): 48–9.

Mackowiak P (1994) Fever: a blessing or a curse? A unifying hypothesis. *Annals of Internal Medicine* **120**: 1037–40.

Peckham CS, Bedford H, Senturia Y et al. (1989) *The National Immunisation Study: Factors Affecting Immunisation Uptake in Childhood*. Action Research, Horsham.

Public Health Laboratory Service (PHLS) (1999) MMR vaccine and autism: no epidemiological evidence for a causal relationship. PHLS, London.

Reynolds JV, O'Farrelly C, Feighery C et al. (1996) Impaired gut barrier function in malnourished patients. *British Journal of Surgery* **83**: 1288–91.

Roberts JV and Bates T (1992) The use of the body mass index in studies of abdominal wound infection. *Journal of Hospital Infection* **20**: 217–20.

Rudd P (1991) Childhood immunisation in the new decade. *British Medical Journal* **302**: 481–2.

Sawyer SM, Bowes G and Phelan PD (1994) Vulvovaginal candidiasis in young women with cystic fibrosis. *British Medical Journal* **308**: 1609–10.

Walker D (1990) Pertussis immunisation: professional attitudes and knowledge. *Health Visitor* **63**: 386–7.

FURTHER READING AND INFORMATION SOURCES

Department of Health (DH) (2006, modified 2007) *Immunisation against Infectious Diseases* (*The Green Book*), Chapter 3. TSO, Norwich. Available www.dh.gov.uk/en/ Policyandguidance/Healthandsocialcaretopics/Greenbook/DH_4097254.

Docherty B and Foudy C (2006) Homeostasis: temperature regulation. *Nursing Times* **102**(16): 20–1.

Male D, Brostoff J, Roth D and Roitt I (2006) *Immunology*, 7th edn. Mosby, Edinburgh.

Martin J (2004) Travel vaccination: an update. *Nursing Standard* **18**(34): 47–53.

National Library for Health – www.library.nhs.uk/.

NHS Immunisation Information – www.immunisation.org.uk.

Nursing Times (2003) Vaccine storage. *Nursing Times* **99**(28): 29.

Pumphery RS (2000) Lessons for management of anaphylaxis from a study of fatal reactions. *Clinical and Experimental Allergy* **30**: 1144–50.

Taylor C (2006) Managing infants with pyrexia. *Nursing Times* **102**(39): 42–3.

CHAPTER 3

The microbiology laboratory

CHAPTER OUTCOMES

After reading this chapter, you should be able to:

➤ State the functions of the hospital microbiology department

➤ Explain what happens when a specimen is processed in the hospital microbiology department

➤ Discuss the role of the health and social care practitioner in safely obtaining good quality specimens for microbiological examination

➤ Identify good practice during specimen handling and storage

Introduction to the microbiology laboratory

Staff in the microbiology department diagnose infection and give advice on the most effective treatment. Their work involves isolating and identifying bacteria and other organisms from specimens of blood, urine, faeces, sputum, pus and cerebrospinal fluid (CSF), and swabs taken from infected sites. Practitioners need to understand the work of the medical microbiology laboratory in order to:

■ Provide information to people in their care about diagnostic tests

■ Collect specimens – success depends on good practice when the person is prepared for the test, when the specimen is obtained and the way in which it is stored and handled before it reaches the laboratory (Higgins, 1994)

■ Understand the findings expressed on laboratory reports.

Developments in technology have paved the way for newer, more rapid ways of performing laboratory tests known as point-of-care or near-patient testing (see below).

PRACTICE APPLICATION 3.1

Point-of-care Testing

Point-of-care testing is particularly used in premises away from laboratories when organisms present in the specimen could perish during transport, especially in situations where people may be reluctant to return for follow-up. In addition, it can help to reduce the prescribing of antibiotics where it is not warranted. The practitioner collects specimens and analyses the results, which are available immediately. For example, a two-minute test can be performed for C reactive protein (CRP) (a marker for inflammation); this is used to identify whether a person with a sore throat or acute cough should receive antibiotics. The results, cross-checked with later laboratory findings, give an accurate and reliable indication of the presence of bacterial infection.

Activity

➤ Find out about the point-of-care testing for infection carried out in your area of practice.

➤ Search the literature for other examples of point-of-care testing for infection. These include influenza viruses, respiratory syncytial virus and antenatal HIV testing.

Diagnostic laboratory services

When a specimen arrives in the laboratory, it is first examined macroscopically and then with a microscope. Detailed identification requires the culture (growth) of the bacteria in a suitable medium. If the specimen has been obtained from a site where other organisms will be present (for example skin or faeces), special techniques are used to isolate those causing infection. Additional biochemical and serological tests may be necessary to confirm the identification. Sensitivity tests are performed to determine the most effective antibiotic.

Following the various examinations and special tests, the laboratory produces a report (Figure 3.1) for the clinician. Urgent, interim results and those of special significance are relayed by telephone, facsimile or email, as are many routine results.

Initial examination

Some information on the nature of the infection can be obtained by an initial inspection: odour and appearance can offer some clues. Foul-smelling, purulent material suggests the presence of anaerobic bacteria (for example *Bacteroides*). CSF or urine that appears cloudy probably contains neutrophils, which indicate active infection. Mucus or blood in a stool suggests dysentery, and many roundworms and the segments of tapeworms are visible to the naked eye.

Microscopic examination

A variety of microscopic techniques are available and some are outlined below.

Wet films

A drop of fluid taken from the specimen is placed on a microscope slide beneath a cover slip and examined at low power (×400). This technique is used to look at:

Patient details in full are needed to identify the patient safely

– always use the unique hospital number

– age may be relevant

– gender may be relevant

Date received in the laboratory (need to know whether the quality of the specimen has been reduced)

Which antimicrobial substances will be effective against the microorganism (S) and those which will not be effective (R)

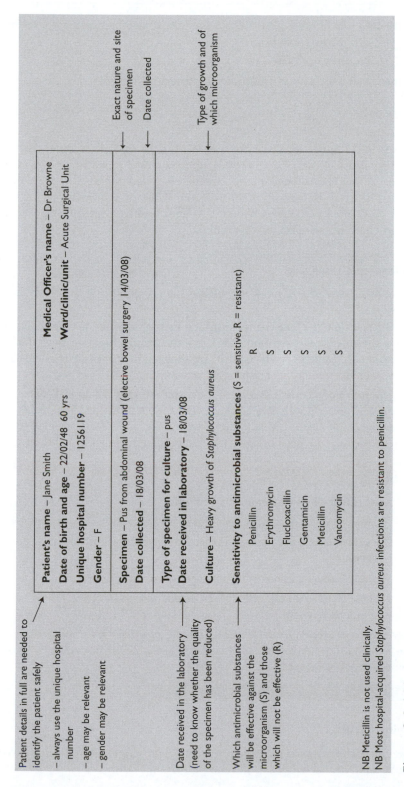

Patient's name – Jane Smith	**Medical Officer's name** – Dr Browne
Date of birth and age – 22/02/48 60 yrs	**Ward/clinic/unit** – Acute Surgical Unit
Unique hospital number – 1256119	
Gender – F	

Specimen – Pus from abdominal wound (elective bowel surgery 14/03/08)

Date collected – 18/03/08

Type of specimen for culture – pus

Date received in laboratory – 18/03/08

Culture – Heavy growth of *Staphylococcus aureus*

Sensitivity to antimicrobial substances (S = sensitive, R = resistant)

Penicillin	R
Erythromycin	S
Flucloxacillin	S
Gentamicin	S
Meticillin	S
Vancomycin	S

Exact nature and site of specimen

Date collected

Type of growth and of which microorganism

NB Meticillin is not used clinically.
NB Most hospital-acquired *Staphylococcus aureus* infections are resistant to penicillin.

Figure 3.1 A laboratory report

- Body fluids – where pus cells or whole organisms may be present, for example, urine, CSF and vaginal secretions
- Faeces, to detect ova or cysts
- Scrapings from hair, skin or nails to detect fungal infection.

Dry films

Dry films provide more detailed information about bacterial infection. A higher magnification is usually necessary (×1000), and stains are added to help to identify the bacteria. A thin film taken from the specimen is added to a microscope slide and the material is 'fixed' by passing it through the flame of a Bunsen burner. Gram staining is most often used (see Chapter 1): Gram-positive organisms appear deep purple, and Gram-negative bacteria stain pink.

Special microscopy techniques

Special techniques are necessary to identify specific bacteria:

1. The **Acid-fast (Ziehl–Neelsen) technique** is used to identify *Mycobacterium* spp. These organisms do not respond well to Gram staining because their thick cell walls are impermeable to the dyes. Instead, they are identified by the acid-fast or acid/alcohol-fast staining technique (see below).
2. **Dark ground microscopy** is used to identify spirochaetes (Chapter 1). These tiny bacteria, which react poorly to traditional staining methods, are best visualized at high magnification against a dark background. Wet films made from a recently collected specimen are used because spirochaetes die rapidly outside the tissues.

INFORMATION BOX 3.1

Acid-fast (Ziehl–Neelsen) staining technique

➤ The smear on the slide is covered with hot carbol fuchsin stain for five minutes

➤ The slide is decolourized with an acid/alcohol solution (hydrochloric acid and ethanol)

➤ The slide is counterstained with methylene blue or malachite green

➤ Acid-fast bacilli (or AFBs) resist decolourization and appear red or yellow on a dark background

NB Acid/alcohol decolourization is used because *Mycobacterium tuberculosis* is distinctive in that it resists decolourization by both acid and alcohol. *M. tuberculosis* is therefore referred to as being acid/alcohol fast.

Identifying bacteria

Many related bacteria appear identical under the microscope. Identification involves growing them in special culture media and performing various tests.

Cultures

Solid media are produced by mixing nutrients with agar. A variety of culture media are used, blood agar being the one most commonly encountered in hospital laboratories. The concentration of different chemicals added to the medium alters its properties so the growth of a particular organism is encouraged while others are suppressed. This makes it easier to identify the pathogen. For example, MacConkey's medium contains a small amount of lactose and a pH indicator. Bacteria able to grow on MacConkey agar and to ferment lactose produce acid, turning the pH indicator red, while species that do not ferment lactose remain colourless.

A special technique is used to inoculate culture media with bacteria taken from the specimen (Figure 3.2).

Introducing the specimen to the
solid medium

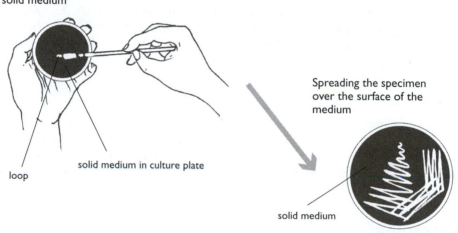

Spreading the specimen
over the surface of the
medium

solid medium in culture plate

loop

solid medium

Figure 3.2 Technique for inoculating a culture medium

Following the inoculation of the culture medium, the specimen is incubated at an appropriate temperature for a certain period of time. Most bacteria able to cause human infection grow steadily at 37 °C, producing visible colonies on the surface of the agar within 24–48 hours (Figure 3.3). However, some bacteria (for example *Myco-bacterium*) grow much more slowly. Such cultures are kept and re-examined for several weeks. If the specimen is likely to contain anaerobes (for example if it arises from a wound), a portion is cultured in a special container free of oxygen (an anaerobic jar).

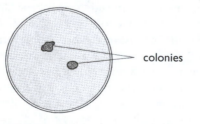

colonies

Figure 3.3 Bacterial colonies

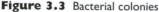

Colonies result when bacteria are cultured on solid media. Each cell multiplies over and over again until a clump visible to the naked eye appears. All the bacteria in the colony are of the same type. The size, colour and shape of colonies vary according to the type of bacteria and can be used to help to identify the different species. For example, *Pseudomonas aeruginosa* produces characteristic green colonies and *Serratia marcescens* red ones. Haemolytic bacteria such as *Streptococcus pyogenes* release enzymes that destroy erythrocytes in blood agar; as a result, each colony becomes surrounded by a clear halo.

Biochemical tests

Biochemical tests are used to confirm the identity of many bacteria. Most tests are designed to detect the presence of specific enzymes and have been developed so that a visible, easily detected change, usually the production of gas or a change in pH, occurs. An indicator incorporated into the medium demonstrates this. *Shigella* species are differentiated by their ability to ferment carbohydrates, releasing bubbles of gas. Commercially prepared kits are available so that biochemical tests can be conveniently performed.

Antibiotic sensitivity

It is vital to establish which antibiotics destroy the pathogen so that the appropriate drug can be prescribed. Antibiotic sensitivity tests are performed by the disc diffusion method. The bacteria are inoculated onto solid media, a paper disc impregnated with different antibiotics is placed over them, and the culture is incubated. Where the bacteria are sensitive to a particular antibiotic, the agar remains clear of growth.

Serological tests

Serological tests are used to identify bacteria based on their immunological reactions. Portions of the specimen containing the organism to be identified are exposed to several different known antibodies, these antibodies being specific to antigens on the surfaces of particular species of bacteria. If the antigens and antibodies belong to the same species, the antibody binds to the bacterial cells, which causes visible clumping (agglutination).

Typing bacteria

During outbreaks, additional, more specialized 'typing' procedures are used to establish whether the same strain is responsible for cross-infection. These tests are usually performed at specialist Health Protection Agency laboratories. Tests distinguish between related strains belonging to the same species by determining their susceptibility to bacteriophages (viruses) or whether they have identical surface antigens. Phage typing is used to identify different strains of meticillin-resistant *Staphylococcus aureus* (MRSA). If all cases are being caused by the same strain, infection must be coming from a common source, which can be identified as a step towards control.

Virology: identifying viral infections

Specimens for virology are transported to the laboratory in a solution containing antibiotics to inhibit bacterial growth. Viral infection is diagnosed by directly detecting the virus particles using the electron microscope, by culture, by serological tests to detect viral antibodies in the patient's blood and by using nucleic acid-based techniques, such as polymerase chain reaction (PCR) or reverse transcriptase-PCR (RT-PCR).

Electron microscopy

Electron microscopy at high magnification is required to visualize virus particles. These are identified according to their characteristic shape once they have been stained. It is possible to identify rotavirus and herpes viruses using the electron microscope. The absence of virus particles in a specimen cannot, however, be taken as conclusive evidence that no infection is present because the particles are minute and, unless present in large numbers, can easily be overlooked.

Viral culture

Viruses cannot be cultured outside living cells. In the laboratory, sheets of cells grown in nutrient medium can be used to culture some viruses. The presence of a particular virus is indicated by the characteristic way in which it changes the shape of the cells.

Serological tests for viruses

Viral infection stimulates the appearance of specific antibodies in the blood, their presence forming the basis of diagnostic testing. The most widely used method is the enzyme-linked immunosorbent assay (ELISA). Specific antigen is mixed with the patient's serum. If the antigen and antibody are from the same virus, they combine. A second antibody attached to the enzyme is added. The conjugate becomes attached to the antibody bound to the original antigen, causing a visible change in the test solution as a result of enzyme action.

Identifying fungal infections

Fungi may be detected in stained films during the routine examination of sputum, swabs and vaginal secretions. Most species will grow in the same types of media as those used to culture bacteria, but apart from a few species that grow quickly (for example *Candida albicans*), colonies do not appear until after the usual incubation period of 24–48 hours. Where fungal infection is suspected, special cultures are set up and examined at intervals of 2–3 weeks. A medium containing antibiotics to inhibit bacterial growth, usually Sabouraud's glucose agar, is used. Identification is generally based on the characteristic appearance of the fungus on the surface of the agar and its microscopic appearance.

Specimens for microbiological examination

The success of diagnostic testing depends on good practice when the patient is prepared, when the specimen is obtained and the way in which it is stored and handled on its way to the laboratory. Practitioners obviously have a vital role to play in ensuring that specimens are obtained correctly and reach the laboratory in good condition. Environmental microbiological sampling is also occasionally undertaken.

Principles of good practice

PRACTICE APPLICATION 3.2

Obtaining Specimens: Ensuring Good Practice

➤ **Obtain informed consent** – explain procedure and obtain informed verbal consent.

➤ **Ensure personal safety** – use of appropriate personal protective equipment (PPE) such as gloves and plastic apron (see Chapter 5).

➤ **Good sampling technique** – the specimen should contain organisms only from the site being investigated; saliva, for example, should not be substituted for sputum.

➤ **Sufficient material should be provided for examination** – for example, rectal swabs should not replace a specimen of faeces because there will be insufficient material for culture.

➤ **Time of collection** – except in an emergency, the specimen should be obtained before antibiotics are given.

➤ **Use the appropriate specimen container** – for example, viruses do not survive well in transport media intended for bacteria.

➤ **Correctly label the specimen and request card** – particular care is needed when patients or residents on the same ward/unit have similar names. Use unique identification, for example bar code or hospital number (see Figure 3.1 above).

➤ **Provide adequate data on the request form** – clinical signs and details of antibiotic therapy (see Figure 3.1 above).

➤ **Transport to the laboratory without delay, at the correct temperature** – wherever possible, specimens should be obtained just before a pick-up is due.

➤ **Complete records** – record the time, date and nature of specimen obtained and when transported to the laboratory in the patient's/client's notes.

(See also Practice Application 3.3, Transporting Specimens Safely, below.)

Collecting different types of specimens

An outline is provided of how some commonly requested specimens are obtained, including, for example, specimens of urine, sputum and stool, and swabs taken from throat, eye and vagina, and so on.

Urine specimens

Urine specimens must be collected as free of contamination as possible. In health, urine is sterile, but it is easily contaminated during collection by contact with the perineum or the hands. Extraneous Gram-negative bacteria multiply rapidly, especially if the specimen is stored, leading to a result that is falsely positive or difficult to interpret.

Collecting a 5–10 ml midstream specimen can reduce the risk of error. Uncircumcised older boys and adult men are instructed or helped to withdraw the foreskin; the urethral meatus is then cleansed with soap and water and the middle portion of the flow collected directly into the sterile receptacle. Collecting an uncontaminated urine specimen from females is never easy, and there are particular problems when the patient is bed-bound or too disorientated to cooperate. The person is required to pass urine with the labia separated, catching the middle part of the stream in the sterile container. The procedure has traditionally involved cleansing the labia and vestibule before obtaining the specimen in a sterile receptacle, but there is little evidence that this procedure yields specimens of any higher quality than when patients have simply passed urine into a clean container. Even without cleansing and collection in a sterile receptacle, most specimens are satisfactory (White, 1992).

For people with a urinary catheter, a fresh specimen is obtained by using a syringe to aspirate urine from the sampling port on the drainage bag tubing. The port is first cleaned with an alcohol swab and allowed to dry. Some drainage systems require a syringe and needle to obtain a sample and great care must be taken to avoid puncturing the drainage tubing with the needle. The drainage apparatus and catheter should never be disconnected to collect a specimen because of the risk of introducing infection. Urine from the drainage bag will not yield satisfactory results because it may be heavily contaminated from environmental sources.

Obtaining uncontaminated specimens from infants is especially difficult. The infant may be held over a sterile container to obtain a 'clean catch' specimen. The least satisfactory method is a bagged sample in which an appropriately sized plastic bag is applied to the perineum. In an emergency, a suitably trained and competent practitioner may obtain a specimen by suprapubic bladder aspiration.

All specimens should be examined within three hours of collection, before any contaminating bacteria not responsible for the infection have had time to multiply, distorting the results. If examination is likely to be delayed, the specimen must be stored at 4 °C until it reaches the laboratory bench. It may, however, be stored at room temperature if a red-topped specimen container is used.

In the laboratory, the specimen is inoculated onto nutrient agar and incubated overnight. The colonies are counted and the number of bacteria present in 1 ml of the urine is calculated the next day. Counts of 10^5 or more organisms per ml suggest that infection is present, especially in the presence of neutrophils. A lower count suggests contamination rather than genuine infection.

Specimens from wounds

Specimen collection from wounds sometimes yields poor results because the swab of pus or exudate dries out and the bacteria are dead before they reach the laboratory.

This especially occurs if the specimen is stored before it is examined. Whenever possible, pus should be aspirated from a wound, or a small portion of excised tissue should be obtained. If swabbing is the only practical method, two or three specimens are better than one: the first can be stained for microscopy, the others used to inoculate the culture medium. Two agar plates are inoculated with the material – one to grow aerobes, the other to grow anaerobes.

Stool specimens

Stool specimens are obtained to identify bacteria (for example *Salmonella* or *Campylobacter*) or viruses (for example rotaviruses) that may be causing infection as well as to identify parasites. Protozoa and the eggs of parasitic worms are always microscopic, but the adult forms of many worms are clearly visible to the naked eye. If their presence is suspected, the specimen should be examined as soon as possible: the ova of parasites survive desiccation and cold, but the worms themselves and protozoa become sluggish on cooling and are more difficult to detect.

Rectal swabs are not acceptable in place of stool specimens because they provide insufficient material for culture. Stools usually contain millions of bacteria, and interpreting the results requires skill. It is not easy to identify those responsible for enteric infection, and several specimens may be necessary before the pathogen is isolated and identified.

Sputum specimens

Sputum is the secretion produced by the mucous membranes lining the lower airways. Its function is to trap inhaled foreign material, including bacteria. About 100 ml are secreted daily, but this is not usually apparent in health, when the sputum is normally swallowed. Excess production occurs when the airways become inflamed. This frequently occurs with infection but, even in the case of severe infection, sputum is often difficult to obtain in sufficient quantity to be examined and cultured. Sputum from an intubated patient is obtained by tracheal aspiration. Others must be encouraged to cough to produce a specimen. Saliva from the oropharynx is frequently sent to the laboratory instead of sputum. The help of a physiotherapist can be enlisted to overcome this difficulty. Many of the organisms responsible for infection of the lower respiratory tract do not survive well outside the host, so specimens should be dispatched to the laboratory immediately.

Throat swabs

Exudate from the throat is obtained by passing the tip of the swab over the tonsils and the posterior pharyngeal wall while the tongue is depressed with a spatula (Figure 3.4). A good source of illumination is necessary to avoid contaminating the swab by contact with the oral mucosa. People usually find this procedure unpleasant and should be warned in advance about the gag reflex. Children may be more cooperative if the help of a parent or carer is enlisted.

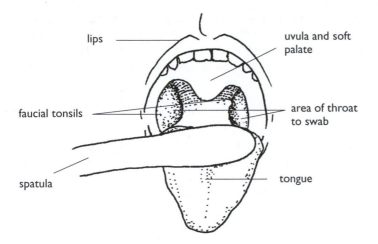

Figure 3.4 Taking a throat swab

Nasal swabs

Nasal swabs are taken with the person's head tilted, rotating the previously moistened swab to ensure that as much secretion as possible is collected. Both nostrils are
swabbed. For infants and very young children, a fine wire swab-holder may be used
instead of a wooden swab-stick. Great care is necessary to avoid damaging the delicate epithelium. When healthy people are screened to exclude staphylococcal
carriage, the tip of the swab is moistened with sterile water because, in health, the
nasal mucosa is usually dry.

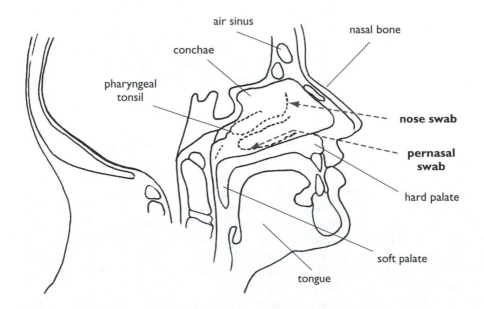

Figure 3.5 Taking a pernasal swab

Pernasal swabs are used to confirm a presumptive diagnosis of pertussis (whooping cough). *Bordetella pertussis* is most readily recovered from the posterior nasopharynx, especially if the specimen is obtained immediately after coughing. The tip of the swab is connected to a fine, flexible wire so that it can be introduced into the space without contamination (Figure 3.5).

Eye swabs

Eye swabs often yield poor results because lysozyme, an antibacterial enzyme naturally present in tears, destroys bacteria. Instead, scrapings from the conjunctiva can be obtained with a plastic loop and inoculated directly onto culture media. This procedure is usually undertaken by staff who have received special training.

Blood cultures

Blood cultures require strict aseptic technique during their collection. Two bottles containing liquid culture media are inoculated, one for aerobic culture and the other for anaerobic culture. The procedure is strictly aseptic to avoid contamination with skin flora. Any patient likely to be septicaemic is very ill, so there should be no delay in sending the specimens to the laboratory: most provide an incubator to receive blood cultures outside normal working hours.

Specimens of cerebrospinal fluid

Cerebrospinal fluid (CSF) is usually obtained by lumbar puncture. This is a highly invasive procedure usually performed on a very sick patient who is likely to be anxious, possibly disorientated and uncooperative. A doctor, assisted by a nurse, undertakes it. The specimen is collected by strict aseptic technique to avoid introducing infection and to prevent the CSF becoming contaminated with skin organisms. Three consecutive tubes are filled with CSF, which must be sent to the laboratory at once. The specimens must be maintained at 37 °C until they are examined, which must occur no later than 2–4 hours after collection.

Vaginal and cervical swabs

Most pathogens recovered from the female genital tract survive poorly in the environment, so contamination is less problematic than with other specimens. Special transport media (Stuart's or Amies' medium) are used. Storage at room temperature may be helpful to the laboratory staff since *Trichomonas vaginalis* will multiply and is more easily detected. When refrigerated, the protozoa become immobile and difficult to detect. *Neisseria gonorrhoeae*, however, survives so poorly outside the tissues that it is advisable for all specimens to be examined immediately when this infection is suspected. Most sexual health clinics (genitourinary medicine) have satellite laboratories so that specimens can be examined at once. It is usual to obtain more than one swab so that culture plates can be inoculated, permitting antibiotic sensitivity testing. This is essential owing to the increasing number of gonococci that have been found to be resistant to penicillin, the drug of choice for this condition.

Environmental sampling

Bacteria are present throughout the environment. Most are not pathogens, those on the floor, walls and so on being unlikely to cause harm. The number of bacteria isolated from a swab will depend on the site sampled. Routine sampling is expensive, time-consuming and (as little is known about the level of contamination that should be taken as unacceptable) uninformative. It is occasionally initiated by the infection control team during an outbreak, when it may help to identify environmental reservoirs or test the efficacy of the ventilation system in a newly commissioned theatre suite, for example. This process involves the use of an air sampler to measure the number of organisms per cubic centimetre of air. Agar 'settle plates' are not a useful substitute because the results are difficult to interpret and may not accurately reflect the level of contamination (Holton and Ridgeway, 1993).

Safe transport of specimens

The safe transport of specimens is vitally important; they should be transported in a way that makes certain that there is no leakage during transit (Department of Health, 2006). Procedures that comply with health and safety legislation are necessary to protect all staff (see below).

PRACTICE APPLICATION 3.3

Transporting Specimens Safely

Specimens must be transported in robust, leak-proof containers, with the request card separate from the specimen container. The outside of the container should not be contaminated with blood or any other body fluid and must not be overfilled: fermentation may occur, especially with faeces, leading to the accumulation of gas and a build-up of pressure sufficient to force off even a tightly fitting lid. Staff handling specimens should be aware of the hazards attached to spillage, they should wear overalls and should know that they must wash their hands frequently, for example after collecting the specimens. Leak-proof trays should be available for transport.

All specimens contain potentially infectious material and therefore present a hazard during transport. In order to reduce the risks to handlers during transport, the use of leak-proof boxes and agreed protocols for dealing with spillages is recommended (Health and Safety Executive, 2003). Biohazard labels are used to indicate to handlers and laboratory staff that a specimen may contain particularly hazardous pathogens. The indications for their use vary between settings. However, they should be applied to specimens that may contain M. tuberculosis or parenterally transmitted viruses, such as hepatitis B and C, or HIV.

The interpretation of laboratory results

Interpreting laboratory reports combines the results of microbiological findings (see Figure 3.1 above) with clinical evaluation. Some of the bacteria isolated may be contaminants or part of the normal flora that do not cause infection at that site. Thus, the diagnosis of infection must also take into consideration the person's signs and symptoms. For example, *Staphylococcus epidermidis* from the skin may contaminate a blood specimen but there will be no evidence of pyrexia.

SELF-ASSESSMENT

1. A high magnification is always needed to observe microbiological specimens. True? or False?

2. State three techniques used to examine microscope slides.

3. Explain why all the bacteria in a colony are of the same type.

4. A specimen of stool, rather than a rectal swab, is required to identify pathogenic bacteria. True? or False?

5. List five points to ensure safe specimen handling and transport.

REFERENCES

Department of Health (DH) (2006) *The Health Act 2006: Code of Practice for the Prevention and Control of Healthcare-associated Infections.* DH, London. Available www.dh.gov.uk.

Health and Safety Executive (HSE) (2003) *Safe Working and the Prevention of Infection in Clinical Laboratories and Similar Facilities.* HSE Books, London.

Higgins C (1994) An introduction to the examination of specimens. *Nursing Times* **90**(47): 29–32.

Holton J and Ridgeway GL (1993) Commissioning operating theatres. *Journal of Hospital Infection* **23**:153–60.

White S (1992) Choosing the right container. *Nursing Times* **88**(6): 64–5.

FURTHER READING AND INFORMATION SOURCES

Gilbert R (2006) Obtaining a midstream specimen of urine. *Nursing Times* **102**(18): 22–3.

Gilbert R (2006) Obtaining a catheter specimen of urine. *Nursing Times* **102**(19): 22–3.

Health and Safety Executive Advisory Committee on Dangerous Pathogens (2005) *Biological Agents: Managing the Risks in Laboratories and Healthcare Premises.* Available www. hse.gov.uk/biosafety/biologagents.pdf.

CHAPTER 4

Antimicrobial drugs

CHAPTER OUTCOMES

After reading this chapter, you should be able to:

➤ Define the terms 'antibiotic', 'bactericidal' and 'bacteriostatic'

➤ State the aims of antibiotic therapy in the treatment of established infection and in chemoprophylaxis

➤ Name the main groups of antibacterial agents and explain how they exert their effects

➤ Discuss the consequences of indiscriminate antibiotic use

➤ Explain the mechanisms that give rise to antibiotic-resistant strains of bacteria

➤ Explain the difficulties associated with the treatment of viral and fungal infections and name the drugs in current use

Introduction to antimicrobial drugs

Antibiotics are, strictly speaking, defined as naturally produced chemicals released by living organisms that are able to inhibit the growth of other organisms. However, the term is now used to refer to any antimicrobial chemotherapeutic agent: those produced naturally, synthetic compounds and the semi-synthetic antibiotics created by modifying natural drugs.

Antibiotics are widely prescribed to treat established infection and as chemoprophylaxis (the prevention of infection by giving antibiotics before signs and symptoms appear; see below) when the risk of developing an infection is significant. Antibiotic use has greatly increased since their introduction; the number of prescriptions in England doubled between 1980 and 1991 (Davey et al., 1996). Healthcare practitioners including those who prescribe need to be able to educate people about antibiotic use and to understand the:

- Aims of antibiotic treatment
- Antibiotic action
- Side-effects
- Dangers of indiscriminate antibiotic use.

Situations in which chemoprophylaxis is appropriate

➤ Colorectal surgery to prevent infection by the normal gut flora, especially anaerobes: metronidazole with gentamicin or a cephalosporin

➤ Orthopaedic surgery to prevent the infection of a prosthesis: flucloxacillin with gentamicin or a cephalosporin

➤ Major cardiac surgery, especially to prevent infection of implanted valve: flucloxacillin with gentamicin or a cephalosporin

➤ Amputation of an ischaemic (insufficient blood supply) limb to avoid the serious risk of infection with *Clostridium perfringens* (bacterium causing gas gangrene): penicillin, or erythromycin for those sensitive to penicillin

➤ Dental treatment for people with a history of infective endocarditis to reduce the risk of streptococcal infection: large dose of amoxicillin immediately before the procedure

➤ Genitourinary and gastrointestinal procedures for people with a history of infective endocarditis: ampicillin and gentamicin

➤ Prevention of streptococcal infection following splenectomy and in sickle-cell disease: amoxicillin

➤ Contacts of patients with meningococcal meningitis: see Chapter 14

➤ Travellers to malaria-endemic regions: see Chapter 14

The purpose of antibiotic therapy

The purpose of antibiotic treatment is to cure the patient or to effect chemoprophylaxis while causing minimum side-effects and discomfort. This is necessary in the case of severe infectious illness but is not considered good practice in the case of trivial infections or if the condition could be caused by a virus against which antibiotics have no effect, for example viral sore throat. In 1998, the Department of Health issued recommendations regarding the use of antibiotics (see below). Unnecessary prescription is dangerous because it promotes the emergence of antibiotic-resistant strains and may cause side-effects (Davies, 1994).

PRACTICE APPLICATION 4.1

Reducing the Inappropriate Use of Antibiotics and Bacterial Resistance

Official guidance was issued to help reduce the bacterial antibiotic resistance (Department of Health, 1998). The main recommendations included:

➤ Not prescribing antibiotics for colds, simple coughs and sore throats caused by viruses

➤ Prescribing antibiotics over the telephone in only exceptional situations

> ➤ Prescribing antibiotics for only three days for uncomplicated cystitis in otherwise healthy women

> ➤ Increasing understanding in professionals and the public about the prescribing of antibiotics

Activity

> ➤ Identify a situation concerning the inappropriate use of antibiotics. Reflect upon the factors involved and consider how a similar incident could be avoided in the future.

Resource

Health Protection Agency – www.hpa.org.uk/infections/topics_az/primary_care_guidance/menu.htm, select *Antibiotic Guidance and References*.

Health and social care practitioners have an important role in educating the general public and junior medical staff with regard to the proper use of antibiotics. The pressure on prescribers to provide antibiotics for patients suffering from minor viral conditions can be very intense. Antibiotic use could be reduced if the public and prescribers had information about conditions in which antibiotics are required. Community nursing staff, practice nurses and those working in walk-in centres and emergency departments are particularly well placed to provide this information for the public. Locally implemented guidelines appear to be effective in reducing the emergence of resistant strains, help reduce the incidence of adverse drug reactions and contribute to cost containment (Alerny et al., 2005). However, recent trends in microbial resistance give cause for concern, for example increasing ciprofloxacin resistance in *Neisseria gonorrhoeae* (Health Protection Agency, 2006).

Historical development of antibiotic therapy

Despite the hazards of side-effects and bacterial resistance, antibiotics still feature among the greatest triumphs of modern medicine. Down the ages, there have been strenuous efforts to control infectious disease, but until the beginning of the 20th century, none were successful. The search to find a cure encompassed every kind of substance imaginable, from toxic chemicals to homemade remedies. Mercury, for example, was used to treat syphilis even though its long-term effects were as severe as the disease itself. A breakthrough at the beginning of the 20th century was made possible because the germ theory of disease had been accepted and advances in the chemical industry permitted the development of previously unknown organic compounds.

The first major advance was made in 1910 by the scientist Paul Ehrlich, who synthesized 605 derivatives of arsenic before isolating neoarsphenamine '606'. This could kill *Treponema pallidum*, although a long course of treatment was necessary to cure syphilis. Nevertheless, for many years it was the main treatment.

Gerhard Domagk made further progress in 1935. His research with dyestuffs yielded a compound able to resolve infection in experimental animals. The active component was sulphanilamide, the forerunner of a group of synthetic drugs called 'sulphonamides'. Over the next 20 years, other sulphonamides became available. Although penicillins eventually superseded these, their success was considerable. However, the sulphonamides were associated with potentially severe side-effects: nausea, rashes and fever. The drugs precipitate out of solution in the urinary tract, leading to obstruction in severe cases. Only a few of the sulphonamides are still used (Table 4.1), having largely been replaced, first by penicillins and then by newer antibiotics.

Table 4.1 Examples of sulphonamides in use

Name of drug	Important properties	Indications
Sulfadiazine (sulphadiazine)		Used to prevent the recurrence of rheumatic fever
Sulfasalazine (sulphasalazine)	Releases sulfapyridine (antibacterial) and 5-aminosalicylic acid (anti-inflammatory drug) in the gut	Inflammatory bowel disease (Crohn's disease, ulcerative colitis). Rheumatoid arthritis
Silver sulfadiazine (sulphadiazine)		Used topically to prevent or treat infection, on burns, abrasions, skin graft donor sites, pressure ulcers and leg ulcers

The discovery of penicillin in 1928 predated Domagk's work. It had been known since the 19th century that fungi could inhibit bacterial growth. The discovery of penicillin, the first naturally occurring antibiotic to be identified, is attributed to Sir Alexander Fleming, working in London. Spores of the fungus *Penicillium notatum* carried by the air currents settled onto a culture that had been inoculated with *Staphylococcus aureus*. The mould took over, producing a chemical that inhibited the growth of the staphylococci. Fleming was unable to isolate the antibiotic produced by *P. notatum*, this being left to Ernst Chain and Sir Howard Florey working in Oxford. The first penicillin was isolated in 1939. The Second World War (1939–45) had provided the impetus for research, leading to the development of commercially available antibacterial agents to treat the large number of infections associated with trauma and communicable diseases among the troops, but penicillin did not become universally available in the UK until the war was over. Throughout the war, the further development of penicillin took place in the USA.

Antibiotics revolutionized the treatment of infection. UK childhood mortality statistics show that in 1940, when the earliest antibacterial agents were just becoming available, 3,000 children per million died of infectious conditions every year. By 1970, the mortality from childhood infectious disease had declined to 450 per million because of the ready availability of treatment. The triumph of antibiotic therapy must, however, be judged in the light of other social and medical advances made towards the end of the 19th and throughout the early 20th century: better social conditions, improved hygiene and immunization programmes. Social historians argue that the development of medicine, despite spectacular advances in the fields of therapeutics and immunology, is insufficient to explain the increase in the rate of infant survival and the decline in mortality that occurred as the 19th century drew to a close. For example, smallpox was conquered and antibacterial drugs became widely available at a time when the health of the nation was already improving, better health occurring secondary to industrial and economic developments such as improved nutrition, education and hygiene. Nevertheless, the contribution of antibiotics should not be underestimated.

The discovery of other antibiotics

Following the widespread, successful use of penicillin, the search commenced for other naturally occurring antibacterial agents. Soil, the normal environment of fungi, was subjected to intensive investigation, leading to the discovery of chloramphenicol, streptomycin and the tetracyclines (1940s), erythromycin and rifampicin (1950s), and gentamicin and sodium fusidate (1960s). The forerunner of the cephalosporin group of antibiotics was isolated from a fungus growing in sewage effluent in 1948. Most of the naturally occurring antibiotics are produced by fungi or *Streptomyces,* a few being made by *Bacillus* spp. and actinomycetes. Each new drug was initially welcomed as a broader spectrum alternative to any of the antibacterials already available, but in reality none has fulfilled these claims, owing to the emergence of antibiotic-resistant strains.

Range of antibiotic action

Antibiotics can be classified according to the type of bacteria against which they act. There are three groups:

1. Drugs active mainly against Gram-positive organisms, for example penicillins and erythromycin
2. Drugs mainly active against Gram-negative organisms, for example colistin and nalidixic acid
3. Broad-spectrum antibiotics active against Gram-positive and Gram-negative organisms, for example tetracyclines, chloramphenicol, ampicillin, cephalosporins and sulphonamides.

There are, however, exceptions. *Neisseria* spp. are Gram negative yet they are usually sensitive to penicillin and erythromycin. The natural susceptibility of many bacteria may be altered by resistance developing through exposure to antibiotics. This occurs much more rapidly with some types of bacteria than others. *Mycobacterium tuberculosis* is able to develop resistance to antibiotics within six weeks, this being the rationale behind the use of combined chemotherapy to treat tuberculosis. Tetracyclines are effective against chlamydias, rickettsiae and mycoplasmas.

Mode of antibiotic action

Antibiotics either kill bacteria or prevent them multiplying:

- **Bactericidal agents** kill bacteria rapidly – for example aminoglycosides, cephalosporins and colistin

- **Bacteriostatic agents** prevent bacteria replicating but do not kill them – for example sulphonamides, tetracyclines and chloramphenicol.

Many antibiotics that operate principally as bacteriostatic agents can become bactericidal in favourable circumstances. Influential factors include the concentration of the drug and the number and type of bacteria present. Where only a few highly sensitive organisms are present and the drug is given in a high dose, an agent such as penicillin that is usually bacteriostatic becomes bactericidal. The mechanisms of antibiotic action are shown in Table 4.2.

Antibiotics exert their effects directly on the bacterial cell wall or penetrate it to disrupt metabolism at the intracellular level. In all bacteria, the cell wall is composed of layers of protein molecules bound together by cross-linkages, but the fine structure depends on whether they are Gram positive or Gram negative, this influencing susceptibility to the different groups of antibiotic. For example, erythromycin penetrates the cell walls of Gram-positive bacteria and is effective in the treatment of some staphylococcal and streptococcal infections, but it has no effect on Gram-negative bacteria.

Table 4.2 Mechanisms of antibiotic action

Action on microorganism	Example
Prevents cell wall formation	Penicillins, cephalosporins, vancomycin
Alters permeability of cell membrane	Antifungals agents, for example amphotericin
Disrupts protein synthesis	Aminoglycosides, tetracyclines, chloramphenicol, erythromycin
Disrupts nucleic acid synthesis	Quinolones
Disrupts cell metabolism	Trimethoprim, sulphonamides

Specific antibiotics: mode of action

Some of the diverse ways in which the different groups of antibiotics exert their effects include:

- **Sulphonamides** have a molecular structure similar to that of a metabolite called 'para-aminobenzoic acid' (PABA) essential for the growth of many bacteria. If a sulphonamide is present, it is absorbed instead of PABA but cannot be metabolized, so the bacteria cease to multiply. This phenomenon is known as 'competitive inhibition'.
- **Trimethoprim** inhibits the action of a bacterial enzyme but has no effect on the corresponding human enzyme. It interferes with the metabolism of folic acid and ultimately prevents the bacteria synthesizing DNA. Trimethoprim and the sulphonamides operate at different points in the same metabolic pathway.
- The **penicillins**, the **cephalosporins** and **vancomycin** inhibit the formation of cross-links between protein molecules in the bacterial cell wall, which gradually weakens, eventually bursting as the cell grows.
- The **tetracyclines, chloramphenicol, streptomycin** and the **aminoglycosides** interfere with protein synthesis within the cell by attaching themselves to the

ribosomes (subcellular organelles concerned with protein synthesis) thus inhibiting protein synthesis and bacterial replication.

- **Quinolones** disrupt the structure of bacterial DNA by inhibiting an enzyme that allows transcription (part of protein synthesis) or DNA replication.

Adverse reactions to antibacterial drugs

Toxicity to antibacterial drugs falls into two broad categories, direct chemical toxicity and superinfection arising through prolonged or inappropriate antibiotic treatment.

Direct chemical toxicity

Direct chemical toxicity can be mediated through side-effects specifically related to the drug. Examples include the nephrotoxic (toxic to renal tubule cells of the kidney) and ototoxic (toxic to cells in the inner ear) action of gentamicin, and the rare depressant effect of chloramphenicol on the bone marrow. These effects are well established, and it is usually possible to find an alternative treatment. If no alternative is readily available, antibiotic assays are required to ensure that the plasma level does not exceed safe limits (see below).

INFORMATION BOX 4.2

Antibiotic assays

Antibiotic assays that measure the concentration of a particular antibiotic in body fluids are necessary in the following circumstances:

➤ To confirm that adequate levels of the antibiotic are being attained in the tissues. This might be necessary in the case of a patient severely ill with meningitis, or when an individual taking an oral drug is known to have impaired absorption from the intestine.

➤ To ensure that the plasma level does not exceed the limits of safety when the patient is receiving a drug with known toxic effects (for example gentamicin).

➤ During the investigation of a new drug. Assay of the body fluids will provide information about absorption, the way in which the drug becomes distributed through the tissues and its rate of excretion.

Additionally, some individuals develop type 1 hypersensitivity (allergic) reactions to particular drugs, often penicillins or cephalosporins (see below). Type 1 hypersensitivity reactions are mediated by IgE (see Chapter 2). The allergen binds to IgE on the surface of the mast cells and basophils, and chemical mediators (for example histamine and bradykinin) are released. Symptoms include nausea, vomiting and diarrhoea if the drug is taken orally, or contact erythema if it is applied topically or injected, and may persist after it is stopped. Anaphylactic shock is a more severe complication, which can be life-threatening (Chapter 2).

PRACTICE APPLICATION 4.2

Hypersensitivity Reactions

It is difficult to predict who will develop a hypersensitivity reaction. Clinical observations suggest that patients with a history of allergy are more susceptible, but all patients should be asked about allergies and sensitivity to drugs before the first dose is administered. A note of any history of allergy or side-effects to drugs should be recorded in the nursing and medical records.

Activity

➤ What protocols exist in your workplace/placement for documenting allergies affecting patients or residents and ensuring that all members of staff are aware?

Superinfection

Superinfection occurs when the body's normal commensal flora is suppressed by antibiotics and replaced by drug-resistant organisms. It may follow treatment with any antibiotic but is most commonly seen with broad-spectrum antibiotics such as the tetracyclines, especially if they are administered for a long time. In the upper respiratory tract, the normal flora is replaced with drug-resistant coliforms (any of the Gram-negative intestinal bacteria such as *Escherichia, Klebsiella, Enterobacter*). Suppression of the normal vaginal flora causes superinfection with yeasts. The normal gut flora is replaced with *Klebsiella, Pseudomonas*, yeasts and staphylococci. Patients complain of a sore mouth, vomiting and diarrhoea, which can lead to non-adherence to a drug regimen.

These problems have been documented since the 1970s, but more recently, superinfection with *Clostridium difficile* has become a major problem. This organism is present as part of the normal gut flora in around 3 per cent of adults (Health Protection Agency, 2007a), but suppression of the gut flora allows it to multiply and release toxins. Large areas of the intestinal epithelium become necrosed, and the patient develops profuse, watery diarrhoea. This condition, known as 'pseudomembranous colitis' (antibiotic-associated colitis), causes ulceration that can lead to potentially life-threatening perforation and peritonitis. During investigations of hospital outbreaks, asymptomatic carriers have been identified (Degl'Innocenti et al., 1989), and the person-to-person spread of clostridia and infection from spores in environmental reservoirs has been documented (Wilcox, 1996). The development of pseudomembranous colitis appears to be exacerbated if patients receive injectable 'third generation' cephalosporins, for example ceftriaxone, that attain high concentrations in the bile, which then delivers them to the gut where they are not fully absorbed. Superinfection with these antibiotics is more marked than that seen with the oral cephalosporins. *C. difficile* superinfection can be treated with vancomycin or metronidazole. A type of *C. difficile* (type 027) that causes severe disease has been identified in the UK. It has been involved in several major outbreaks with associated deaths in English hospitals. The spread of *C. difficile* can be prevented by isolation, meticulous attention to handwashing and by ensuring that the environment does not become contaminated with spores spread from infected individuals (symptomatic or asymptomatic) (see below).

PRACTICE APPLICATION 4.3

Preventing the Spread of *Clostridium difficile*

Preventive measures include:

➤ The isolation of patients with diarrhoea to stop cross-infection and environmental contamination

➤ Wearing plastic aprons and gloves for any contact with faeces and during environmental cleaning procedures

➤ Thorough handwashing by staff and visitors following any patient contact is required because alcohol gels do not kill spores (Department of Health, 2007)

➤ Handwashing by patients both before and after meals

➤ The proper disposal of used linen in red alginate bags

➤ Frequent changes of bed linen – at least every 24 hours

➤ The proper disposal of waste in yellow bags for incineration

➤ High standards of environmental cleaning, using chlorine disinfectants (Department of Health, 2007). Frequent monitoring

➤ Avoiding the transfer of patients between wards and to or from other hospitals

➤ Thorough environmental cleaning to remove spores once the patient is free from infection

➤ Liaison with the infection control team

➤ Informing and educating all concerned

Activity

➤ Find out about the prevalence of *C. difficile* in your workplace/placement. What protocols exist to prevent its spread?

Bacterial resistance to antibiotics

Antibiotic-resistant microorganisms are defined as those not inhibited or killed by antibiotics at the drug concentration achieved in the body after a therapeutic dose. This is not a recent phenomenon: Ehrlich, working in the early 1900s, noticed that neoarsphenamine had to be administered in an increasing dose because the treponemes gradually became less susceptible. The first major concern was expressed by Miles (1944), who predicted that the incidence of drug-resistant organisms, particularly Gram-negative bacteria, might increase as more patients received sulphonamides and penicillin to treat Gram-positive infections. These fears were confirmed three years later when Florey et al. (1947) reported that 50 per cent of traumatic wounds treated in hospital became colonized with coliforms, the major predisposing factor being antibiotic treatment. The ability of *Pseudomonas* to cause cross-infection in critical care units soon became apparent, a situation further exacerbated by the introduction of broad-spectrum antibiotics (Colebrook et al., 1948).

Staphylococci first became significant as nosocomial pathogens during the 1940s, replacing streptococci, which had previously been responsible for most cases of cross-infection. Penicillin-resistant strains were first reported during the 1950s. The new synthetic penicillins initially helped to control the problem, but strains resistant to meticillin (methicillin) were reported before the end of the decade (Shanson, 1985). Meticillin itself is not used therapeutically because its oral absorption is poor, but meti-cillin resistance is of enormous clinical significance because meticillin-resistant strains of bacteria are inevitably also resistant to cloxacillin, flucloxacillin and the cepha-losporins. New synthetic antibiotics at first brought about a dramatic improvement in the treatment of infection. The disappearance of meticillin-resistant *Staphylococcus aureus* (MRSA) during the 1970s was greeted with complacency, which evaporated in the 1980s when persistent outbreaks of MRSA were reported worldwide (Cafferkey et al., 1985). The control of MRSA is now regarded as one of the major challenges facing infection control experts (Cox et al., 1995).

Enterococci are an increasingly common cause of infection in hospitalized patients (Beaumont, 1998). Over the past decade, there has been a worrying escalation in the development of multiresistant strains of enterococci. Many enterococci, espe-cially *Enterococcus faecium*, are now resistant to vancomycin – so-called vancomycin-resistant enterococci (VRE) or glycopeptide-resistant enterococci (GRE) (Chapter 1). Treatment options are extremely limited, and bacteraemia caused by VRE/GRE carries a high mortality rate. VRE/GRE are discussed further in Chapter 6.

A further hazard for vulnerable patients in intensive care settings is infection with *Acinetobacter*. This aerobic bacterium can develop resistance to many antibiotics and is responsible for a wide range of infections, for example pneumonia and wound infection. *Acinetobacter* is spread via the hands of staff, on which it is capable of surviving for some time. The organism also thrives in damp conditions such as humidification devices. It is vital, therefore, that equipment is stored dry.

Bacterial resistance may be described as high level when the drug is completely ineffective, or partial when a high tissue concentration can still be effective. This may not, however, be feasible, for example if the drug is toxic if given in a high dose. Gentamicin is nephrotoxic (toxic to the kidney) in high doses and is there-fore not suitable for patients with renal impairment. Bacterial resistance to anti-bacterial drugs falls into two broad categories: intrinsic resistance and acquired resistance. Antibiotic-resistant bacteria are an increasing problem in both hospital and the community (see below).

INFORMATION BOX 4.3

Antibiotic-resistant bacteria in hospital and the community

Antibiotic resistance is recognized as a major problem in hospital because broad-spectrum antibiotics are commonly prescribed for the critically ill, contributing to the well-documented problems of superinfection and cross-infection. Antibiotic resistance is, however, not a problem restricted to hospitals. Patients who become colonized in hospital may continue to carry antibiotic-resistant strains of bacteria and cause problems when they are readmitted. Infection control procedures have now become necessary in community settings, such as nursing homes, to help to contain the spread (Cox et al., 1995). Antibiotics are also prescribed very widely for people with minor infections, both systemically and as topical creams, ointments and powders. People who use these unsupervised at home may not recognize the dangers presented to the environment if antibiotics are spilled and may unknowingly contribute to the emergence of resistance by failing to complete a course of medication, exposing the bacteria to subclinical doses. Practitioners in general practice have a role educating the public about the safe use of antibiotics, and antibiotic policies should be implemented in community settings as well as in hospitals (see Practice application 4.1 above).

Intrinsic resistance

Intrinsic resistance is the innate property of the organism determined by the structure of the cell wall. Gram-positive bacteria are more susceptible to antibiotics than Gram-negative bacteria because their cell walls are less complex and lack the natural sieve effect against large antibiotic molecules that is shown by Gram-negative organisms. This explains why *Pseudomonas aeruginosa* has always been resistant to flucloxacillin.

Acquired resistance

High levels of antibiotic prescribing are linked to increased resistance among bacteria recovered from the hospital environment, which may contribute to cross-infection (Dancer et al., 2006). Bacteria become resistant either by spontaneous chromosomal mutation and selection, or by the transfer of a plasmid carrying genes that code for antibiotic resistance.

Mutation is the chance genetic change in one cell resulting in the synthesis of an altered protein. Mutation is often lethal but occasionally results in a bacterium able to withstand the action of a particular antibiotic better than its parent cell. When exposed to the antibiotic to which it has become resistant, the mutant will have obvious advantages over the rest of the bacterial population and will be free to multiply without competition for nutrients and space. The indiscriminate use of antibiotics promotes the multiplication of antibiotic-resistant mutants that then spread to other people by cross-infection.

Plasmid transfer occurs by conjugation, transformation or transduction (Chapter 1). Transformation does not appear to be clinically important in the dissemination of resistance. However, streptococci, staphylococci and clostridia readily undergo conjugation, and transduction plays an important role in the transmission of resistant genes between staphylococci and *Streptococcus pyogenes*.

Factors contributing to bacterial resistance include:

- The misuse of antibiotics in chemoprophylaxis. Antibiotics should be restricted to those cases in which the advantages outweigh the risks (see Information box 4.1 above).
- Employing antibiotics used to treat systemic infection in topical preparations. This practice promotes plasmid-mediated resistance in the normal skin flora.

■ Adding antibiotics to animal feeds, which is still common in some countries.

Principles of antibiotic therapy

The following principles ensure adequate treatment for the individual and reduce the exposure of organisms to antibiotics, promoting resistance:

■ The use of antibiotics should be restricted to occasions when they are genuinely necessary. They should not be used for trivial infections or viral infections.

■ Antibiotic chemoprophylaxis should be reserved for people identified as being at risk of developing bacterial infection known to present a specific threat (see Information box 4.1 above), and not used as part of a blanket policy. Chemoprophylaxis is no substitute for good infection prevention and control practice.

■ Treatment should be based on a sound bacteriological diagnosis, specimens being obtained for laboratory examination if possible before the first dose of antibiotic is administered.

■ Broad-spectrum antibiotics are not indicated for infections against which an antibacterial drug with a more specific range could be used.

■ Antibiotics should be administered for a full therapeutic period (usually a minimum of three days). If the person's condition has not responded to treatment towards the end of this time, the following possibilities should be considered:

  ■ The bacteria are resistant to the antibiotic and further specimens must be sent to the laboratory

  ■ The drug is not reaching the organisms because they are sheltered in an abscess or a blood clot; further investigation is required

  ■ The person has not been taking the drug, and the possibility of non-concordance and the reasons for it must be explored.

■ Antibiotics used in preparations for topical application should not be the same as those used to treat systemic infections. Antibiotics commonly used in topical preparations include mupirocin, colistin and bacitracin.

■ The spillage of antibiotic solutions and powders should be avoided because exposure may induce hypersensitivity reactions in some people.

■ Antibiotic policies should be adopted in hospital and general practice.

Antibiotic policies

Policies have been developed to encourage the efficient, safe and economical use of antibiotics, their purpose being to reduce the emergence of antibiotic-resistant strains. In most hospitals, a local formulary is drawn up to reserve the use of particular drugs. Most local policies adopt the following general format:

■ A section that includes a single member of each of the main groups of antibiotic. Each of these can be prescribed without a formal procedure and is held as ward stock.

- A reserve section containing alternatives, including the most newly developed antibiotics. These are not usually prescribed without liaison with the infection control team and are not held as ward stock.

Policies need regular updating and reviewing to take account of new drugs and changing patterns of microbial behaviour. The purpose of an antibiotic policy is to limit prescription to just a few antibiotics so that bacteria lack the opportunity to develop resistance. The decision to prescribe any other antibiotic is usually taken between the doctor and medical microbiologist.

Main groups of antimicrobial drugs

There are several distinct groups of drugs that have antimicrobial actions. Some of these groups are described below but readers should always consult an up-to-date national formulary (for example *British National Formulary*) and the manufacturer's product information before prescribing, dispensing or administering the drug.

Penicillins

Penicillins (Table 4.3) belong to the beta-lactam group of antibiotics, their molecular structure including the beta-lactam ring – the part exhibiting antibacterial properties (Figure 4.1). Penicillins are still effective against many common pathogens and, apart from their ability to induce hypersensitivity reactions in susceptible individuals, are generally less toxic than many of the other antibiotics currently in use. Their value has, however, been seriously undermined by the ability of many bacteria to synthesize beta-lactamase (penicillinase) enzymes. These degrade the beta-lactam ring so that it becomes ineffective. Ninety per cent of staphylococci and many *Escherichia coli* are now resistant to penicillin.

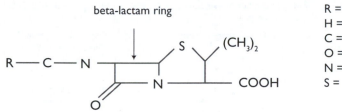

R = variable side chains
H = hydrogen
C = carbon
O = oxygen
N = nitrogen
S = sulphur

Figure 4.1 The beta-lactam antibiotics

Clavulanic acid is a naturally occurring beta-lactamase compound. It has little antibacterial activity when used alone but is a powerful inhibitor of many of the beta-lactamase enzymes and can be combined with other antibiotics to destroy strains that would otherwise show resistance. Amoxicillin combined with clavulanate is prescribed as Augmentin®; ticarcillin combined with clavulanate is prescribed as Timentin®.

Table 4.3 Examples of the penicillins

Drug	Indications	Comments
Benzylpenicillin	Diphtheria, syphilis, endocarditis, meningitis	Parenteral
Phenoxymethylpenicillin (penicillin V)	Streptococcal sore throats, respiratory infections. Prophylaxis against streptococcal infection in sickle-cell disease, post splenectomy and rheumatic fever	Oral
Broad spectrum		
Ampicillin	Pneumonia, bronchitis, ear infection, urinary infection	Oral
Amoxicillin (amoxycillin)	Pneumonia, bronchitis, urinary infection. Prophylaxis against endocarditis	Oral, parenteral, well absorbed
Antipseudomonal		
Ticarcillin with clavulanic acid (Timentin®)	Gram-negative organisms including *Pseudomonas aeruginosa, Bacteroides, Proteus* spp.	Parenteral
Piperacillin with a beta-lactamase inhibitor	Systemic Gram-negative sepsis and anaerobic infection	Parenteral
Beta-lactamase resistant		
Flucloxacillin	Staphylococcal infection (tissue, bone, joint)	Oral, parenteral
Mecillinams		
Pivmecillinam hydrochloride	Gram-negative organisms including *Escherichia coli, Enterobacter, Klebseilla, Salmonella*	Oral

Table 4.4 Examples of the cephalosporins

Drug	Indications	Comments
Oral		
Cefalexin, cefadroxil, cefradine (mainly replaced by newer drugs)	Moderately severe infections. Active against Gram-positive but less effective for Gram-negative infection	First generation. Wide spectrum, good oral absorption
Cefaclor	Urinary and respiratory infections	Second generation. Wider spectrum, active orally
Cefpodoxime proxetil	Respiratory infections	Third generation. More resistant to beta-lactamase
Parenteral		
Cefuroxime	Respiratory, urinary, some types of meningitis and septicaemia. Surgical prophylaxis. Active against *Haemophilus influenza*. Single dose for gonorrhoea	Second generation. Wide range of activity. Also given orally
Cefotaxime*, ceftazidime and ceftriaxone	Greater effect against Gram-negative infections. Urinary and respiratory infections *Cefotaxime is used for some types of meningitis	Third generation. May cause superinfection

Cephalosporins

The cephalosporins (Table 4.4) are chemically related to the penicillins as they also contain the beta-lactam ring. Thus, they share many of the properties of the penicillins: they may cause hypersensitivity reactions, and resistance may develop if the bacteria can produce beta-lactamase enzymes. The extended-spectrum beta-lactamase (ESBL)-producing *E. coli* is resistant to several antibiotics, notably the cephalosporins (Health Protection Agency, 2007b). It has, however, been possible to produce different 'generations' of cephalosporins to achieve a wider antibacterial spectrum than is possible with the penicillins, and resistance is less marked. The newer cephalosporins are valuable in the treatment of septicaemia and other severe infections. Cefotaxime can be used to treat meningitis because when the membranes are inflamed it crosses the blood–brain barrier effectively. The chief drawbacks associated with the cephalosporins are their comparatively high cost compared with other antibiotics, and superinfection, which develops because no individual member of the group has a complete antibacterial spectrum.

Aminoglycosides

The aminoglycosides (Table 4.5) are a group of bactericidal antibiotics effective against a wide range of Gram-negative aerobic bacteria. They are also effective against many Gram-positive bacteria, although not to the same extent as many other antibiotics. Their range of action can be extended by combining treatment with other antibacterials (for example cephalosporins). The aminoglycosides are associated with a number of potentially severe and highly undesirable side-effects, inducing renal and auditory impairment. Patients should have their blood level of the drug monitored to ensure that a toxic concentration is not reached, and diuretics should if possible be avoided.

Table 4.5 Examples of the aminoglycosides

Drug	Indications	Comments
Gentamicin	Serious Gram-negative infection	Parenteral. Assay needed
Tobramycin Netilmicin	Gentamicin-resistant organisms	
Amikacin	Gentamicin-resistant organisms	See gentamicin
Neomycin	Usually topical use only. Also used to reduce the numbers of bacteria in the gut in patients with liver failure, or prior to large bowel surgery	Toxic if absorbed
Streptomycin	Tuberculosis	Only used in the UK if the organism is resistant to isoniazid

Tetracyclines

The tetracyclines are broad-spectrum antibiotics whose use has declined in recent years, as bacterial resistance has increasingly become a problem. They are, however, still used to treat genitourinary, respiratory and dermatological infections and periodontal disease (Table 4.6). One of their chief advantages is that they are effective against chlamydial, rickettsial and *Mycoplasma* infections against which other antibiotics would have no action. Caution must be exercised when the tetracyclines are prescribed because they may be deposited in developing bones and teeth, and can have a teratogenic effect (see below). Patients taking tetracyclines may complain of gastrointestinal upsets resulting from superinfection, and existing renal failure may be exacerbated.

Tigecycline is the only example of a new class of glycylcycline antibacterials; it is related to the tetracyclines. It is effective against Gram-positive and Gram-negative organisms including some antibiotic-resistant strains, such as MRSA and VRE/GRE.

Table 4.6 Examples of the tetracyclines

Drug	Indications	Comments
Tetracycline oxytetracycline, minocycline and doxycycline	Respiratory, genital infections, skin infections, acne, oral infections, periodontal disease	Superinfection. Renal failure exacerbated

---

INFORMATION BOX 4.4

Safer use of tetracyclines

The deposition of tetracycline in developing bones and teeth can occur both before birth and during childhood, and can result in staining of the teeth and bone deformities. These potential problems can be avoided by ensuring that tetracyclines are not prescribed during pregnancy, during lactation or for children under the age of 12 years.

Macrolides

The macrolides include erythromycin, the most commonly prescribed member of the group, and a number of newer drugs, including telithromycin, clarithromycin and azithromycin. Erythromycin is a bacteriostatic drug, first introduced in 1952, effective in the treatment of Gram-positive infections including *Legionella* and *Mycoplasma* infections. Erythromycin is useful for patients who are allergic to penicillin because its range of action is similar. Unfortunately, bacteria readily become resistant. Clarithromycin and azithromycin can be used in the treatment of infection with the protozoan *Toxoplasma gondii*.

Antituberculosis drugs

Treatment with antituberculosis drugs is complicated by the lack of compliance and the emergence of multidrug resistant tuberculosis (MDR-TB) and more recently extensively drug-resistant tuberculosis (XDR-TB) (Chapter 14). The effectiveness of medication depends on prescribing drugs that are still able to destroy the mycobacteria, and on ensuring patient adherence. Examples of antituberculosis drugs include isoniazid, rifampicin, ethambutal, pyrazinamide, amikacin, capreomycin and so on. In the UK, the treatment of TB caused by non-resistant organisms has an initial phase during which four drugs are used, and a continuation phase when two drugs are used (see below).

■ PRACTICE APPLICATION 4.4 ■

Treatment of Tuberculosis

The treatment of TB is complex; therefore it is important that practitioners can explain it to patients to ensure their adherence to treatment regimens.

Activity

Access the resources below and find answers to the following questions:

➤ Why are four drugs used in the initial phase?

➤ Which drugs are used in the initial and continuation phases?

➤ When might longer courses of treatment be needed?

Resources

Beckford-Ball J (2006) NICE guidelines to improve TB management and prevention. *Nursing Times* 102(19): 19–20.

British National Formulary (2008) – www.bnf.org.

National Institute for Health and Clinical Excellence (NICE) (2006) *Tuberculosis – Clinical Diagnosis and Management of Tuberculosis, and Measures for its Prevention and Control.* Clinical guideline 33. Available www.nice.org.uk.

Antituberculosis drugs have a number of toxic side-effects that may be serious, including disturbed gastrointestinal and hepatic function. This and the length of treatment reduce adherence to the regimen. According to the National Institute for Health and Clinical Excellence (2006), drug administration three times per week should be considered for people having directly observed therapy.

Examples of other antimicrobial drugs

An outline of some other antimicrobial drugs is provided below.

Chloramphenicol

Chloramphenicol is a broad-spectrum antibiotic that acts in a similar way to the tetracyclines. It is potentially a very valuable drug as it is absorbed readily from the gastrointestinal tract and crosses the blood–brain barrier into the cerebrospinal fluid. However, highly toxic, albeit rare, effects on the bone marrow, which reduce the leucocyte count to a dangerously low level, limit its usefulness. Prescription is limited to those patients for whom a useful alternative is not available. Chloramphenicol is sometimes used to treat typhoid and paratyphoid fevers and *Haemophilus influenzae* meningitis because of its ability to cross the blood–brain barrier.

Clindamycin

Clindamycin is used to treat staphylococcal infections involving the bones and joints, and severe intra-abdominal sepsis. Its value is reduced by its tendency to cause super-infection, leading to *C. difficile* infection (see above).

Co-trimoxazole: trimethoprim and sulfamethoxazole (sulphamethoxazole)

Like the sulphonamides, trimethoprim interferes with bacterial metabolism by disrupting the production of folic acid. The combination of a sulphonamide and trimethoprim is very effective because it prevents bacterial division and is also bactericidal. Co-trimoxazole is effective against the same range of organisms as the sulphonamides: *Haemophilus influenzae* and *Salmonella*. It has been widely and successfully used to treat chronic bronchitis, urinary infections, *Pneumocystis jiroveci* (previously known as *Pneumocystis carinii*) infections in the immunocompromised and occasionally salmonellosis, but its usefulness is restricted by the number of side-effects that can occur. For example, nausea, vomiting and, more rarely but also more seriously, blood disorders and Stevens–Johnson syndrome, characterized by a rash with bullae (fluid-filled blisters over 5 mm in diameter), fever and ulceration of the mouth. This latter condition can be fatal.

Trimethoprim can be used on its own and has superseded co-trimoxazole in the treatment of urinary tract infections because it causes fewer side-effects.

Fucidic acid

Fucidic acid is a narrow-spectrum antibiotic able to penetrate all tissues, especially bone. It is used mainly to treat penicillin-resistant staphylococcal infection, for example in osteomyelitis. Bacterial resistance may develop rapidly, a problem overcome by the simultaneous administration of another antibiotic. Side-effects involve the gastrointestinal system and the liver.

Glycopeptides: vancomycin and teicoplanin

Vancomycin is effective against most Gram-positive bacteria and is of particular value in the treatment of resistant strains such as MRSA. It may be given orally to treat pseudomembranous colitis, and by slow intravenous infusion: if it is given too quickly, the patient may develop a sensitivity reaction characterized by hypotension (low blood pressure) and the appearance of a rash over the face and trunk. The side-effects of vancomycin – ototoxicity and nephrotoxicity – are severe. Plasma assays are essential during treatment.

Teicoplanin is similar to vancomycin but is associated with fewer side-effects. It has been used to control MRSA.

Linezolid (an oxazolidone)

Linezolid is an antibacterial drug, which can be effective in Gram-positive infections such as MRSA and VRE/GRE. It can cause serious side-effects.

Metronidazole

Metronidazole was originally introduced as an antiparasitic drug but is also highly effective in the treatment of anaerobic infections arising after gynaecological and gut surgery, and in the treatment of pseudomembranous colitis. Side-effects are uncommon, but patients taking metronidazole at home are advised to avoid alcohol because of possible interactions. Metronidazole is also used in combination with other drugs to eradicate *Helicobacter pylori*, the organism implicated in the aetiology of gastritis and peptic ulceration.

Nitrofurans

Nitrofurantoin is the only member of this group still in routine use. It has a fairly wide antibacterial spectrum, becomes concentrated in the urine and is effective in the treatment of urinary tract infections. It has few side-effects, but nausea is sometimes reported. Nitrofurantoin is not suitable for patients with impaired renal function because accumulation to toxic levels will occur. It may also cause gastrointestinal upsets.

Polymyxins

Colistin is active against Gram-negative bacteria, including *Pseudomonas*. It is not absorbed orally but is used to destroy the skin and gastrointestinal flora of severely immunocompromised patients. If administered by injection, it causes severe toxic effects involving the neurological system, vertigo and muscle weakness. Colistin and polymyxin B are also used topically.

Quinolones

The quinolones operate by interfering with an enzyme essential for the division of bacterial cells. They are a rapidly expanding group of synthetic antibacterial agents that include nalidixic acid, ciprofloxacin, levofloxacin and ofloxacin. Ciprofloxacin is effective against a wide range of bacteria, although it is generally less successful for Gram-positive infections. It can be used to treat infections resistant to the older antibacterial drugs and as chemoprophylaxis for people who have been in contact with meningococcal meningitis. Adverse reactions include gastrointestinal upsets and rashes. Nalidixic acid is effective against most Gram-negative urinary pathogens apart from *Pseudomonas*. It concentrates in the urine and is valuable in the treatment of urinary tract infection because its action is not affected by urinary pH. Resistance develops rapidly. Occasional toxic reactions include urticarial rashes and gastrointestinal disturbances.

Quinupristin and dalfopristin

The streptogramin antibacterial drugs quinupristin and dalfopristin combined are used in serious Gram-positive infections, which do not respond to other drugs, for example MRSA and vancomycin-resistant *Enterococcus faecium*. It is administered intravenously into a central vein.

Antiviral drugs

Treating viral infections is difficult because:

- Viruses are minute, intracellular particles so it is difficult for drugs to reach and attack them
- Infection is usually well established before symptoms appear
- Many of the agents currently used have severe toxic side-effects.

Several different drug groups are used in the management of serious viral infections (Table 4.7). For example, nucleoside reverse transcriptase inhibitors, protease inhibitors and non-nucleoside reverse transcriptase inhibitors are all used for HIV/AIDS disease, and interferons and monoclonal antibodies in viral hepatitis.

Table 4.7 Examples of antiviral drugs

Drug	Indications and comments
Aciclovir	Local and systemic herpes simplex and varicella-zoster infections. It can be given topically, orally or by slow intravenous infusion. Renal function must be carefully monitored
Amantidine	Prophylaxis against the influenza type A virus
Amprenavir	A protease inhibitor. Used in HIV/AIDS
Didanosine	A nucleoside reverse transcriptase inhibitor. Used for HIV/AIDS
Efavirenz	A non-nucleoside reverse transcriptase inhibitor. Used in HIV/AIDS
Foscarnet	Used for cytomegalovirus (CMV) infection. Can cause renal damage
Ganciclovir	Serious CMV infections in immunocompromised patients. Bone marrow suppression is a serious and potentially life-threatening side-effect
Lamivudine	Viral hepatitis, hepatitis B
Interferons, for example peginterferon alfa-2a	Viral hepatitis, hepatitis B and C
Oseltamivir	Prevents replication of influenza A and B viruses
Palivizumab	Monoclonal antibody used for infection with the respiratory syncytial virus (RSV)
Ribavirin (tribavirin)	Used for infection with the RSV. Used in combination with other drugs for chronic hepatitis C infection
Ritonavir	A protease inhibitor. Used for HIV/AIDS
Zanamivir	Prevents replication of influenza A and B viruses
Zidovudine (azidothymidine, AZT)	A nucleoside reverse transcriptase inhibitor. Used for HIV/AIDS. Bone marrow suppression is a severe side-effect

Antifungal drugs

Most serious fungal infections warranting treatment occur in patients who are immunocompromised, especially if they have received powerful broad-spectrum antibiotics resulting in superinfection. Examples of the main antifungal drugs currently available are indicated in Table 4.8.

Table 4.8 Examples of antifungal drugs

Drug group and examples	Indications	Comments
Polyenes		
Nystatin	Oral and vaginal candidiasis	Topical application. Too toxic for parenteral use
Amphotericin	Systemic and topical fungal infection	Oral, topical and parenteral. Severe toxic effects: fever, hypokalaemia (abnormally low level of potassium in the blood) and nephrotoxicity
Imidazoles		
Clotrimazole	Topical fungal infections	
Ketoconazole	Systemic fungal infections, resistant infections of the skin and mucosae, gastrointestinal tract, vagina, etc.	Not as effective as amphotericin. Hepatic toxicity (toxic to liver cells)
Miconazole	Topical fungal infections	
Triazoles		
Fluconazole	Include vaginal and mucosal candidiasis; invasive infections with candida and cryptococcus; prophylaxis in immunocompromised individuals; fungal infections such as tinea pedis	Oral, parenteral
Itraconazole	As above. Plus nail infections, histoplasmosis, aspergillosis	Oral, parenteral
Other antifungal drugs		
Griseofulvin	Dermatophyte fungal infection	Oral. Concentrates in keratin so is the drug of choice for intractable fungal infection of the skin
Flucytosine	Systemic yeast infection	Oral and parenteral. Not effective against *Aspergillus* or dermatophytes

SELF-ASSESSMENT

1. A bactericidal agent kills bacteria. True? or False?

2. Give an example of a situation in which chemoprophylaxis is appropriate.

3. Staphylococci are usually resistant to penicillin. True? or False?

4. Which of the following bacteria exhibit a high level of intrinsic resistance to many antibiotics?

   (a) staphylococci
   (b) *Pseudomonas*
   (c) *Streptococcus pyogenes*
   (d) *Klebsiella aerogenes*

5. Which of the following drugs contain a beta-lactam ring in their structure?

   (a) macrolides
   (b) cephalosporins
   (c) penicillins

(d) aminoglycosides

6. Which of the following are effective against *Chlamydia*?

   (a) macrolides
   (b) cephalosporins
   (c) tetracyclines
   (d) aminoglycosides

7. When does superinfection arise?

8. Why are virus infections difficult to treat?

REFERENCES

Alerny C, Campany D, Monterde J et al. (2005) Impact of local guidelines and an integrated dispensing system on antibiotic prophylaxis quality in a surgical centre. *Journal of Hospital Infection* **60**: 111–17.

Beaumont G (1998) Resistance movement. *Nursing Times* **94**(37): 69–75.

Cafferkey MT, Coleman D, McGrath B et al. (1985) *Staphylococcus aureus* in Dublin. *Lancet* **2**: 705–8.

Colebrook L, Duncan JM and Ross WP (1948) The control of infection in burns. *Lancet* **1**: 893.

Cox RA, Mallaghan C, Conquest C et al. (1995) Epidemic methicillin resistant *Staphylococcus aureus*: controlling the spread outside hospital. *Journal of Hospital Infection* **29**: 107–19.

Dancer SJ, Coyne M, Robertson C et al. (2006) Antibiotic use is associated with resistance of environmental organisms in a teaching hospital. *Journal of Hospital Infection* **62**: 200–6.

Davey PG, Bax RP and Reeves D (1996) The growth of the use of antibiotics in the community in England and Scotland in 1980–1993. *British Medical Journal* **312**: 613–14.

Davies J (1994) Antibiotic resistance and the dissemination of resistance genes. *Science* **264**(5157): 375–82.

Degl'Innocenti R, De Santis M, Berdondini I et al. (1989) Outbreak of *Clostridium difficile* diarrhoea in an orthopaedic unit: evidence by phage typing for cross infection. *Journal of Hospital Infection* **13**: 309–14.

Department of Health (DH) (1998) *The Path of Least Resistance. Report on the Impact of Clinical Prescribing on Antibiotic Resistance* (98/361). Standing Medical Advisory Committee, DH, London.

Department of Health (DH) (2007) *A Simple Guide to* Clostridium difficile. Available www. dh.gov.uk.

Florey ME, Ross R and Turton EC (1947) Infection of wounds with Gram-negative organisms: clinical manifestation and treatment. *Lancet* **2**: 855–61.

Health Protection Agency (HPA) (2006) *Trends in Antimicrobial Resistance in England and Wales (2004–2005)*. Available www.hpa.org.uk/.

Health Protection Agency (HPA) (2007a) *Clostridium difficile:* Frequently asked questions. Available www.hpa.org.uk/topics/index.htm.

Health Protection Agency (HPA) (2007b) Press statement *Infections caused by ESBL-producing E. coli*. Available www.hpa.org.uk/.

Miles AA (1944) Epidemiology of wound infection. *Lancet* 1: 809–14.

National Institute for Health and Clinical Excellence (NICE) (2006) *Tuberculosis – Clinical Diagnosis and Management of Tuberculosis, and Measures for its Prevention and Control.* Clinical guideline 33. Available www.nice.org.uk.

Shanson DC (1985) Control of a hospital outbreak of methicillin-resistant *Staphylococcus aureus*: the value of an isolation ward. *Journal of Hospital Infection* **6**: 285–92.

Wilcox M (1996) Cleaning up *Clostridium difficile* infection. *Lancet* **348**: 767–8.

FURTHER READING AND INFORMATION SOURCES

British National Formulary (2008) Available www.bnf.org.uk/.

Guven GS and Uzun O (2003) Principles of good use of antibiotics in hospitals. *Journal of Hospital Infection* **53:** 91–6.

Price MF, Dao-Tran T, Garey KW et al. (2007) Epidemiology and incidence of *Clostridium difficile*-associated diarrhoea diagnosed upon admission to a university hospital. *Journal of Hospital Infection* **65**(1): 42–6.

Watkins S and Ames J (2006) Interventions to reduce *Clostridium difficile* infection. *Nursing Times* **102**(49): 30–1.

PART II

Principles of Infection Prevention and Control

CHAPTER 5

Infection control policies in healthcare settings

CHAPTER OUTCOMES

CHAPTER OUTCOMES

After reading this chapter, you should be able to:

➤ Outline risk management in controlling infection

➤ Discuss the role of the hands in cross-infection and the steps taken to reduce the transmission of microorganisms via this route

➤ Define the terms 'cleaning', 'disinfection' and 'sterilization', giving examples of when each procedure would be appropriate and the most suitable method for the task

➤ Outline strategies used to manage waste materials in hospital and community premises

➤ State the measures taken to decontaminate laundry

➤ Debate the role of personal protective equipment (PPE) in the prevention of infection

➤ List the special precautions taken to control infection in theatres and other high-risk units

➤ Discuss effective policies for patient isolation

Introduction to strategies that prevent infection

The strategies that prevent infection fall into three categories:

■ **Individual patient/resident care** – identifying factors that increase susceptibility to infection or constitute an infection risk and delivering the appropriate care tailored to meet individual need.

■ **Policies and procedures** – to reduce the risk of infection to all the patients/residents and staff in the hospital, community healthcare setting or the person's home where they are implemented, for example cleaning policies, antibiotic policies (Chapter 4), handling and disposal of sharps (Chapter 12) and standard (universal) blood and body fluid precautions/principles (Chapter 12). The resources and tools provided in *Saving Lives: Reducing Infection, Delivering Clean and Safe*

Care (Department of Health, 2007a) are designed to assist NHS Trusts to apply the code of practice for preventing and controlling healthcare-associated infections (HCAIs), as required by the Health Act 2006 (Department of Health, 2006).

■ **Public health measures** – policies to promote the health of the entire community, for example the notification of infectious diseases to the Health Protection Agency, immunization programmes (Chapter 2) and the inspection of premises where food is produced or sold.

Tackling HCAI is a priority for health workers (Jenkinson et al., 2006).

Risk factors associated with hospital admission and in other healthcare settings

Risk factors (Chapter 2) when people are admitted to hospital include:

■ Shared facilities
■ Contact with different members of staff carrying microorganisms, especially antibiotic-resistant strains
■ Mass-produced food
■ Physical and psychological stress, which reduces resistance to infection, very sick and long-stay patients being at particular risk.

Very sick patients are handled more often, and by a larger number of people, undergo more invasive procedures (mechanical ventilation and catheterization, for example) and are more likely to receive antibiotics.

Long-stay patients have a greater exposure to the hospital flora. They are more likely to succumb to infection and to operate as reservoirs of antibiotic-resistant hospital strains, presenting an infection risk to others.

Members of the infection control team (Chapter 6) play an important role when modern hospitals are planned and built in order to reduce risks of HCAI by ensuring that sufficient isolation rooms and other facilities are incorporated into the design (Wilson and Ridgeway, 2006).

In the past, emphasis was placed on preventing infection in inpatient settings. Although this remains of key importance, there is now a clear need to reduce HCAI in primary care and community settings, in line with the move of healthcare beyond traditional hospital boundaries in the UK (see below).

┌─ PRACTICE APPLICATION 5.1 ─

Infection Control in Non-hospital Settings

The number of chronically ill and older people is increasing. Many live in care/nursing homes and are also at risk of infection (Ward, 2001).

Activity

➤ Read the article by Ward (2001) and then identify the factors in your workplace/placement that increase the risk of infection.

> ➤ Consider the key topics suggested by Ward (2001) for inclusion in an
> infection control policy – compare the list with those in the policy in your
> workplace/placement.
>
> **Resource**
>
> Department of Health (DH) (2006) *Infection Control Guidance for Care Homes*. DH,
> London. Available www.dh.gov.uk.

The importance of preventing the spread of infection in healthcare settings

In 2000, the National Audit Office (2000) highlighted the extent of the problems faced by the NHS in relation to HCAI. This report supported the findings of research by Plowman et al. (2001), which pointed out the economic consequences of HCAI to the NHS and to patients and their families. Collectively, these reports drew attention to the increasing profile of infection control since the early 1990s, both politically and economically. Infection control has become part of the clinical governance framework in both acute and primary care (Health Service Circular, 1999). The chief medical officer's report, *Winning Ways: Working Together to Reduce Healthcare-Associated Infection in England* (Department of Health, 2003), acknowledged that infection control had previously been of low priority in the NHS to the detriment of patient care, and it contained a range of strategic drivers and clinical recommendations intended to increase the status of infection control.

Policies and procedures to prevent infection

In hospital and community settings, infection prevention and control policies should address levels of risk and the following areas, including standard (universal) precautions/principles:

- Policies for the use of cleaning agents, disinfection and sterilization, including guidance on the use of equipment such as autoclaves
- The disposal of clinical waste
- The disposal of soiled laundry
- The isolation of potentially infectious patients
- Standard (universal) precautions/principles:
  - Environmental cleaning
  - The use of personal protective equipment (PPE)
  - Fundamental hygiene, including handwashing and decontamination
  - Proper handling and disposal of sharps; including procedures to be followed in the case of accidents, especially needlestick injury and exposure to blood and body fluids.

Pratt et al. (2007) stress the importance of good hospital hygiene as part of the strategy for preventing HCAI in acute hospitals.

Standard and high-risk situations

Until recently, the healthcare environment was not considered to contribute greatly to infection rates. However, it is now increasingly recognized that the environment may influence infection rates, although the extent of its influence is hard to determine (Patel, 2004) (see below).

PRACTICE APPLICATION 5.2

How Clean is the Healthcare Setting?

Consider a particular healthcare setting, for example your workplace/placement or one that you use, or visit.

Activity

➤ Assess the standard of general cleanliness – is it appropriate for the setting?

➤ What potential hazards can you identify?

The healthcare environment consists of everything on the premises: all fixtures, fittings, equipment, patients and staff. It is possible to differentiate between two settings – those where the risk of infection is exceptionally high and extraordinary precautions are necessary (theatres and critical care units), and all others, where hazards certainly exist but are not of the same magnitude. However, the same principles of infection prevention are vital everywhere. The general principles include:

■ Providing an environment hostile to the growth and multiplication of microorganisms: clean, dry, well ventilated and with good lighting, as the ultraviolet rays in sunlight destroy bacteria

■ Protecting susceptible people/sites from contamination, for example by dressing wounds and employing isolation precautions to protect immunosuppressed patients

■ Containing sources of infection: avoiding spillage and using colour-coded systems for waste disposal, for example

■ Decontamination.

Situations where the risk of contamination and subsequent infection is high are given below.

INFORMATION BOX 5.1

Situations in which risk of contamination is high

➤ Situations in which there is potential for contact with organic waste, for example blood, body fluids, waste food, raw food and cleaning fluid

➤ Handling materials that have been in contact with an infected site, for example soiled dressings, sharps, linen, body fluids and laboratory specimens

➤ The immediate environment of patients who are infectious

> ➤ The immediate environment of highly susceptible patients, for example critical care units, neonatal units, burns units and theatres

Risk management

Risk management (Figure 5.1) may be effectively incorporated into programmes designed to control infection. Risk management is a systematic process of identifying and analysing the accepted risks that may occur in a given situation, deciding the action required and evaluating the potential and actual risks (Department of Health, 1993a), thus providing a mechanism for reducing risk of infection and avoiding economic loss. It is necessary because of the need to provide safe and effective health services and the increasing number of claims made against healthcare providers and the cost of court settlements. Its objectives are to minimize the number of risks occurring, to enhance quality of care and to reduce costs to the organization. It has been known for decades that many items of equipment in the clinical environment may become heavily contaminated. These include:

- Baths
- Bedclothes
- Bedpans and commodes
- Catheter drainage bags
- Flannels
- Hoists
- Mattresses
- Urinals
- Washbowls.

There is recent clear evidence that a wide range of healthcare equipment is contaminated and can operate as a potential source of HCAI (Schabrun and Chopchase, 2006).

IDENTIFYING THE RISK
depends on a knowledge of:

- The nature of the service provided in a particular setting
- The equipment and supplies required
- The legislation and regulations affecting provision
- The potential liability that may be incurred (based on previous reports or audit)

⬇

ANALYSING ACTUAL AND POTENTIAL RISKS

- Likelihood of risk
- Severity (from previous claims)
- Previous trends of occurrence
- The cost of eliminating or reducing risk
- Deciding whether any immediate action is required

⬇

IDENTIFYING POSSIBLE RISK SOLUTIONS

- Dispense with the procedure
- Implement new protocols/new equipment (staff training being necessary)
- No immediate action necessary

⬇

MONITORING/EVALUATING

- The number and nature of accidents
- The number and nature of injuries
- The number of claims

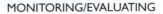

Figure 5.1 The risk management process

Decontamination

Decontamination is achieved at three levels:

- Cleaning
- Disinfection
- Sterilization.

Each level becomes progressively more effective but also more expensive, more diffi-cult to perform and more likely to damage the item concerned. Considerable time and money can be spent performing unnecessary rituals (Axnick and Yarborough, 1984), which is not acceptable in the present cost-conscious climate of healthcare. Thus, the method of decontamination chosen should not be more complex or expensive than necessary. In addition to expense, other important factors to consider include the nature of the item to be decontaminated and the circumstances in which decontamination will be performed. Key questions to ask are:

- **How soon will recontamination occur?**

Some items become recontaminated so rapidly that the need for disinfection must be carefully evaluated. Floors, drains, sluice hoppers and toilets fall into this cate-gory and for this reason until recently cleaning rather than routine disinfection was the recommended approach to decontamination. However, with the increased emphasis on hospital cleanliness, some infection control teams are reviewing their recommendations.

- **Will the equipment withstand the procedure chosen?**

Metal surfaces are corroded by hypochlorite disinfectants and delicate equipment will not withstand autoclaving. Even when sterility is essential, some other method must be chosen.

- **Will contact with the cleaning or disinfecting agent be possible for long enough?**

Disinfectants require time to take effect, the length of time varying between differ-ent agents.

Cleaning the environment

Cleaning maintains the appearance, structure and efficient functioning of the clinical environment and its contents. It contributes to infection control by reducing the number of microorganisms present and preventing their transfer (see below). The safe removal of cloths, mop heads and cleaning fluids is essential as they may become heavily contaminated, inefficient practices leading to the redistribution of microor-ganisms. These may also be spread if the cleaning materials are used again without decontamination. In the clinical environment, cleaning is a skilled activity under-taken by domestic staff who should receive special training. Good practice includes:

- The use of disposable cloths

- Autoclaving equipment when possible
- Storing equipment (for example mops and buckets) clean and dry between uses
- Damp-dusting to avoid the dispersal of microorganisms into the air
- Avoiding splashes to reduce risks of contamination and accidents (for example falls on slippery floors)
- Drying surfaces after damp-cleaning as moisture supports the growth of bacteria
- Regularly changing the cleaning solution.

INFORMATION BOX 5.2

Outline policy for good cleaning practice

➤ Use a new cleaning solution for each task, checking that it is of the required dilution

➤ Apply it evenly to all surfaces, ensuring that all equipment (for example mops and wipes) is clean and dry before use. Avoid applying excess solution, as it can seep into joins and cracks, thus damaging equipment, and it makes drying more difficult

➤ Change the solution at regular intervals during cleaning to prevent the accumulation of bacteria, leading to recontamination

➤ Allow sufficient time for the solution to penetrate surface soiling

➤ Dispose of solution without splashing to prevent environmental contamination. Use a sluice hopper rather than washbasins adjacent to clinical areas

➤ Dry the surface thoroughly as bacteria thrive in moisture and slippery surfaces are dangerous

➤ Wash the hands

The National Patient Safety Agency (2007) has recently issued a document that sets out a standard colour-coding system for hospital cleaning materials and equipment (see below).

PRACTICE APPLICATION 5.3

Colour-coding for Cleaning Materials and Equipment

The National Patient Safety Agency recommends that a national colour-coding scheme be adopted by NHS organizations in England and Wales.

Activity

Using the Safer practice notice No. 15 (2007), answer the following questions

➤ What are the advantages of adopting a standard colour-coding scheme?

➤ Which cleaning materials/equipment should be colour-coded?

➤ How many colours are there in the scheme; which area is designated red in the coding and which is blue?

> **Resource**
>
> National Patient Safety Agency (NPSA) (2007) *Colour Coding for Hospital Cleaning Materials and Equipment.* Safer practice notice No. 15. NPSA, London. Available www. npsa.nhs.uk/.

In hospital, nurses or technicians are responsible for looking after equipment that is too delicate or expensive for domestic staff to handle and for items directly involved in patient care that need regular cleaning to avoid heavy contamination. In many community settings (health centres and family planning clinics, for example), nurses take responsibility for the routine cleaning and decontamination of all clinical equipment.

The precleaning of instruments is essential before disinfection or sterilization as the first step in decontamination. All items should be washed in warm water and detergent using a brush, and then thoroughly rinsed. Care is necessary as brushing can produce contamination through aerosols or splashing. Brushes must be sterilized every day and stored dry. Staff should use PPE such as plastic aprons and gloves appropriate to the cleaning tasks.

Clinical equipment should be stored clean and dry wherever possible. Soaking in disinfectant solutions is poor practice as the fluid is rapidly inactivated by organic matter and becomes heavily contaminated, setting up a reservoir of infection (Burdon and Whitby, 1967).

Disinfection

Disinfection is the destruction of vegetative microorganisms but not their spores. Infection is likely to supervene when a large number of microorganisms is present. The aim of disinfection is to reduce this number to a level below the infective dose. 'Safe' levels of microorganisms are likely to vary according to circumstance. This will depend on:

- **The patient** – Someone who is very sick will be more susceptible. A level of bacteria that would not be harmful to a healthy individual might, for example, cause a fatal infection in a child with leukaemia.
- **The virulence** – Some species of microorganism are more readily destroyed than others. The spores of Gram-positive bacteria (such as *Bacillus* and *Clostridium*) are particularly resistant.

It is difficult and expensive to destroy all the microorganisms present, so a compromise is usually reached by attempting to destroy most of them, bearing in mind the limitations of the chosen method. There are two methods: heat and chemical disinfection.

Heat disinfection (pasteurization)

Heat disinfection is the method of choice. It is rapid, cheaper than chemical disinfection and more easily controlled. Microorganisms vary considerably in their ability to withstand high temperatures, but nearly all species of clinical significance are destroyed by exposure to moist heat between 50 and 70 °C for 20–30 minutes. The current recommendation is 65 °C for 10 minutes, 71 °C for 3 minutes or 80 °C for 1 minute (Department of Health, 1993b); spores are more resistant to heat and some will not be destroyed. The disinfection temperature and time commonly used ranges from 60 °C for 10 minutes to 80 °C or above for one minute. Extra time is needed for cold instruments to reach the disinfection temperature and to become cool enough for handling afterwards.

In hospital, nurses are unlikely to be responsible for heat disinfection, but in community settings they may be required to operate hot-water disinfectors. The correct procedure involves:

- Precleaning all items
- Placing them on the tray within the disinfector, completely covering them with water and ensuring that no air bubbles are trapped
- Checking that the hot-water disinfector is not overloaded
- Ensuring that the water returns to the boil for at least five minutes after the items have been added, using a timer for accuracy
- Raising the tray holding the items with clean forceps
- Placing the items on a clean surface and leaving them covered while they cool
- Storing clean items in a dry, clean container
- Changing the water in the boiler daily.

Cleaning and disinfection are often combined in dishwashers, washing machines and bedpan washers. Most of the contaminants are removed by the mechanical action of cleaning, those remaining being destroyed by heat (see below).

INFORMATION BOX 5.3

Maintaining equipment

Maintaining equipment in good working order is of paramount importance in the successful control of infection. Bedpan washers and macerators pose special problems. Surveys have shown that a high proportion do not function adequately (Block et al., 1990), typical problems including poor water pressure, blockage by solid material, attachment to pipes of the wrong size and lack of drainage. Breakdown is common and has been implicated as one of the factors contributing to outbreaks of HCAI infection (Curie et al., 1978). This problem is most acute when patients are immunocompromised (Chadwick and Oppenheim, 1994). Macerators may create aerosols when the lid is slammed and may leak if overfilled, thereby causing environmental contamination. Routine maintenance checks are necessary for all equipment.

Chemical disinfectants

The ideal disinfectant is effective, does not damage equipment or harm people and is inexpensive. No chemical incorporating all these properties exists, and the entire process of chemical disinfection is at best an uncertain process. Many chemical disinfectants are toxic, corrosive, unstable in solution and readily deactivated by organic matter, plastics, rubber, detergents and hard water. When there is no alternative to chemical disinfection, compromise is required, taking into consideration the factors that determine the effectiveness of chemical disinfectants. These include:

- **Satisfactory contact** – Disinfection is not possible unless the solution has direct and complete contact with all surfaces. Precleaning, complete immersion and expelling trapped air bubbles are important precautions
- **Avoiding neutralization** – Hard water, plastic, rubber, organic waste and many detergents reduce the effectiveness of many chemical disinfectants
- **Concentration** – A solution reconstituted below the recommended strength will not be fully effective, while higher concentrations are not necessarily more efficacious but are a waste of resources. For example, 100 per cent alcohol evaporates too rapidly to disinfect
- **Stability** – Dilutions may deteriorate with age. The expiry date on the container must be checked before use
- **Speed of action** – Some chemical disinfectants destroy microorganisms more readily than others. Hypochlorites and alcohol act rapidly; glutaraldehyde disinfects slowly
- **Range of action** – Chemical disinfectants do not all destroy the same range of microorganisms. Consideration must be given to the pathogens likely to be present
- **Cost** – Using a chemical disinfectant inappropriately is expensive and inefficient, for example chlorhexidine is too expensive and has too narrow a spectrum for satisfactory use as an environmental disinfectant.

Soaking equipment in disinfectant is poor practice as solutions may support the growth of Gram-negative bacteria, leading to heavy contamination (Burdon and Whitby, 1967).

Clear soluble phenolics

Clear soluble phenolics are suitable as environmental disinfectants at concentrations of 1–2 per cent. They are toxic and corrosive but stable in solution, are not easily neutralized, are cheap and destroy a wide range of microorganisms, although not spores or viruses.

Hypochlorites

Hypochlorites are marketed at different solutions, expressed as parts per million (ppm) of available chlorine (Table 5.1). Hypochlorites destroy a wide range of microorganisms and are effective against the hepatitis B and human immunodeficiency viruses. Their activity is reduced in the presence of organic matter. They are corrosive at concentrations necessary for environmental disinfection.

Table 5.1 Hypochlorites and their uses at different dilutions

Uses	Dilution (%)	Available chlorine (ppm)
Blood/body fluids	1.0	10,000
General environmental use	0.1	1,000
Infant feeding equipment	0.0125	125

Milton (125–140 ppm) can be safely used in food preparation and to clean infant feeding bottles, but articles should not be left soaking because the solution is readily neutralized by organic matter. The contamination of feeds may occur in hospital milk kitchens (Ayliffe, 1970); this may be avoided by heat sterilization or purchasing commercially prepared feeds.

Glutaraldehyde

Glutaraldehyde is a highly toxic chemical that may be used to decontaminate expensive, precision items, principally fibreoptic endoscopes that would be damaged by heat or more corrosive chemicals. Disinfection is achieved after a contact time of 20 minutes. Prolonged contact of three hours or more will destroy spores, acid-fast bacilli (AFBs) and viruses, achieving sterilization. The use of glutaraldehyde, however, has serious health and safety issues (see below).

INFORMATION BOX 5.4

Glutaraldehyde: health and safety

Glutaraldehyde is a respiratory sensitizer and exposure to its vapour or mist is linked to the development of occupational asthma (Health and Safety Executive, 1998/2005). A maximum exposure level was set in 1999 and this is part of the Control of Substances Hazardous to Health (COSHH) Regulations, but there is no safe limit. Glutaraldehyde must be used in accordance with guidelines produced by the Health and Safety Executive and the Department of Health, and must conform to the relevant COSHH Regulations.

Web-based information provided by the Health and Safety Executive (2007) recommends that, whenever possible, a substitute disinfectant should be used in place of glutaraldehyde and if it is used, this must be justified. Where a substitute solution is not possible, glutaraldehyde vapour/mist should be contained within enclosed equipment, or staff should use a respirator of the correct type. Health surveillance must be provided for staff who work with glutaraldehyde.

Resource

Health Service Circular (HSC) (1998) *Glutaraldehyde*, HSC 1998/208. DH, London. Available www.dh.gov.uk.

Alcohol

Alcohol (isopropanol or ethanol) in 70 per cent solution is suitable to rapidly disinfect physically clean surfaces and clinical equipment (dressing trolleys and thermometers, for example). It evaporates quickly, leaving the surfaces dry, and penetrates organic matter poorly. Alcohol destroys most viruses but not spores. A contact time of at least two minutes is necessary to destroy HIV (Hanson et al., 1989). Alcohol is convenient because it can be incorporated into sprays, impregnated into swabs or combined with emollients into handrubs.

Chlorhexidine

Chlorhexidine is formulated to disinfect human tissue. It is a non-toxic, non-corrosive but relatively expensive fluid, more effective against Gram-positive than Gram-negative bacteria. It continues to destroy organisms for some time after application (Russell and Day, 1993). Chlorhexidine has slight activity against AFBs but does not destroy spores. It is readily inactivated by organic matter and chemicals. Its expense and narrow range of bactericidal activity make it unsuitable for environmental use. It is incorporated into alcoholic handrub and is sometimes used preoperatively as a skin antiseptic.

Iodophors

Iodophors (povidine iodine) have a broader spectrum than chlorhexidine and destroy spores.

Hexachlorophane

Hexachlorophane is used as a skin antiseptic, especially on neonatal units. It destroys bacteria and some viruses but not spores. Once extremely popular, it is now used with caution following reports of central nervous system damage to infants.

Quaternary ammonium compounds

Quaternary ammonium compounds destroy most Gram-positive and -negative bacteria, but not AFBs or spores. Organic matter and many other chemicals rapidly inactivate these compounds. The most widely used member of the group is cetrimide, which has natural detergent properties. It is sometimes used as a wound disinfectant. Cetrimide and chlorhexidine are marketed in combination as a wound and skin disinfectant.

Hydrogen peroxide

Hydrogen peroxide is now being tested to explore its effectiveness as an agent to decontaminate rooms and equipment. It is used as a 5 per cent dry fume released by a programmed device. In tests it appears to have good sporicidal effectiveness (Andersen et al., 2006). It may be valuable when rooms need terminal decontamination after patients with MRSA have been discharged (French et al., 2004).

Disinfectant policies

A typical hospital disinfectant policy will include:

- A detergent for general domestic purposes
- A phenolic for 'heavy' environmental use
- A hypochlorite for situations where contamination with blood or body fluids is possible
- Isopropanol 70 per cent for cleaning physically clean clinical equipment
- A system for the decontamination of endoscopes and other precision equipment. (See above for the problems associated with the use of glutaraldehyde, which should be avoided where possible.)

The number of agents used is generally limited both for simplicity and because large quantities can be purchased more cheaply on contract. Staff training is important to the success of the policy, and auditing is recommended (Coates and Hutchinson, 1994).

Hand hygiene

The hands are the main vectors of infection in hospital wards (Reybrouck, 1983), strains colonizing patients' skin and nurses' hands invariably being the same. Rates of infection and colonization have fallen following the introduction of stringent hand decontamination protocols (Casewell and Phillips, 1978). The aim of hand hygiene is to remove transient microorganisms before their transfer to susceptible patients. Cross-infection is possible as the member of staff moves from one patient/resident to another or handles different sites on the same person (for example giving an injection after bed-bathing). Hands should be decontaminated frequently both between people and between sites. Gloves (see Chapter 12) give added protection in situations where heavy contamination occurs (such as attending a person who is incontinent or changing stoma bags) and washing is unlikely to remove the bacteria effectively (Kjolen and Andersen, 1992). Decontamination is still necessary because gloves may puncture or leak (Kotilainen et al., 1990). Even if they remain intact, hands can become contaminated during removal of the gloves.

Hand decontamination

Hand decontamination is recommended:

- Between each direct patient/resident contact
- Before aseptic procedures
- After handling patients/residents
- After handling any items that are or could be soiled
- Before handling food
- As soon as the hands become visibly soiled.

Soap, antiseptics and alcoholic handrubs containing 60–70 per cent ethanol or isopropanol are available. It is difficult to demonstrate that one particular product destroys more organisms than another. Laboratory studies to test bactericidal effectiveness are performed under tightly controlled conditions that allow comparisons but do not necessarily reflect the clinical situation. When soap is used, the mechanical action of washing and drying removes microorganisms. Antiseptics destroy organisms, providing the contact time is sufficient, which it is often not.

An effective technique for handwashing is described below.

PRACTICE APPLICATION 5.4

Handwashing Technique

An effective handwashing technique (Figure 5.2) incorporates the following:

➤ Using elbow- or foot-operated taps to avoid transferring organisms either to the clean hands when the tap is switched off or to the next person

➤ Using the product from a dispenser as bar soap may be heavily contaminated with Gram-negative rods. Dispensers should not be 'topped up' as this introduces the risk of contamination (Gould and Chamberlain, 1997)

➤ Moistening the hands before the agent is added. This helps to reduce contact with harsh chemicals that can damage the skin

➤ Vigorously rubbing all the surfaces (dorsum, palm and interdigital spaces) with lather for at least 10 seconds. This is often poorly executed (Gould and Ream, 1993)

➤ Thorough drying as damp hands transfer bacteria more readily than dry ones (Gould, 1984), and residual dampness contributes to soreness

➤ Disposal of the paper towel into a bin without touching the lid, in order to avoid recontamination

The choice of hand decontamination depends on the type of activity undertaken and the susceptibility of the patient/resident:

- **Soap** is adequate for most routine tasks (for example helping patients/residents with hygiene, and bed-making)
- **Antiseptics** are recommended before invasive procedures (such as urinary catheterization and tracheobronchial suction)
- **Handrubs** are recommended by manufacturers for application to physically clean hands but are not otherwise suitable because they have no detergent properties and will not remove grime. They are often routinely used in critical care units when invasive procedures are frequently performed because they give added protection to conventionally washed hands.

I

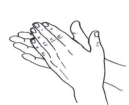

Palm to palm

2

Right palm over left dorsum,
left palm over right dorsum

3

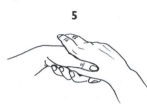

Palm to palm, fingers
interlaced

4

Fingers to
opposing palms

5

Rotational rubbing of right
thumb clasped over left palm

6

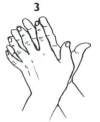

Rotational rubbing
backwards and forwards
with fingers of right
hand in palm of left
and vice versa

7 Hands and wrists rubbed until end of 30-second period

Figure 5.2 Hand decontamination technique

When using a handrub for decontamination, the correct technique involves the following steps:

- Dispense 3 ml of solution into the cupped hands
- Massage thoroughly until no trace of moisture remains
- Take particular care to contact all hand surfaces with handrub. Alcohol lacks viscosity and this may result in insufficient contact.

The advantages of using a handrub include:

- **Reduced damage to the skin** – This increases compliance. Emollients may be incorporated to further reduce dryness and soreness, both well-documented hazards of frequent decontamination (Kownatzki, 2003).
- **Increased bactericidal effectiveness** – Dry, cracked skin increases the number of bacteria present because they are more difficult to dislodge by the friction of conventional washing. This defeats the aim of decontamination.
- **Convenience** – The hands are decontaminated more often when handrub is available at the bedside, especially when the workload is high and valuable time would be expended making trips to the nearest sink (Voss and Widmer, 1997).

In the UK, hand hygiene is currently receiving a great deal of interest. A major initiative called the 'cleanyourhands' campaign was launched across NHS hospitals in England and Wales during 2004 by the National Patient Safety Agency to help reduce infection rates (Storr, 2005). However, there is emerging evidence that overreliance on alcohol handrubs is contributing to the increase in the incidence of *Clostridium difficile* because alcohol is neither sporicidal nor able to remove spores from hands by the friction that would occur with traditional washing (Gould et al., 2007).

Care of the hands is important in reducing infection. Using a good-quality hand cream from a tube reserved for individual use, as communal dispensers can become contaminated, can reduce soreness and dryness induced by frequent decontamination. Cuts and abrasions should be covered with waterproof dressings in order to avoid the risk of parenterally transmitted infection. Septic lesions must be occluded to prevent cross-infection. Advice from the occupational health department should be sought, and antibiotics may have to be prescribed. Wearing rings is not advisable as this encourages the growth of Gram-negative bacteria on the underlying skin (Hoffman et al., 1985); an optimal handwashing technique is required to remove these organisms (Jacobson et al., 1985). The nails should be kept short, as bacteria beneath them are leached out by sweating after gloves have been worn so more are present on the surface of the hands, contributing to the risk of cross-infection (Peireira et al., 1990). There is no clear evidence that wearing nail polish is associated with an increased risk of causing HCAI, but it seems likely that other forms of 'nail art' may pose a threat (Jeanes and Green, 2001). The frequency, appropriateness and technique of hand decontamination can be monitored by periodic auditing.

Sterilization

Sterilization is the destruction of all microorganisms and spores. It is necessary when the small number surviving disinfection would be able to establish infection, either because the organisms themselves are highly virulent or because the patient is very susceptible. Situations in which sterilization is necessary include:

- Equipment that will be used to breach the body's natural barriers to infection, for example surgical instruments, urinary catheters, injection needles and intravenous fluid sets
- Dressing materials and topical applications in contact with areas of the body that would normally be free of microorganisms
- Situations in which contamination is possible with a large number of bacterial spores, for example exposure to *Clostridium* spp. or *Bacillus anthracis*
- Equipment that has been in contact with extremely virulent pathogens, for example in the viral haemorrhagic fevers.

Sterilization is rarely absolute, and quality control is essential to ensure that adequate numbers of microorganisms and spores are destroyed.

Items marked for single use, such as syringes, lancets and so on, should be just that – they must not be reused (see below).

PRACTICE APPLICATION 5.5

Single-use Devices

The range of products marketed for single use is increasing; they are convenient, especially in hospitals, busy clinics and domiciliary settings. The Consumer Protection Act 1987 would be contravened if an item marked for single use only was recycled.

Activity

➤   Access the resources below and consider the advice about the reuse of single-use devices in relation to the practices in your workplace/placement.

Resources

Medicines and Healthcare Products Regulatory Agency (MHRA) (2006) *Single-use Medical Devices: Implications and Consequences of Reuse*, DB2006(04). MHRA, London. Available www.mhra.gov.uk.

Wilkinson E (2006) The implications of reusing single-use medical devices. *Nursing Times* 102(45): 23–4.

Methods of sterilization

The various methods used to sterilize items are outlined below. Chemicals such as ethylene oxide are used to sterilize items that will be damaged by high temperature. Radiation is used commercially to sterilize single-use items such as syringes or needles. Methods that involve heat are described below in more detail.

INFORMATION BOX 5.5

Methods of sterilization

➤   **Heat**
Dry heat – incineration, hot-air ovens, infrared convectors
Moist heat under pressure – autoclaves

➤   **Radiation**
Ultraviolet irradiation
X-rays
Gamma rays

➤   **Chemicals**
Ethylene oxide gas
Formaldehyde gas
Glutaraldehyde solution (see above)

➤   **Filtration**
Filters to remove all vegetative bacteria, spores and viruses from commercially prepared solutions

Dry heat sterilization is possible at 160 °C for 60 minutes or for shorter periods at higher temperatures. It is suitable only for items that are very heat resistant; this excludes plastics, rubber and many fabrics. The items are placed in a hot-air oven after precleaning. Ovens should be fan assisted to ensure an even distribution of heat to all items. Items enter cold so heating time must be added to the period of sterilization.

Autoclaving employs moist heat (steam under pressure) to sterilize. It is more efficient than dry heat because steam penetrates fabrics and porous objects rapidly, a property enhanced by increased pressure. In the autoclave, air is removed by suction to create a vacuum before the steam enters, thus ensuring contact with every surface; failure of contact results in failure of sterilization. Sterilization is achieved at:

- 121 °C for 15 minutes
- 126 °C for 10 minutes
- 134 °C for 5 minutes.

In hospital, equipment is autoclaved in large batches by technicians. In outpatient departments, where the same small items of equipment are required in rapid succession, and in clinics in the community, nurses may have to operate the autoclaves. The procedure involves:

- Precleaning all items.
- Arranging them within the autoclave. They should not touch one another because this could impede steam penetration. Hinged instruments should be opened to allow the maximum exposure of all surfaces, and items should not be wrapped or placed inside one another.
- Items should be removed from the autoclave by sterile forceps and placed in a sterile container.
- They should be used as soon as possible. Resterilization is necessary if they are not used within three hours.
- Autoclaves should be serviced on a regular basis in line with the timing recommended by the manufacturer.
- Routine testing to ensure efficient function should be performed at least weekly, recording the results in a logbook.
- Small autoclaves of the type used in primary care are not suitable for sterilizing porous loads (such as dressings or fabrics).

Disposing of waste, dealing with laundry and other contaminated items

This section outlines the policies that reduce the infection risks that arise from waste, laundry and other items.

Waste disposal policies

Waste forms part of the hospital and care environment and contains potentially pathogenic material. Inappropriate handling or disposal may lead to environmental contamination or a reduction in socially acceptable or aesthetic standards. To avoid this problem, waste must be contained in colour-coded bags (Health Services Advisory Committee, 1987):

- **Black bags** – for normal household waste
- **Yellow bags** – for clinical waste to be incinerated
- **Light blue/transparent bags** (with light blue inscriptions) – waste to be autoclaved before disposal.

In addition, glass and aerosols are disposed of in specific bins and colour-coded bins are provided for cytotoxic waste and other drugs (Royal College of Nursing, 2005).

High-risk clinical waste is autoclaved before incineration. There is no advantage in double-bagging (Maki et al., 1986).

Waste awaiting collection must be stored in a secure, washable, covered area to discourage the attention of drug misusers and pests (rodents or feral cats). This is much easier on hospital or nursing/care home premises than when people are nursed at home. The amount of waste generated in hospital is enormous, but, as more acutely sick people are cared for at home and in other community settings, the disposal of clinical material from community premises will increase, giving rise to new problems of storage, collection and transport. Under the Environmental Protection Act 1990, a duty of care has been placed on those dealing with waste, who must prevent:

- Waste causing environmental pollution or harm to human health, secure packaging being essential at all times
- Handling by those unauthorized to receive waste. Controlled waste should only be dealt with by a registered waste carrier or someone holding a disposal licence. When waste is transferred, a transfer note describing the contents should be given to the recipient, and labelled to identify the source.

There is considerable legislation, both domestic and that resulting from European Union Directives, which regulates the disposal of clinical waste (see below).

PRACTICE APPLICATION 5.6

Clinical Waste

Consider the types of clinical waste created in your practice and the related local policies.

Activity

- ➤ Identify those that contain potentially pathogenic material.
- ➤ What arrangements exist for its collection from the premises?
- ➤ Identify the current legislation that covers clinical waste.
- ➤ Who in the organization is responsible for ensuring that practices conform to the relevant legislation?

Laundry policies

Laundry falls into three categories (Department of Health, 1995):

1. Used (soiled and fouled)
2. Infected
3. Heat-labile fabrics such as wool and synthetic materials.

Linen is considered to be infected only if it has been used by patients who have or are suspected of having an enteric infection, hepatitis, open pulmonary tuberculosis, HIV or any of the notifiable diseases (Chapter 14). In this case, it should be placed directly into a water-soluble bag without sorting. This bag is sealed and placed within a red laundry bag. A national colour code is recommended for linen bags and their containers:

- **A white bag** – used (soiled and fouled) linen; to be laundered at 65 °C for 10 minutes or 71 °C for 3 minutes
- **A water-soluble bag enclosed in a red bag** – infected, heavily bloodstained linen; washing times and temperatures as above
- **White bags with a prominent orange stripe** – heat-labile fabrics damaged by thermal disinfection; to be laundered at 40 °C.

The holding area where linen is stored before collection must be dry and covered. In the laundry, dirty and infected linen should be received separately and dealt with in a machine designated for its use.

Staff uniforms and workwear

In conjunction with other initiatives to deal with HCAIs, the Department of Health (2007b) published *Uniforms and Workwear: An Evidence Base for Developing Local Policy.* This provides guidance covering all aspects of uniform and workwear, including:

- Laundering uniforms at the hottest temperature compatible with the fabric
- Not wearing white coats when giving patient care
- Short sleeves for uniform and workwear to facilitate effective handwashing.

Many health workers in the UK launder their own uniforms in domestic washing machines, often at 40 °C. Tumble-drying and ironing are necessary to remove vegetative bacteria (Patel et al., 2006).

Crockery and cutlery

Crockery and cutlery should be heat disinfected. In ideal circumstances, this will involve removal from the clinical area to a central kitchen and processing in a dishwasher operating at a minimum temperature of 60 °C, with a final rinse at a minimum temperature of 82 °C.

Personal protective equipment

PPE should:

- Protect clothing from contamination by pathogens that could subsequently be transferred to other people, from patient/resident to practitioner or vice versa
- Prevent the direct transfer of pathogenic organisms from patient/resident to practitioner or vice versa
- Prevent clothing becoming soiled, wet or stained.

In the past, the use of PPE appeared to have been given undue emphasis in infection control programmes. Today, research findings suggest that clothes are of secondary importance to hands in the dissemination of infection and that applying evidence-based practice to the use of PPE could save considerable time and money. There are, however, situations in which adequate protection is necessary, and the regulations of the Health and Safety Executive (1993) require employers to provide it, to ensure that staff are instructed in the correct use of PPE and to ensure that it is worn appropriately.

The use of gloves is discussed in Chapter 12.

Aprons, gowns and tabards

Research concerning PPE for use in theatres and burns units has now become specialized, resulting in the manufacture of sophisticated garments (Mackintosh, 1982). Their use in these settings is justified because patients are particularly vulnerable. However, in the wards, the hazards of airborne spread from skin scales on clothes have been exaggerated, and less expensive precautions are usually sufficient for most patients (Rahman, 1985).

Plastic aprons are more suitable than cotton gowns as cotton weave is permeable and plastic aprons carry fewer bacteria than cotton ones because they cannot adhere readily to cold, slippery surfaces and they dry out quickly. Plastic aprons are cheap and should be used as intended by the manufacturers – being discarded between patients/residents or after activities that may result in heavy soiling (Curran, 1991).

Tabards worn to cover the uniform in child health areas are usually made of cotton. They should be changed daily, being laundered at 65 °C for at least 10 minutes or at 71 °C for at least 3 minutes to achieve adequate disinfection (Department of Health, 1995).

Surgical masks

Most studies to evaluate the effectiveness of surgical masks have been performed either by analysing postoperative infection rates or by laboratory studies. Early simulation tests to examine the risk of contamination after sneezing, coughing and speech indicated that paper masks were superior to fabric ones (Madsen and Madsen, 1967). Even if they incorporate filters, their efficiency is imperfect because bacteria-laden particles can escape around the sides (Davis, 1991). The routine use of masks outside theatre is unnecessary and, except in high-risk situations such as orthopaedic surgery or burns units, masks may eventually be abandoned (Tunevall, 1991). The same number of bacteria is shed into the environment whether masks are worn properly to cover both nose and mouth, or leave the nose exposed (Berger et al., 1993).

Hair covering

Hair is a source of staphylococci, but disposable hair coverings have no effect on bacterial air counts under ventilated conditions (Humphreys et al., 1991). There is now some suggestion that the use of headgear by non-scrubbed staff could be abandoned. However, it seems advisable for the surgeon and his or her assistants to cover their hair because of their close proximity to the operative field. Hair coverings are of no value on wards. Cross-infection is possible when staff suffer from scalp infections, but in these circumstances they should not be at work.

Overshoes

Overshoes contribute to the risk of infection rather than help to prevent it. Bacteria from the floor are seldom responsible for infection, but handling footwear without washing the hands provides a route for cross-infection (Carter, 1990). 'Sticky mats' outside theatres or isolation cubicles are of no value (Meddick, 1977).

Theatre precautions

The operating theatre is a special high-risk environment because the body's tissues are exposed, vastly increasing the opportunity for infection. In wards, bacteria are not disseminated to any great extent via the airborne route, but in theatre airborne staphylococci can cause wound infections, especially during lengthy procedures and orthopaedic surgery (Ayliffe and Lowbury, 1982). The insertion of an orthopaedic prosthesis poses a special risk because the operation is usually lengthy and complex, and because a small number of bacteria are able to cause deep-seated infection within the implanted device (Whyte et al., 1990).

Staff and patients are the main source of airborne bacteria in theatre. During walking, for instance, 10^4 skin scales are shed per minute, about 10 per cent of which carry clusters of bacteria of sufficient number to generate infection (Hambraeus, 1988). The bacteria usually settle onto drapes and are transferred into the open wound on instruments and via the hands. Ventilation is important to reduce postoperative infection (see Chapter 8), to maintain a comfortable working environment for staff and to disperse anaesthetic gases. This is reflected in the prominence afforded to ventilation systems in theatre design and to the conduct recommended for staff during surgical operations.

Reducing the risks of infection in theatre

Infection risks in theatre are controlled by:

- Maintaining the environment through regular cleaning and safety checks
- Precautions taken by staff, especially when surgery is in progress

- The design of the operating theatre suite, especially the demarcation between clean and dirty areas.

The environment

Risks associated with the operating theatre environment can be minimized by, for example:

- Thorough cleaning of the theatre daily
- Damp-dusting floors and surfaces between cases and removal of any visible soiling and spillage of blood or body fluids
- Ensuring, when possible, that 'dirty cases', such as drainage of an abscess, are at the end of a theatre list
- Switching on the ventilation system daily before the list commences. Hospital engineers must check, and arrange servicing of, the system at the intervals set out in the manufacturer's documentation.

Staff precautions and conduct during surgery

Staff precautions include:

- Gowns and overshoes (note the comments made above regarding their effectiveness) are required by all visitors to the theatre suite
- Theatre staff should wear:
  - filter masks
  - shoes reserved for use in theatre
  - trouser suits (or dresses) changed at least daily
  - hair covering by scrubbed staff
  - sterile gowns worn by scrubbed staff
  - sterile gloves, worn by all scrubbed staff and changed whenever there is evidence of puncture, or between certain stages of some procedures
- Illness among staff (for example boils, diarrhoea and vomiting) should be reported to the occupational health department.

The correct conduct during operations includes:

- Aseptic technique must be strictly observed
- Movement within theatre needs to be kept to a minimum to keep the number of airborne particles to a minimum
- The number of people in the operating room should be as low as possible: a viewing gallery should be available for educational purposes
- Incidents and breaches in asepsis should be monitored
- The infection rate of clean wounds should be monitored (see Chapter 8).

Requirements for theatre suite design

It is conventional for the theatre suite to be divided into four zones (Medical Research Council, 1962). These are:

- The **aseptic zone** – the operating room and the layout room
- The **clean zone** – the anaesthetic rooms and scrub area
- The **protective zone** – the reception area and changing facilities
- The **disposal zone** – where the sluice is situated.

The zonal layout focuses attention on the importance of good practice and helps to prevent the entry of an excessive number of people (Humphreys et al., 1991).

The requirements for the design of theatre suites include:

- Division into 'clean' and 'dirty' zones is considered
- Doors should be self-closing; windows should be hermetically sealed and accessible for cleaning
- Floors should be durable, easily cleaned and free of horizontal ledges
- Ventilation systems should comply with official recommendations (Department of Health and Social Security, 1983). This involves:
  - Ensuring that the air source is as far as possible from sources of bacterial contamination and protected from the weather
  - Ensuring that there is a pressure gradient from the sterile to all other areas so that air moves from the cleanest to the least clean areas and corridors
  - Ensuring that the air filters are correctly sited and sealed to prevent air escaping around the sides.

In the UK, official guidelines have been developed to direct the microbiological commissioning and monitoring of operating theatres (Hoffman et al., 2002).

Isolation policies

Isolation was introduced as a method of preventing the spread of infection in hospitals early in the 20th century. Special fever hospitals were built to accommodate those with infectious disease. In general hospitals, the lack of cubicles on long 'Nightingale' wards was compensated for by the erection of physical barriers and by staff wearing the full range of PPE. Physical barriers served mainly to remind staff to take 'barrier nursing' precautions, but these were distressing to patients and the complicated rituals performed were often superfluous to requirements. They were practised in view of the widely held belief that infectious particles could easily become airborne and be readily transferred to other patients. It has gradually become apparent that most infections are transmitted primarily in body secretions and that the hands, and to a lesser extent other fomites, rather than airborne spread, are the route of transmission. In most cases, airborne transmission, if it occurs at all, takes place over a relatively short distance.

Isolation policies designed to contain infection have become much simplified, falling into two main categories – disease-specific isolation precautions and isolation based on categories of infection. Appropriate isolation precautions, along with standard precautions/principles, are used in infection prevention and control.

Disease-specific isolation precautions

Disease-specific isolation precautions involve breaking the chain of infection by taking precautions specific to the particular infection. For example, in the case of enteric organisms such as *Salmonella*, spread by the faecal-oral route, precautions would include wearing PPE when handling excreta and washing the hands after patient contact. Operating this system when an infectious patient is admitted would involve routine assessment to establish:

- The probable cause of infection.
- The mechanism of dissemination.
- Articles likely to become heavily contaminated that could readily transmit infection and that would require careful disposal or decontamination.
- The need for a single room. A single room might be desirable but not practical; an older patient with an infected pressure ulcer might become confused if nursed in isolation, even if visited frequently by the nurse: the experience of isolation can itself be distressing (Knowles, 1993).
- Any other circumstances peculiar to that individual. A person with HIV does not need to be isolated but may prefer privacy, especially during terminal care, with close friends and family in constant attendance.
- The susceptibility of other patients and staff. Precautions required where immunosuppressed patients are nursed will not be appropriate on a general ward.

Disease-specific isolation is cost-effective as it eliminates unnecessary rituals and the wasteful use of equipment such as masks, which are usually unnecessary. The disadvantage is that all nurses need a very good knowledge of the way in which each type of infection is spread. Non-specialist nurses frequently do not have this information, so for the system to operate successfully, there must be good communication with the infection control team, with opportunities for regular updating (Gould, 1985). Additional problems occur when the infection is difficult to diagnose or it becomes apparent that the patient has been carrying an infectious organism for some time.

Categories of isolation

With this system, patients are assigned to a particular category of isolation according to the mode of transmission of the organism involved. A system of colour-coded cards provides guidelines for specific source isolation (Control of Infection Group, Northwick Park Hospital, 1974). This approach is effective if staff and visitors follow the instructions but can be criticized for a number of reasons:

- It results in mechanistic, task-oriented care, not in keeping with the spirit of person-oriented, individualized care
- It is necessary to display the instruction card on the door of the person's room. The precise nature of the infection is not disclosed, but it will be immediately apparent to any casual observer that he or she has an infection.

For people carrying parenterally transmitted infections, the card system is redundant. Isolation in a single room is not usually necessary for those carrying such infections because their carrier status should be irrelevant if standard (universal) precautions/principles are taken, and labelling people breaches confidentiality.

Protective isolation

Protective isolation is required for patients with a high risk of developing infection because they are immunocompromised. This includes patients with prolonged neutropenia (reduction in the number of neutrophils circulating in the blood, usually defined as less than $1.0 \times 10^9/l$) caused by chemotherapy for leukaemia, lymphoma and bone marrow transplantation. For these patients, infection can be life-threatening. Initially the focus was on the provision of a 'germ-free' environment in a specialist unit, with sterile food and contact only with fully gowned staff. This was distressing for patients and their families, expensive, time-consuming and not always effective as it focused on the exclusion of extrinsic organisms spread by cross-infection from other people. However, considerable risk comes from the patient's own flora, especially the gastrointestinal tract, and a germ-free state is not attainable. Today, stringent precautions are reserved for patients undergoing bone marrow transplantation. For other patients, a less stringent approach, possibly outside specialist transplant units, is recommended (Fenelon, 1995).

Simple protective isolation

Single room accommodation is unlikely to have a protective effect but may help by reminding staff and visitors that special precautions are required, and may be appreciated owing to the considerable stress experienced by patients (Knowles, 1993). There is no reason to exclude visitors unless they have an infection, and providing they will not have contact with the patient, there seems no logical reason for them to wear protective clothing.

Handwashing should be thorough (see above) before patient contact to reduce the risk of cross-infection.

PPE is of secondary importance to handwashing in the prevention of cross-infection but is of value in preventing the patient's own flora gaining access to a vulnerable site. Gloves and aprons used during contact with blood and body fluids should be changed before contact with a wound or any invasive device, and the hands should be washed.

Food contains organisms that are not harmful if their numbers are small. Salads are a well-known source of Gram-negative bacteria that may be a threat to immunocompromised patients, and raw food may harbour *Listeria*. Eggs, as a possible source of *Salmonella*, should be thoroughly cooked.

Invasive procedures are a major threat to immunosuppressed patients as they have a very high rate of bacteraemia (bacteria in the blood). Today, good protocols for care exist, which are particularly important for these patients (see Chapters 7, 8, 9 and 10).

Staff who are pregnant should not have contact with immunosuppressed patients who may be carrying a large number of organisms that could damage the fetus.

Critical care units

Patients in critical care units, for example intensive, neonatal units, are immunocompromised and at high risk of infection. Particular care must thus be taken with hand hygiene. In some units, theatre dress is worn by staff with direct patient contact, and in the past it has been common policy to insist that all visitors wear a gown or a plastic apron. This does not, however, contribute to the prevention of infection (Haque and Chagla, 1989).

■ SELF-ASSESSMENT ■

1. Decontamination is achieved at three levels – cleaning, disinfection and sterilization. True? or False?

2. Which items in the clinical environment may become heavily contaminated?

3. Chemical disinfection is superior to disinfection by heat. True? or False?

4. Chlorhexidine is effective against:
   (a) Gram-positive bacteria
   (b) spores
   (c) viruses
   (d) *Mycobacterium tuberculosis*

5. Handwashing is necessary:
   (a) before aseptic procedures
   (b) after handling patients
   (c) after handling items that are or could be soiled
   (d) before handling food

6. Hands are the most likely way to disseminate infection. True? or False?

7. Sterilization is achieved at 121 °C moist heat for 15 minutes. True? or False?

8. When might protective isolation be used?

■ REFERENCES ■

Andersen BM, Rasch M, Hochlin K et al. (2006) Decontamination of rooms, medical equipment and ambulances using an aerosol of hydrogen peroxide disinfectant. *Journal of Hospital Infection* **62:** 149–55.

Axnick KJ and Yarborough M (1984) *Infection Control: An Integrated Approach.* Mosby, Toronto.

Ayliffe GA (1970) Contamination of infant feeds in a Milton milk kitchen. *Lancet* **1**: 559–60.

Ayliffe GA and Lowbury EJ (1982) Airborne infection in hospital. *Journal of Hospital Infection* **3**: 217–40.

Berger SA, Kramer M, Nagar H et al. (1993) Effect of surgical mask position on bacterial contamination of the operative field. *Journal of Hospital Infection* **23**: 51–4.

Block C, Baron O, Bogkowski B et al. (1990) An in-use evaluation of polypropylene versus steel bedpans. *Journal of Hospital Infection* **16**: 331–8.

Burdon DW and Whitby JL (1967) Contamination of hospital disinfectants with *Pseudomonas* species. *British Medical Journal* **2**: 153–4.

Carter R (1990) Ritual and risk. *Nursing Times* **86**: 63–4.

Casewell MW and Phillips I (1978) Epidemiological patterns of *Klebsiella* colonisation and infection in an intensive care unit. *Journal of Hygiene* **80**: 295–300.

Chadwick PR and Oppenheim BA (1994) Vancomycin-resistant enterococci and bedpan washer machines. *Lancet* **344**: 685.

Coates D and Hutchinson DN (1994) How to produce a hospital disinfection policy. *Journal of Hospital Infection* **26**: 57–68.

Control of Infection Group, Northwick Park Hospital (1974) Isolation system for general hospitals. *British Medical Journal* **2**: 41–6.

Curie K, Speller DC, Simpson RA et al. (1978) A hospital epidemic caused by gentamicin-resistant *Klebsiella aerogenes*. *Journal of Hygiene* **80**: 115–23.

Curran E (1991) Protecting with plastic aprons. *Nursing Times* **87**(38): 64–8.

Davis WT (1991) Filtration efficiency of surgical face masks: the need for meaningful standards. *American Journal of Infection Control* **19**: 16–18.

Department of Health (DH) (1993a) *Risk Management in the NHS*. HMSO, London.

Department of Health (DH) (1993b) *Guidance on Decontamination: Sterilisation, Disinfection and Cleaning of Medical Equipment*. HMSO, London.

Department of Health (DH) (1995) *Hospital Laundry Arrangements for Used and Infected Linen*, HSG (95)18. DH, London. Available www.dh.gov.uk.

Department of Health (DH) (2003) *Winning Ways: Working Together to Reduce Healthcare Associated Infection in England* (Chief Medical Officer). DH, London. Available www.dh.gov.uk.

Department of Health (DH) (2006) *The Health Act 2006: Code of Practice for the Prevention and Control of Healthcare-associated Infections*. DH, London. Available www.dh.gov.uk.

Department of Health (DH) (2007a) *Saving Lives: Reducing Infection, Delivering Clean and Safe Care*. Available www.dh.gov.uk.

Department of Health (DH) (2007b) *Uniforms and Workwear: An Evidence Base for Developing Local Policy*. Available www.dh.gov.uk.

Department of Health and Social Security (DHSS) (1983) *Ventilation of Operating Departments: A Design Guide*. HMSO, London.

Fenelon LE (1995) Protective isolation: who needs it? *Journal of Hospital Infection* (Supplement) **30**: 218–22.

French GL, Otter JA, Shannon KP et al. (2004) Tackling contamination of the hospital environment by methicillin-resistant *Staphylococcus aureus* (MRSA): a comparison between conventional terminal cleaning and hydrogen peroxide vapour decontamination. *Journal of Hospital Infection* **57**: 31–7.

Gould DJ (1984) The significance of hand drying in the prevention of infection. *Nursing Times* **80**(47): 33–5.

Gould DJ (1985) Isolation procedures in one health district. *Nursing Times* **81**(7): 47–51.

Gould DJ and Chamberlain A (1997) The use of a ward-based educational teaching package to enhance nurses' compliance with infection control procedures. *Journal of Clinical Nursing* **6**(1): 55–67.

Gould DJ and Ream E (1993) Assessing nurses' hand decontamination performance. *Nursing Times* **89**(25): 47–50.

Gould DJ, Hewitt-Taylor J, Drey N et al. (2007) The cleanyourhands campaign: critiquing policy and evidence base. *Journal of Hospital Infection* **65**: 95–101.

Hambraeus A (1988) Aerobiology of the operating suite. *Journal of Hospital Infection* (Supplement A) **11**: 68–76.

Hanson PJ, Gor D and Jeffries DJ (1989) Chemical inactivation of HIV on surfaces. *British Medical Journal* **298**: 862–4.

Haque KN and Chagla AH (1989) Do gowns prevent infection in neonatal intensive care units? *Journal of Health Hospital Infection* **14**: 159–62.

Health and Safety Executive (HSE) (1993) *Personal Protective Equipment at Work Regulations: Guidance on Regulations*. HSE, Leeds.

Health and Safety Executive (HSE) (1998/2005) *Respiratory Sensitizers and COSHH: Breathe Freely*. An employers' leaflet on preventing occupational asthma. HSE, London. Available www.hse.gov.uk/pubns/indg95.pdf.

Health and Safety Executive (HSE) (2007) Healthcare workers. Glutaraldehyde. Available www.hse.gov.uk/asthma/healthcare.htm.

Health Service Circular (HSC) (1999) *Clinical Governance in the New NHS*, HSC 1999/065. DH, London. Available www.dh.gov.uk.

Health Services Advisory Committee (1987) *Recommendations for the Disposal of Waste*. HSE/Environment Agency, London.

Hoffman PN, Cooke EM, McCarville MR et al. (1985) Micro-organisms isolated from skin under wedding rings worn by hospital staff. *British Medical Journal* **290**: 206–7.

Hoffman PN, Williams J, Stacey A et al. (2002) Microbiological commissioning and monitoring of operating theatre suites. *Journal of Hospital Infection* **52**(1): 1–28.

Humphreys H, Russell HJ, Marshall HJ et al. (1991) The effect of surgical headgear on bacterial counts. *Journal of Hospital Infection* **19**: 175–80.

Jacobson G, Thiele JE, McCune JH et al. (1985) Handwashing, ringwearing and number of microorganisms. *Nursing Research* **34**: 186–8.

Jeanes A and Green J (2001) Nail art: a review of current infection control issues. *Journal of Hospital Infection* **49**: 139–42.

Jenkinson H, Wright D, Jones M et al. (2006) Prevention and control of infection in non-acute healthcare settings. *Nursing Standard* **20**(40): 56–63.

Kjolen H and Andersen BM (1992) Handwashing and disinfection of heavily contaminated hands; effective or ineffective? *Journal of Hospital Infection* **21**: 61–71.

Knowles HE (1993) The experience of infectious patients in isolation. *Nursing Times* **89**(30): 53–6.

Kownatzki E (2003) Hand hygiene and skin health. *Journal of Hospital Infection* **55**: 239–45.

Kotilainen HR, Avato JL and Gantz NM (1990) Latex and vinyl non-sterile examination gloves: status report on laboratory evaluation of defects by physical and biological methods. *Applied Environmental Microbiology* **56**: 1627–30.

Mackintosh CA (1982) A testing time for gowns. *Journal of Hospital Infection* **3**: 5–8.

Madsen P and Madsen R (1967) A study of disposable surgical masks. *American Journal of Surgery* **114**: 431–5.

Maki DG, Alvardo C and Hassemer C (1986) Double-bagging items from isolation rooms is unnecessary as an infection control measure: a comparative study of surface contamination with single and double bagging. *Infection Control* **7**: 535–7.

Meddick MM (1977) Bacterial contamination control mats: a comparative study. *Journal of Hygiene* **79**: 133–40.

Medical Research Council (MRC) (1962) Design and ventilation of operating room suites for control of infection and for comfort. *Lancet* **2**: 945–51.

National Audit Office (NAO) (2000) *The Management and Control of Hospital Acquired Infection in Acute NHS Trusts in England*. NAO, London. Available www.nao.org.uk/.

Patel S (2004) The impact of environmental cleanliness on infection rates. *Nursing Times* **100**(1): 32–4.

Patel S, Murray-Leonard J and Wilson AP (2006) Laundering of hospital staff uniforms at home. *Journal of Hospital Infection* **62**: 89–93.

Peireira LJ, Lee GM and Wade FJ (1990) The effect of surgical handwashing routines on the microbial counts of operating room nurses. *American Journal of Infection Control* **18**: 354–64.

Plowman R, Graves N, Griffin MA et al. (2001) The rate and cost of hospital-acquired infections occurring in patients admitted to selected specialities of a district general hospital in England and the national burden imposed. *Journal of Hospital Infection* **47**(3): 198–209.

Pratt RJ, Pellowe CM, Wilson JA et al. (2007) epic2: National evidence-based guidelines for preventing healthcare-associated infections in NHS hospitals in England. *Journal of Hospital Infection* **65** (Supplement 1): S1–S64. Available www.epic.tvu.ac.uk.

Rahman M (1985) Commissioning a new hospital isolation unit and assessment of its use over five years. *Journal of Hospital Infection* **6**: 65–70.

Reybrouck G (1983) The role of hands in the spread of nosocomial infections. *Journal of Hospital Infection* **4**: 103–11.

Royal College of Nursing (RCN) (2005) *Good Practice in Infection Prevention and Control: Guidance for Nursing Staff*. RCN, London.

Russell AD and Day MJ (1993) Antibacterial activity of chlorhexidine. *Journal of Hospital Infection* **25**: 229–38.

Schabrun S and Chopchase L (2006) Healthcare equipment as a source of nosocomial infection: a systematic review. *Journal of Hospital Infection* **63**: 239–45.

Storr J (2005) The effectiveness of the national *cleanyourhands* campaign. *Nursing Times* **101**(8): 50–1.

Tunevall TG (1991) Post-operative wound infections and surgical masks: a controlled study. *World Journal of Surgery* **15**: 383–8.

Voss A and Widmer AF (1997) No time for handwashing? Handwashing versus alcoholic rub: can we afford 100% compliance? *Infection Control and Hospital Epidemiology* **18**: 203–8.

Ward D (2001) Infection control policies in nursing homes. *Nursing Standard* **15**(46): 40–4.

Whyte W, Hamblen DI and Kelly IG (1990) An investigation into occlusive polyester surgical clothing. *Journal of Hospital Infection* **15**: 363–74.

Wilson AP and Ridgeway GL (2006) Reducing hospital-acquired infection by design: the new University College London Hospital. *Journal of Hospital Infection* **63**: 264–9.

▓▓▓▓▓▓ FURTHER READING AND INFORMATION SOURCES ▓▓▓▓

Department of Health (DH) (2007) *Clean, Safe Care: Reducing MRSA and Other Healthcare Associated Infections*. Available www.clean-safe-care.nhs.uk.

Health and Safety Executive – www.hse.gov.uk.

Infection Control Nurses' Association/Royal College of Nursing (2003) *Infection Control Guidance for General Practice*. ICNA, Bathgate.

Infection Protection Society (IPS) incorporating Infection Control Nurses' Association – www.ips.uk.net.

Jeanes A (2005) Using alcohol products. *Nursing Times* **101**(28): 28–9.

Medicines and Healthcare Products Regulatory Agency (MHRA) – www.mhra.gov.uk/.

National Institute for Health and Clinical Excellence (NICE) (2003) *Infection Control*,

Prevention of Healthcare-associated Infection in Primary and Community Care. Clinical guideline 2. NICE, London. Available www.nice.org.uk/.

National Patient Safety Agency (NPSA) (2004) *Clean Hands Help to Save Lives.* Patient safety alert No. 4. NPSA, London. Available www.npsa.nhs.uk/.

NHS Estates (2004) *The NHS Healthcare Cleaning Manual.* DH, London.

Pellowe CM, Pratt RJ, Harper P et al. (2003) Evidence-based guidelines for preventing healthcare-associated infections in primary and community care in England. *Journal of Hospital Infection* **55** (Supplement): S2–S53.

CHAPTER 6

Preventing infection in healthcare settings

CHAPTER OUTCOMES

After reading this chapter, you should be able to:

➤ Explain what is meant by 'healthcare-associated infection'

➤ Discuss the problems of healthcare-associated infection for healthcare providers and from the patient's/resident's perspective

➤ State which infections occur most commonly in healthcare settings

➤ Discuss the approaches taken to monitor, prevent and control infection in healthcare settings

➤ List the main groups of bacteria responsible for infection in healthcare settings and suggest the most effective control methods in each case

➤ Outline the role of the infection prevention and control team and committee

Introduction

Healthcare-associated infection (HCAI) is infection not present or incubating at the time of admission or healthcare intervention (Bennett and Brachman, 1979). It is not a new phenomenon, but the types of infection that commonly occur in healthcare settings have changed dramatically since the second half of the 18th century when HCAI first attracted attention.

The significance of healthcare-associated infection

Today the cost of HCAI in financial terms is considerable – to the government and hence to taxpayers and to patients/residents. Hospital stay is usually increased, so 'hotel' costs often represent a substantial proportion of the additional expenditure. However, people with infections require more drugs (antibiotics and analgesia), more dressings and more nursing time, whether they are in hospital or have returned to the community. In addition, patients face major inconvenience and distress while the waiting lists for elective procedures build up (Plowman et al., 2001). Thus, the need to develop effective control measures is now fully acknowledged by health service policy-makers, and in recent years, a number of attempts have been made to quantify the risk of developing HCAI as the first step towards preventing it. Increasing age is a risk factor for infection and older adults form a high proportion of the hospital population. According to the Health Protection Agency (2007a), over 75 per cent of *Clostridium difficile*, meticillin-resistant *Staphylococcus aureus* in the bloodstream and surgical site infections occur in patients aged 65 years or older.

These control measures include the assessment of risk factors for HCAI and the actions required to reduce or control the risks (Sud and Gorman, 2007). Hospital infection rates can be regarded as a marker of quality and can be used for the purposes of auditing and contract specification (Royal College of Nursing, 1994). In England, recent legislation in the Health Act (Department of Health, 2006) sets out the responsibilities for NHS Trusts and health professionals in respect of HCAIs. The Department of Health (2007) publication *Saving Lives: Reducing Infection, Delivering Clean and Safe Care* assists NHS Trusts to discharge their responsibilities in respect to the provisions of the Health Act 2006.

In England, the current health regulator, the Healthcare Commission, monitors standards of safety, infection control and cleanliness as part of its remit. However, legislation is planned that will create an integrated health and adult social care regulator in 2008. The new body, to be known as the Care Quality Commission, will result from a merger of the Healthcare Commission, the Mental Health Act Commission and the Commission for Social Care Inspection.

The extent of healthcare-associated infection

The extent of the problem can be estimated by prevalence or incidence surveys (Chapter 14).

Prevalence surveys

Prevalence studies conducted in 1980 showed that 9.2 per cent of hospital inpatients developed HCAI, the most common being urinary tract infection (Meers et al., 1981). Over the years, the percentage of inpatients developing HCAI has not changed much; the second prevalence study undertaken in 1993/4 showed 9 per cent of patients had an infection (Emmerson et al., 1996). A summary of the third national prevalence study carried out in 2006 indicates that 8.2 per cent of patients had a HCAI (Hospital Infection Society/Infection Control Nurses Association, 2007).

Incidence surveys

Incidence studies are more expensive and difficult to conduct than prevalence studies and are usually conducted on a smaller scale. They indicate that, overall, the rate of HCAI is 6 per cent. This figure is probably more accurate than statistics derived from prevalence data because patients who have developed infection generally stay in hospital longer, overestimating the true rate.

Monitoring healthcare-associated infection

HCAI infection can be monitored by surveillance or audit.

Surveillance

Surveillance consists of the routine collection and analysis of infection rates with feedback to staff (Hay, 2006). It gives infection control teams greater insight into the patterns of infection in healthcare settings, drawing early attention to potential outbreaks. Feedback helps to reduce infection by stimulating the examination of local practices to identify areas in which remedial action should be taken and encouraging the most appropriate use of resources. The value of surveillance was first demonstrated in the United States, where hospitals cannot be licensed without evidence that effective infection control policies are operating. A major study in the US involving 338 hospitals, the Study of the Efficacy of Nosocomial Infection Control project, revealed that surveillance with feedback to clinical staff could reduce HCAI by 32 per cent; in hospitals without surveillance, the infection rate was higher (Haley et al., 1985).

In the UK, the Public Health Laboratory Service, which is now part of the Health Protection Agency, established a Nosocomial Infection Surveillance Unit, and in 1997, the unit launched the Nosocomial Infection National Surveillance Scheme (NINSS). The NINSS is now called the Surgical Site Infection Surveillance Service (SSISS) and provides confidential data to hospitals so that infection control teams and clinicians can benchmark their own infection rates from year to year with anonymized data from other hospitals. This enables each hospital to undertake surveillance targeted at a specific area or patient group. The success of an infection control activity can be examined by benchmarking the numbers of cases before and after the intervention.

Audit

Audit is another approach to infection control, often introduced at a local level. The audit cycle involves making systematic quantifiable comparisons between existing practice and explicit, agreed standards in order to highlight areas in which improvements could be made (Glover, 1992; Figure 6.1). It involves the systematic critical analysis of the quality of care and should include:

- Procedures used to diagnose and treat patients
- The use of resources
- The resulting outcome and quality of life for the patient.

HCAI is a prime target for audit because it affects all three selection criteria (French, 1993). Effective methods of auditing using this approach have been developed (Millward et al., 1993).

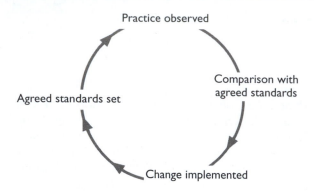

Figure 6.1 The audit cycle

The auditing of infection control initiatives can be expensive and time-consuming if it involves obtaining and processing microbiological samples. An alternative approach is to audit the documentation concerned with infection prevention (French, 1993). Factors to be taken into consideration include:

- Whether written documents exist for a given procedure (see below)
- Their acceptability
- Whether hospital practice adheres to the guidelines
- Whether there is any demonstrable alteration in HCAI after introducing the new guideline or following a training programme to increase staff awareness of the established documentation.

In addition, many infection control teams are concerned about the distribution and behaviour of particular pathogens responsible for a high proportion of all infections occurring in hospital.

INFORMATION BOX 6.1

Suggested documentation for infection control audit

- ➤ Care of urinary catheters
- ➤ Care of intravenous lines
- ➤ Staff occupational health policies (immunization programmes for hepatitis B and rubella, and screening after exposure to patients with tuberculosis)
- ➤ Disposal of contaminated waste
- ➤ Disinfectant policies
- ➤ Prevention of Legionnaire's disease
- ➤ Antibiotic policies
- ➤ Control of meticillin-resistant *Staphylococcus aureus* bacteraemias
- ➤ Control of outbreaks of *Clostridium difficile*

Pathogens causing healthcare-associated infection

This section covers infections caused by bacteria most commonly responsible for HCAI.

Staphylococcal infection

Coagulase-producing organisms may cause staphylococcal infections; the enzyme coagulase clots plasma when the bacteria are grown on solid culture media. The bacterium known as *Staphylococcus aureus* may also be meticillin resistant. Other staphylococci causing infection, for example *Staphylococcus epidermidis*, are not coagulase producers.

Staphylococcus aureus

Staphylococcus aureus is a Gram-positive bacterium that produces coagulase. It is carried in the nose, throat, axillae, toe webs and perineum of 30–50 per cent of healthy people without causing clinical infection. Asymptomatic carriage is clinically significant because the bacteria can be transferred to susceptible sites (for example from the nose to a wound) or from a fit asymptomatic individual to someone less healthy who will succumb to clinical infection.

Staphylococcus aureus is the most common cause of pyogenic (pus-forming) infection, causing a range of infections that includes boils, abscesses, septic fingers, styes, impetigo (inflammatory skin condition with pustules) and sticky eyes in neonates. Transmission is through contact, mainly via hands. In hospital, *Staphylococcus aureus* causes serious wound infections, bronchopneumonia, osteomyelitis (inflammation of bone marrow, usually caused by bacterial infection) and endocarditis (inflammation of the endothelial tissue that lines the heart and covers the heart valves). Some strains produce toxins that cause extensive cellular damage. For example, staphylococcal toxins cause the toxic shock syndrome (TSS) associated with the use of vaginal tampons and in other situations. The main method of epidemiological typing used to identify whether a cluster of staphylococcal infections originate from a common source is 'phage typing'. This has revealed outbreaks in intensive care and burns units.

Meticillin-resistant staphylococcal infection

Meticillin-resistant *Staphylococcus aureus* (MRSA) causes the same range of infections as meticillin-sensitive *Staphylococcus aureus*, is disseminated in the same way and is not usually more virulent. Most people become asymptomatic carriers and never develop clinical infection, especially if they are healthy. However, they operate as reservoirs and are therefore a risk to seriously ill patients. MRSA has become a cause for great concern because it is extremely difficult to eradicate. Skin lesions such as chronic wounds or cannula insertion points can become heavily colonized, so are particularly likely to operate as reservoirs. The risk of developing clinical MRSA infection is greater among older, more debilitated individuals. In a recent study, 80 per cent of people dying after MRSA infection were aged over 70 years of age (Health Protection Agency, 2007b). Factors that encourage the dissemination of MRSA through a population of hospital patients include the prescription of two or more antibiotics to individual patients and poor infection control precautions, such as substandard handwashing (Casewell, 1986). MRSA can spread between hospitals when staff and patients are moved between sites. MRSA is not just a problem in hospital; patients with MRSA who are discharged to nursing/care homes or their own homes should be managed according to national guidelines (Patel, 2007).

Epidemic meticillin-resistant *Staphylococcus aureus* (EMRSA) spreads more easily than other strains of MRSA and appears to colonize skin and mucous membranes more readily (French et al., 1990). The first strain, EMRSA-1, was isolated in 1984 (Marples et al., 1985), 16 strains now having been reported in the UK. EMRSA-1 and EMRSA-3 caused large outbreaks in the 1980s and contributed to a number of deaths, but they seldom affected healthy people and never spread beyond one or two NHS regions (Marples and Reith, 1992). The other strains caused fewer problems and are now seldom a source of infection, with the exception of EMRSA-14 and EMRSA-16, first isolated in 1991–92. These have become widely disseminated in hospitals and have been detected in the community, particularly in residents in nursing homes (Cox et al., 1995).

A more recent development has been the emergence of a vancomycin-resistant strain of MRSA; it was first detected in 2002 in the United States where three cases have been reported (Health Protection Agency, 2004). Vancomycin-intermediate *Staphylococcus aureus* (VISA), also known as glycopeptide-intermediate *S. aureus* (GISA), strains with reduced susceptibility to vancomycin have been detected in several countries including the UK (Coia et al., 2006).

Guidelines for controlling MRSA

Guidelines for controlling MRSA in the UK have been developed and revised by Coia et al. (2006) for the Joint Working Party of the British Society for Antimicrobial Chemotherapy, the Hospital Infection Society and the Infection Control Nurses Association (see below). The guidelines detail the actions designed to control MRSA in hospital, such as MRSA surveillance, eradication of nasal and skin carriage in some patient groups and standard infection control precautions, including single-room isolation or cohorting, handwashing facilities and an appropriate level of cleaning (Coia et al., 2006).

The Report of a combined working party of the British Society for Antimicrobial Chemotherapy and the Hospital Infection Society (1995) provides separate guidance for the management of MRSA in the community, and Patel (2007) stresses that the guidelines for hospitals are not suitable for use in community settings and vice versa. The joint working party (Coia et al., 2006) recommends that more research needs to be undertaken in order to generate guidelines for managing MRSA in community settings.

In many other countries, a much more proactive approach has been taken to controlling MRSA. In some countries in Continental Europe, a 'search and destroy' strategy is used and infected and colonized patients are routinely isolated (Wertheim et al., 2004). This appears to have been effective because rates of infection are generally lower than in the UK.

▬ PRACTICE APPLICATION 6.1 ▬

Managing MRSA in Diverse Settings

Healthcare settings have different levels of risk in respect to MRSA. For example, a mental health unit may be minimal risk, whereas an orthopaedic ward or intensive care unit is considered high risk. Therefore it is vital that the level of intervention is appropriate for the level of risk.

Activity

➤ Consider the level of risk in your workplace/placement.

➤ Access the current guidelines (Coia et al., 2006), then select and read about a particular activity, for example surveillance, screening or isolation.

➤ Consider the policy in your workplace/placement – how similar is it to the guidelines?

Treatment of MRSA

The drug of choice against MRSA (Chapter 4) is the glycopeptide vancomycin, patients who experience toxic effects being given teicoplanin (Daum et al., 1990). Combined therapy may be tried if single therapy has not been effective. Rifampicin and sodium fusidate may be effective together. Other drugs that may be used for particular types of MRSA infection include linezolid, quinupristin combined with dalfopristin, and tigecycline. Topical mupirocin is usually used to eradicate skin and nasal carriage in both patients and staff, but other drugs, such as cream containing chlorhexidine and neomycin, are needed for mupirocin-resistant MRSA.

It is important to keep MRSA in perspective, remembering that most carriers never develop clinical infection. Nevertheless, the control of this organism is likely to remain an infection control challenge for some time, especially as strains of vancomycin-resistant MRSA, VISA (GISA) and mupirocin-resistant MRSA have emerged and are becoming more widespread.

Coagulase-negative staphylococci

Numerous species of staphylococci are unable to produce coagulase and are therefore described as coagulase-negative staphylococci (CNSs). The most well-known example of this group is *Staphylococcus epidermidis*, which is a skin commensal. As the ability to secrete coagulase is one of the factors contributing to the pathogenic potential of *Staphylococcus aureus*, CNSs were once believed to have low pathogenicity. However, these bacteria produce extracellular slime that enables them to adhere to plastic and metal surfaces. Once they become covered with slime, they are protected from the host defences and multiply, establishing a focus of infection. CNSs are associated with an increasing incidence of infections involving peritoneal dialysis catheters, prosthetic heart valves and orthopaedic implants. If they gain access to the bloodstream via intravascular devices, they cause septicaemia. Infections are difficult to eradicate because CNSs are naturally resistant to many antibiotics (Harmory and Parisi, 1987). In some cases, it can be difficult to determine whether CNSs are behaving as contaminants or are clinically significant (Martin de Nicolas et al., 1995).

Clostridium difficile

C. difficile is a Gram-positive, spore-forming bacillus, which is able to form toxins that cause diarrhoea, ranging from mild to severe and life-threatening (Chapter 4). The toxins disrupt the ecology of the normal bowel flora. This usually occurs after the patient has received broad-spectrum antibiotics, especially ampicillin, clindamycin or the cephalosporins (Starr, 2005). The terms 'antibiotic-associated diarrhoea or colitis', or 'pseudomembranous colitis' are also used.

Other risk factors include increasing age, co-morbid conditions and prolonged hospital stay. *C. difficile* is the most common cause of infectious diarrhoea in hospital patients and can result in high levels of morbidity and mortality, contributing to the escalating costs of healthcare, especially in services for older people (Price et al., 2007). Symptoms usually start when the patient is taking antibiotics, but can be delayed for weeks or months. As a result, the condition may not be diagnosed until after the patient has returned to the community. Symptoms frequently return after treatment, probably because spores persist in the gut. Diagnosis is confirmed by the presence of the bacteria and its toxin in the faeces. It has been estimated that about 5 per cent of adults in the community and 20 per cent of those hospitalized are carrying *C. difficile.* In the UK, the incidence is rapidly increasing. Transmission can occur from patient to patient, via the hands of health workers and from environmental reservoirs, including equipment such as bedpans and urinals contaminated with spores, which are able to survive for months. Several outbreaks have occurred, attracting criticism in the media. The use of alcohol handrubs may be exacerbating spread: none of the products commonly used to decontaminate hands destroy spores effectively, but traditional washing and drying probably helps to remove them mechanically, in contrast to the use of a rapidly evaporating alcohol handrub.

Mandatory reporting of *C. difficile* is now required in the UK. Other important infection control precautions include isolation of patients excreting toxin-producing strains of *C. difficile* while they are experiencing diarrhoea, the use of protective clothing and strict attention to hand hygiene. Antibiotic policies to control the use of broad-spectrum antibiotics and early discontinuation of antibiotics are important factors in control.

Streptococcal infection

Streptococci are Gram-positive, chain-forming cocci classified into the Lancefield groups A–S.

Group A beta-haemolytic streptococcus

Group A beta-haemolytic streptococcus (*Streptococcus pyogenes*) is responsible for serious infections – pharyngitis, skin infections and puerperal fever (Ayton, 1981). The bacteria can spread through the tissues by releasing toxins, thus generalized infection may result. Scarlet fever is pharyngitis with a rash induced by the release of toxin. The toxins may also induce hypersensitivity reactions, for example glomeru-lonephritis and rheumatic fever that develop up to four weeks after the infection.

Group A haemolytic streptococci were the first bacteria identified as a source of HCAI (nosocomial infection) and were responsible for major outbreaks in burns units and maternity and surgical wards between 1930 and 1950. The development of serological typing techniques revealed that cross-infection was common. Person-to-person transmission has been well documented. The bacteria are carried in the nasopharynx of 6–8 per cent of the general population, mostly children, carriers dispersing them by coughing, sneezing and talking. The droplets dry out, heavily contaminating the environment.

Following the introduction of penicillin, the incidence of streptococcal infection declined. Most strains are still sensitive, and until recently Group A streptococci remained a comparatively rare cause of infection, although its incidence is now increasing in hospital and in the community. Older people, especially those with serious underlying medical conditions, are most at risk, and there appears to be substantial risk of transmission in hospitals as well as the community (Davies et al., 1996). Screening staff to exclude carriers, isolating infected patients until antibiotic therapy has become effective and environmental cleaning to remove reservoirs are recommended to control outbreaks (Sarangi and Rowsell, 1995).

Group B streptococci

Group B streptococci (GBS) are commensals in the gut and vagina. GBS are oppor-tunists and can cause life-threatening meningitis, pneumonia and septicaemia in the newborn if contamination occurs during delivery (see below); it also causes infec-tion in older adults and in people with chronic diseases that include diabetes.

INFORMATION BOX 6.2

Group B streptococci, pregnancy and newborns

GBS is a common cause of meningitis and septicaemia in newborns; the disease may be early-onset (during the first week of life), or late-onset, occurring when the infant is between a week and some months of age.

Many women are asymptomatic carriers of GBS, although it may cause urinary tract infection (UTI). Carrier status can be confirmed by obtaining vaginal and rectal swabs between 35 and 37 weeks' gestation; routine screening is offered in the US. Women who test positive for GBS are routinely given antibiotics during labour; they should also commence antibiotics if the membranes rupture before labour starts. Women who have had a UTI caused by GBS, or have previously had a baby affected by GBS disease should also receive antibiotics during labour. Other situations where there is a high risk of vertical transmission include preterm labour, elevated temperature during labour and a prolonged time with ruptured membranes, when antibiotics should be given.

Viridans group

The viridans group of streptococci are commensals but are well known for their ability to cause infective endocarditis in patients with previously damaged heart valves, gaining access to the bloodstream after dental treatment.

Pneumococcus

The pneumococcus (*Streptococcus pneumoniae*) is a commensal in the respiratory tract. It causes a range of serious infections, including otitis media (inflammation of the middle ear), pneumonia and meningitis (inflammation of the meninges – membranes covering the brain and spinal cord). Some strains have become resistant to penicillin, and cross-infection has been attributed to a failure to identify and isolate infected patients and carriers.

Enterococci

Enterococci are Gram-positive bacteria; they are harmless bowel commensals of humans and many animals. They are weak pathogens that colonize hosts without causing symptoms much more frequently than causing obvious infection, although faecal carriage can persist for months or years (Roghmann et al., 1997). Enterococcal gastrointestinal infection is characterized by diarrhoea.

There are several species of enterococci, but *Enterococcus faecalis* accounts for the vast majority of isolates. Most of the remaining species in humans are *Enterococcus faecium*. Enterococci are present in the faeces of most healthy individuals, but they can cause serious infections in vulnerable patients who are more susceptible, especially those with indwelling devices (Chadwick et al., 1996). Enterococci cause a wide range of infections, including septicaemia, endocarditis, wound infections, UTIs and, infrequently, pneumonia. Most enterococcal infections have occurred in specialist units including intensive care, renal, haematology and liver (Gray and George, 2000). Infections caused by enterococci are treated with glycopeptide antibiotics, such as vancomycin. However, glycopeptide-resistant enterococci (GRE) (also known as vancomycin-resistant enterococci –VRE) emerged in the 1980s and have since been the cause of outbreaks within a single hospital and between hospitals following the transfer of patients (Livornese et al., 1992).

Most infections with GRE occur in specialist units where very ill patients are exposed to a wide range of different antibiotics, promoting the survival of antibiotic-resistant strains. Enterococcal resistance to glycopeptide antibiotics is extremely worrying because it can spread to other highly pathogenic bacteria via plasmids (Tenover et al., 2004) (Chapter 1).

Enterococci can be transmitted between patients, particularly during outbreaks (Gray and George, 2000). As well as the presence of enterococci in the stools, various sites can be colonized, including the skin, throat, perineum, vagina, wounds, urine and vascular catheter sites (Bonten et al., 1996). GRE is not usually a risk to healthy people living at home, in care homes or nursing homes, or residential accommodation who do not have wounds or invasive devices, and neither is it a risk to health workers. Thus far, there are no reports of health workers being the source of colonization or infection to susceptible patients/residents (Cookson et al., 2006).

Enterococci are able to survive for several days on various surfaces (Noskin et al., 1995) and very high levels of contamination occur when patients with symptomatic infection have diarrhoea (Weber and Ruatala, 1997). In common with other HCAIs, the hands of healthcare practitioners are involved in the transmission of GRE, but equipment, such as thermometers, has also been implicated in its spread (Weber and Rutala, 1997). Defective bedpan washers have been a source of enterococci (Chadwick et al., 1996). People who have asymptomatic colonization with enterococci do not seem to cause the high levels of environmental contamination that occur close to patients with enterococcal infection (Gray and George, 2000).

Outbreaks of GRE are increasing in number (Humphreys, 2006). Significant contributory factors include poor bed management, particularly the pressure to keep acute beds open, the transfer between wards, units and hospitals of patients infected or colonized with enterococci and an inability to implement strict and rigorous infection control precautions with high standards of environmental cleanliness (Humphreys, 2006).

Guidelines to control the spread of GRE have been developed by the Hospital Infection Society and the Infection Control Nurses' Association (Cookson et al., 2006) (see below). Although patients carrying GRE asymptomatically do not usually need antibiotic treatment, it may be prudent to mark their notes, because of the long-term nature of faecal carrier status (Roghmann et al., 1997) and the frequency of readmissions or daycare, such as ongoing renal dialysis, in this patient group. Strict antibiotic control is accepted as being very important in preventing the spread of GRE (Barrett, 2004).

▬ PRACTICE APPLICATION 6.2 ▬

Controlling the Spread of GRE

In the *Guidelines for the Control of Glycopeptide-resistant Enterococci in Hospitals* (Cookson et al., 2006), the importance of infection control measures (for example handwashing, isolation of patients and environmental cleaning) is emphasized.

Activity

➤ Access the guidelines and read the section covering 'infection control measures'.

➤ Consider the extent to which these measures are followed in your workplace/placement.

➤ Discuss with your mentor how compliance with hand hygiene recommendations could be improved.

The GRE working party recommends that infection control teams should consider the costs and risks of infection control procedures and balance them alongside the potential benefits whenever cases of GRE or outbreaks arise. The authors defend this approach on the grounds that enterococci are not highly virulent and usually cause serious infection only among immuncompromised patients. The GRE working party recommends a risk assessment approach. Patients with diarrhoea should be nursed in single rooms or cohorted if possible. Patients without symptoms do not require isolation, but gloves and aprons should be worn for contact with faeces and urine (Gray and George, 2000).

Gram-negative infections

Increasing colonization and infection by coliform bacteria and other Gram-negative bacteria such as *Pseudomonas* followed the initial conquest of nosocomial staphylococcal infection in the 1960s. The important Gram-negative bacteria include:

- *Pseudomonas*
- *Klebsiella*
- *Escherichia coli*
- *Proteus.*

Coliforms (a general term covering intestinal bacteria) survive in minute traces of moisture – on the hands (Burke et al., 1971), on patients' skin (Montgomerie and Morrow, 1980) and on articles that come into direct contact with patients (Sanderson and Weissler, 1992). Coliforms had previously been considered to have very low pathogenic potential, but it soon became apparent that cross-infection could readily occur in acute and long-stay wards, contributing significantly to morbidity and mortality, especially among the critically ill (Swiatlo et al., 1987). Coliforms are naturally resistant to many antibiotics, and the prevention of infection depends on adhering to the fundamental principles of infection control, especially handwashing, as environmental contamination readily occurs and reservoirs of infection may develop (Garland et al., 1996). The bacteria may ascend to the bladder, colonize the gut and appear in the faeces, and can be transferred from the oropharynx to the lower respiratory passages, causing pneumonia.

Infection prevention and control services

The Cooke Report (Department of Health and Social Security, 1988) recommended the provision of an infection control committee, an infection control nurse in all hospitals providing acute services, and the management of infection outbreaks. This was updated in 1995 to include guidance on routine surveillance and information for purchasers (Department of Health/Public Health Laboratory Service, 1995). Further changes emphasized the importance of effective prevention including the creation of the post of 'director of infection prevention and control' (Department of Health, 2003).

The role of infection prevention and control services in hospital

The infection prevention and control team is responsible for, and reports appropriately on, all aspects of the surveillance, prevention and control of infection in hospital. Its role is to implement an annual programme and policies of infection control, and to offer a 24-hour service to prevent and control infection, providing advice and education to all staff. The infection control doctor and specialist nurse are key members of the team.

The role of the specialist nurse

The specialist nurse is responsible for implementing the recommendations of the infection prevention and control team on a day-to-day basis. This involves liaising with staff at all levels and establishing educational programmes, in addition to collecting surveillance data and ensuring that the annual programme is implemented. Some Trusts have established link nurses at ward level to facilitate liaison between the clinical areas and the infection prevention and control team. They have an important role in providing early information to curtail possible outbreaks, and in drawing attention to changes in practice or equipment that may have implications for infection (Teare and Peacock, 1996).

The infection prevention and control committee

An infection prevention and control committee should cover every hospital (see below). Membership should include an infection control doctor and specialist nurse, and a typical committee would include representatives from the following departments/organizations:

- clinical audit and effectiveness
- microbiology department
- Primary Care Trust
- Health Protection Agency
- occupational health department
- pharmacy
- hotel services
- sterile services
- estates
- all directorates
- a medical and surgical consultant and
- the infectious diseases physician if there is one.

A series of subcommittees, such as an outbreaks subcommittee, deal with specific areas.

■ PRACTICE APPLICATION 6.3 ■

Infection Prevention and Control Committee

One function performed by the committee is the ratification of all polices that deal with infection prevention and control.

Activity

➤ Identify the responsibilities and functions of the committee in your workplace/hospital placement.

➤ Which departments in the hospital and which community organizations are represented on the committee?

Infection control policies, guidelines and standards

In England, the Department of Health and other agencies, such as the National Patient Safety Agency, publish a range of policy documents on issues related to HCAI. These take the form of reports, safety bulletins, codes of practice and health notices sent as recommendations. Guidance is sought from experts including medical microbiologists, specialist nurses and pharmacists before publication and in response to specific enquiries from manufacturers. The information is implemented locally according to requirements. The key elements of an effective infection control policy are outlined below.

INFORMATION BOX 6.3

Key elements of an effective infection control policy

To be effective, a policy must fulfil the following criteria, as identified by Simpson (1991):

➤ The objectives should be clearly expressed

➤ The information should be easy to understand

➤ The information should be easy to find (for example with adequate cross-referencing when necessary)

➤ The information should be practical, as compliance with complicated, time-consuming procedures will be poor

➤ The necessary equipment must be readily available

SELF-ASSESSMENT

1. Surgical wound infections are the most common HCAI. True? or False?

2. Surveillance of HCAIs is conducted at national level in the UK. True? or False?

3. Explain why MRSA is a particular infection control problem in hospitals.

4. *Staphylococcus epidermidis* is coagulase positive. True? or False?

5. Why is strict antibiotic control so important in preventing the spread of GRE?

6. Coliforms are naturally resistant to many antibiotics. True? or False?

7. List five individuals/departments/organizations typically represented on the infection prevention and control committee.

REFERENCES

Ayton M (1981) An outbreak of streptococcal infection in a children's ward. *Nursing Times* **77**(10): 13–15.

Barrett SP (2004) Debate – guidelines for GRE control – the case for optimism. *Journal of Hospital Infection* **57**(4): 285–9.

Bennett JV and Brachman PS (1979) *Hospital Infections*. Little, Brown, Boston.

Bonten M, Hayden MK, Nathan C et al. (1996) Epidemiology of colonisation of patients and environment with vancomycin-resistant enterococci. *Lancet* **348**: 1615–19.

Burke JP, Ingall D, Klein JO et al. (1971) *Proteus mirabilis* infections in a hospital nursery traced to a human carrier. *New England Journal of Medicine* **284**: 115–21.

Casewell MW (1986) Epidemiology and control of 'modern' methicillin-resistant *Staphylococcus aureus*. *Journal of Hospital Infection* (Supplement A) **7**: 1–11.

Chadwick PR, Chadwick CD and Oppenheim BA (1996) Report of a meeting on the epidemiology and control of glycopeptide-resistant enterococci. *Journal of Hospital Infection* **33**: 89–92.

Coia JE, Duckworth GJ, Edwards DI et al. (2006) for the Joint Working Party of the British Society of Antimicrobial Chemotherapy, the Hospital Infection Society, and the Infection Control Nurses Association. Guidelines for the control and prevention of meticillin-resistant *Staphylococcus aureus* (MRSA) in healthcare facilities. *Journal of Hospital Infection* **63** (Supplement): S1–S44. Available www.his.org.uk/resource_library.cfm.

Cookson BD, Macrae MB, Barrett SP et al. (2006) Guidelines for the control of glycopeptide-resistant enterococci in hospitals. *Journal of Hospital Infection* **62:** 6–21. Available www.his.org.uk/resource_library.cfm.

Cox RA, Mallaghan C, Conquest C et al. (1995) Epidemic methicillin-resistant *Staphylococcus aureus*: controlling the spread outside hospital. *Journal of Hospital Infection* **29**: 107–19.

Daum TE, Schaberg DR, Terpinning MS et al. (1990) Increasing resistance of *Staphylococcus aureus* to ciprofloxacin. *Antimicrobial Agents and Chemotherapy* **34**: 1862–3.

Davies HD, McGeer A, Schwartz B et al. (1996) Invasive group A streptococcal infections in Ontario, Canada. *New England Journal of Medicine* **335**: 547–54.

Department of Health (DH) (2003) *Winning Ways: Working Together to Reduce Healthcare Associated Infection in England* (Chief Medical Officer). DH, London. Available www.dh.gov.uk.

Department of Health (DH) (2006) *The Health Act 2006: Code of Practice for the Prevention and Control of Healthcare-associated Infections*. DH, London. Available www.dh.gov.uk.

Department of Health (DH) (2007) *Saving Lives: Reducing Infection, Delivering Clean and Safe Care*. DH, London. Available www.dh.gov.uk.

Department of Health/Public Health Laboratory Service (DH/PHLS) (1995) *Hospital Infection Control: Guidance on the Control of Infection in Hospitals*. DH/PHLS, London.

Department of Health and Social Security (DHSS) (1988) *Hospital Infection Control. Guidance on the Control of Infection in Hospitals Prepared by the Joint DHSS/PHLS Hospital Infection Working Group* (Cooke Report). HMSO, London.

Emmerson AM, Enstone JE, Griffin M et al. (1996) The second National Prevalence Survey of Infection in Hospitals – overview of the results. *Journal of Hospital Infection* **32**: 175–90.

French GL (1993) Closing the loop: audit in infection control. *Journal of Hospital Infection* **24**: 301–8.

French GL, Cheng AF, Ling JL et al. (1990) Hong Kong strains of methicillin-resistant and methicillin-sensitive *Staphylococcus aureus* have similar virulence. *Journal of Hospital Infection* **15**: 117–25.

Garland SM, Mackay S, Tabrizi S et al. (1996) Pseudomonas outbreak associated with a contaminated blood gas analyser in a neonatal intensive care unit. *Journal of Hospital Infection* **33**: 145–51.

Glover S (1992) *Making Medical Audit more Effective.* Joint Centre for Education in Medicine, London.

Gray JW and George RH (2000) Experience of vancomycin-resistant enterococci in a children's hospital. *Journal of Hospital Infection* **45**: 11–18.

Haley RW, Cuylver DH and White JW (1985) The efficacy of infection surveillance and control programs in preventing nosocomial infection in US hospitals. *American Journal of Epidemiology* **121**: 182–205.

Harmory BH and Parisi JT (1987) *Staphylococcus epidermidis*: a significant nosocomial pathogen. *Journal of Hospital Infection* **15**: 59–74.

Hay A (2006) Audit in infection control. *Journal of Hospital Infection* **62**: 270–9.

Health Protection Agency (HPA) (2004) A third case of vancomycin-resistant MRSA in the United States. *CDR Weekly* **14**(18). Available http://www.hpa.org.uk/cdr/archives/archive04/news/news1804.htm.

Health Protection Agency (HPA) (2007a) *Surveillance of Healthcare Associated Infections Report.* Available www.hpa.org.uk/.

Health Protection Agency (2007b) *National Confidential Study of Deaths Following Meticillin Resistant* Staphylococcus aureus *(MRSA) Infection.* Available www.hpa.org.uk/.

Hospital Infection Society/Infection Control Nurses Association (HIS/ICNA) (2007) *Summary of Preliminary Results of The Third Prevalence Survey of Healthcare Associated Infections in Acute Hospitals* (for England) (2006). Available www.his.org.uk/.

Humphreys H (2006) Implementing guidelines for the control and prevention of meticillin-resistant *Staphylococcus aureus* and vancomycin-resistant enterococci: how valid are international comparisons? *Journal of Hospital Infection* **62**: 133–5.

Livornese LL, Dias S, Samel C et al. (1992) Hospital-acquired infection with vancomycin-resistant *Enterococcus faecium* transmitted by electronic thermometers. *Annals of Internal Medicine* **117**: 112–16.

Marples RR and Reith S (1992) Methicillin-resistant *Staphylococcus aureus* in England and Wales. *Communicable Disease Report* **2**(3): R25–R29.

Marples RR, Richardson JF, de Saxe MJ (1985) Bacteriological characters of strains of *Staphylococcus aureus* submitted to a reference laboratory related to methicillin-resistance. *Journal of Hygiene* **96**: 217–23.

Martin de Nicolas MM, Vindel A and Saez-Nieto JA (1995) Epidemiological typing of clinically significant strains of coagulase-negative staphylococci. *Journal of Hospital Infection* **29**: 35–43.

Meers PD, Ayliffe GA, Emmerson AM et al. (1981) Report of the National Survey of Infection in Hospitals. *Journal of Hospital Infection* **2**: 23–8.

Millward S, Barnett J and Thomlinson DA (1993) Clinical infection audit programme: evaluation of an audit tool used by infection control nurses to monitor standards and assess staff training. *Journal of Hospital Infection* **24**: 219–32.

Montgomerie JZ and Morrow JW (1980) Long-term pseudomonas colonisation in spinal injury patients. *American Journal of Epidemiology* **112**: 508–17.

Noskin GA, Stosor V, Cooper I et al. (1995) Recovery of vanocomycin-resistant enterococci on finger tips and environmental surfaces. *Infection Control and Hospital Epidemiology* **16**: 577–81.

Patel S (2007) Managing MRSA in hospital and in the community. *Nursing Times* **103**(10): 48–9.

Plowman R, Graves N, Griffin MA et al. (2001) The rate and cost of hospital-acquired infections occurring in patients admitted to selected specialities of a district general hospital in England and the national burden imposed. *Journal of Hospital Infection* **47**(3): 198–209.

Price MF, Dao-Tran T, Garey KW et al. (2007) Epidemiology and incidence of *Clostridium difficile*-associated diarrhoea diagnosed upon admission to a university hospital. *Journal of Hospital Infection* **65**: 42–6.

Report of a combined working party of the British Society for Antimicrobial Chemotherapy and the Hospital Infection Society (1995) Guidelines on the control of methicillin-resistant *Staphylococcus aureus* in the community. *Journal of Hospital Infection* **31**(1): 1–12.

Roghmann M, Qaiyumi S, Johnson JA et al. (1997) Recurrent vanocomycin-resistant *Enterococcus faecium* bacteraemia in a leukaemia patient who was persistently colonized with vanocomycin-resistant enteococci for two years. *Clinical Infectious Diseases* **24**: 514–15.

Royal College of Nursing (RCN) (1994) *Guidelines on Infection Control in Hospital.* RCN, London.

Sanderson PJ and Weissler S (1992) Recovery of coliforms from the hands of nurses and patients: activities leading to contamination. *Journal of Hospital Infection* **21**: 85–93.

Sarangi J and Rowsell R (1995) A nursing home outbreak of Group A streptococcal infection: case control study of environmental contamination. *Journal of Hospital Infection* **30**: 162–4.

Simpson RA (1991) Using guidelines, policies and standards. Are we in control? *Journal of Hospital Infection* (Supplement A) **18**: 99–105.

Starr J (2005) *Clostridium difficile*-associated disease diarrhoea: diagnosis and treatment. *British Medical Journal* **331**: 498–501.

Swiatlo E, Kocka C, Chittom AL et al. (1987) Survey of multiply resistant *Providenti stuartii* in a chronic care unit. *Journal of Hospital Infection* **9**: 182–90.

Sud H and Gorman J (2007) A nurse-led initiative to reduce levels of HCAIs in hospital. *Nursing Times* **103**(14): 30–1.

Teare EL and Peacock A (1996) The development of an infection control link-nurse programme in a district general hospital. *Journal of Hospital Infection* **34**: 267–78.

Tenover FC, Weigel LM, Appelbaum PC et al. (2004) Vancomycin-resistant *Staphylococcus aureus* isolate from a patient in Pennsylvania. *Antimicrobial Agents and Chemotherapy* **48**: 275–80.

Weber DJ and Rutala WA (1997) Role of environmental contamination in the transmission of vancomycin-resistant entrerococci. *Infection Control and Hospital Epidemiology* **18**: 306–9.

Wertheim HF, Vos MC and Boelens HA (2004) Low prevalence of methicillin-resistant *Staphylococcus aureus* (MRSA) at hospital admission in the Netherlands: the value of search and destroy and restrictive antibiotic use. *Journal of Hospital Infection* **56:** 321–5.

▓▓▓▓▓▓▓ FURTHER READING AND INFORMATION SOURCES ▓▓▓▓▓▓

Department of Health (DH) (2006) *Infection Control Guidance for Care Homes.* DH, London. Available www.dh.gov.uk.

Department of Health (DH) (2007) *Clean, Safe Care: Reducing MRSA and other Healthcare-associated Infections. A National Update.* DH, London. Available www.dh.gov.uk.

Infection Control Nurses' Association/Royal College of Nursing (ICNA/RCN) (2003) *Infection Control Guidance for General Practice.* ICNA, Bathgate.

Infection Protection Society incorporating Infection Control Nurses' Association – www.ips.uk.net.

National Institute for Health and Clinical Excellence (NICE) (2003) *Infection Control, Prevention of Healthcare-associated Infection in Primary and Community Care.* Clinical guideline 2. NICE, London. Available www.nice.org.uk/.

National Patient Safety Agency (NPSA) (2004) *Clean hands help to save lives.* Patient safety alert No. 4. NPSA, London. Available www.npsa.nhs.uk/.

NHS Estates (2004) *The NHS Healthcare Cleaning Manual.* DH, London.

Nye KJ, Leggatt VA and Watterson L (2005) Provision and decontamination of uniforms in the NHS. *Nursing Standard* **19**(33): 41–5.

Pellowe CM, Pratt RJ, Harper P et al. (2003) Evidence-based guidelines for preventing healthcare-associated infections in primary and community care in England. *Journal of Hospital Infection* **55** (Supplement 2): S2–127.

Pratt RJ, Pellowe CM, Wilson JA et al. (2007) epic2: National evidence-based guidelines for preventing healthcare-associated infections in NHS hospitals in England. *Journal of Hospital Infection* **65** (Supplement 1): S1–S64. Available www.epic.tvu.ac.uk.

Royal College of Nursing (RCN) (2005) *Good Practice in Infection Prevention and Control: Guidance for Nursing Staff.* RCN, London.

PART III

Applying Knowledge to Practice

PART III

CHAPTER 7

Urinary infection and catheterization

CHAPTER OUTCOMES

After reading this chapter, you should be able to:

➤ Define the terms 'bacteriuria', 'biofilm' and 'encrustation' and explain how these occur

➤ State the usual reasons for urinary catheterization and justify why they are necessary in particular circumstances

➤ Suggest feasible alternatives to urinary catheterization

➤ List the organisms commonly responsible for urinary infection

➤ State the complications associated with urinary catheterization and urinary infection, explain how they arise and make recommendations for clinical practice

➤ Describe different methods for auditing the management of people who have indwelling urinary catheters

Introduction: urinary infection and catheterization

Urinary infection accounts for 19.7 per cent of all HCAIs in acute hospitals and, to understand the relative importance of urinary infection, it should be remembered that surgical site infection (wound infection), which receives substantial publicity, represents 13.8 per cent of HCAIs (Hospital Infection Society/Infection Control Nurses Association, 2007). Urinary infection is usually associated with catheterization (catheter-associated urinary tract infection – CAUTI), especially long-term catheterization of people in nursing homes (Pellowe and Pratt, 2004). Apart from the considerable discomfort to patients/residents and the cost implications, urinary infection can cause serious side-effects, including septicaemia and death.

The use of urinary catheters

A high proportion of patients/residents will have catheters. Urinary catheterization may be:

■ Short term (1–7 days)

■ Medium term (8–28 days)

■ Long term (more than 28 days)

■ Intermittently to relieve urinary retention in the person with an atonic bladder or paraplegia. Self-catheterization, as a clean procedure, is often performed by this client group, both in hospital and at home.

The average length of time for a catheter to remain in situ during short-term hospital use is 4 days (Crow et al., 1986). Four per cent of patients nursed at home use catheters (Roe, 1989), the average period of catheterization for this client group being 4 years, although catheterization for up to 17 years has been recorded (Roe and Brocklehurst, 1987).

Urinary tract infection (UTI) and urinary catheterization

Infection arising from urethral catheterization represents a considerable nursing challenge. Infection is a major complication, significant because of its frequency and the seriousness of associated side-effects.

Urinary infection may result from a small inoculum of bacteria since the bladder has little defence against invading pathogens (Stickler and Chawla, 1987). Risk is increased by the presence of an indwelling urethral catheter because it operates as a foreign body, interfering with the normal process of the flushing effect that eliminates bacteria from the healthy bladder (Falkiner, 1993). Infections related to urinary catheterization represent the most frequent and intractable infection control problem in hospital, likely to increase as the population ages. The bacterial strains responsible are frequently antibiotic resistant. The move towards community care will not necessarily reduce the emergence of antibiotic resistance, as many people nursed at home and in other community settings require intermittent admission to undergo particular procedures, exposing them to hospital pathogens.

The risk of CAUTI is greatest for those with severe underlying illness and increases with the length of use. Up to half of all catheterized patients develop bacteriuria (the presence of bacteria in the urine), 100,000 pathogens in 1 ml of freshly voided urine representing an infection (Trilla et al., 1991). CAUTI contributes directly to further morbidity and may result in mortality. Bacteraemia (the presence of bacteria in the blood) may develop and in some cases this is fatal. The best way to prevent urinary infection is to avoid catheterization (see below) or, if it is inevitable, to remove the catheter as soon as possible. Regular reviews of the need for a urinary catheter avoid its unnecessary use (Saint et al., 2005). In a university hospital, daily reminders by nurses to doctors to remove unnecessary catheters significantly reduced the length of time the catheter was in place in two out of the five areas studied (Crouzet et al., 2007).

INFORMATION BOX 7.1

Alternatives to indwelling urinary catheters

Possible alternatives include:

➤   condom drainage systems

➤   incontinence aids and garments

➤   intermittent catheterization.

A careful assessment of individual patient/client need, coupled with a choice of appropriate equipment from the wide range now commercially available, enhances the quality of care. Such alternatives may not, however, necessarily be associated with a reduction in infection rates; in patients with spinal cord injuries, colonization by Gram-negative bacteria of various body sites and UTI may still occur with condom drainage systems (Montgomerie and Morrow, 1978).

Organisms responsible for urinary infection

Organisms responsible for urinary infection are mainly Gram-negative bacilli such as *Escherichia coli* (*E. coli*), *Klebsiella* and *Proteus*, but some Gram-positive organisms may also be responsible, for example *Staphylococcus epidermidis*, *Staphylococcus aureus* and *Enterococcus faecalis*. Although the extended-spectrum beta-lactamase (ESBL)-producing *E. coli* can cause UTI, it is only rarely responsible for simple cystitis (inflammation of the bladder) (Health Protection Agency, 2007).

The ability to attach to the mucosa of the urinary tract enhances virulence. Most *E. coli* urinary infections are caused by a few serotypes carrying a particular surface antigen (antigen K), which appears to offer protection against phagocytes. Certain strains of *Proteus* are particularly successful as urinary pathogens because pili enable them to attach to the host's epithelium. They are thus less easily dislodged, ascend the ureters and cause acute pyelonephritis (inflammation of the renal pelvis and functional part of the kidney). In future, it may be possible to avoid infection by reducing their adherence to the bladder epithelium. Cranberry juice reduces adherence (Beachy, 1981; Sobota, 1984), but further controlled trials are needed to test its effectiveness in preventing infection. The success of *Staphylococcus epidermidis* as a urinary pathogen is related to its ability to adhere to plastic surfaces (Pascual et al., 1993).

Some bacteria which contaminate urine float freely in suspension. Others adhere to surfaces, where they deposit extracellular secretions forming a 'biofilm' (a layer of microorganisms and proteins) on the sides of the catheter and drainage apparatus (Mulhall, 1991). This eventually forms a glycocalyx (protein and sugar coating), which becomes cemented into position, contributing to the problem of encrustation.

Complications secondary to CAUTI

The complications that are secondary to CAUTI include:

■ Encrustation

- Blockage
- Leakage
- Pain and discomfort.

All the above are related to infection and to each other.

Encrustation

Encrustation affects 16–28 per cent of people with a urinary catheter. Bacteria collecting on the surfaces of the catheter and drainage apparatus secrete extracellular products to form a biofilm (Mulhall et al., 1993). Surfaces in direct contact with the urethral and bladder epithelia are protected by a mucus layer that prevents the deposits of adherence (Kunin et al., 1987). Encrustations consist of calcium and magnesium salts precipitated as large crystals and smaller, powdery deposits. Infection with *Proteus* is particularly likely to cause encrustation because members of this genus secrete an enzyme, urease, that acts on urea to produce ammonium ions (electrically charged particles). The resulting highly alkaline urine favours the formation of insoluble salts, which precipitate from solution.

Blockage

Blockages develop when mineral salts occlude the eyes of the catheter as the sequel to encrustation (see below).

PRACTICE APPLICATION 7.1

Managing Catheter Blockage

Catheter blockage is a common occurrence in 40–50 per cent of people who are catheterized long term (Getliffe, 2003a). It is possible to identify those at risk of recurrent catheter blockage. The results of a prospective longitudinal study with 47 catheterized patients nursed in the community provided firm evidence that catheter blockage was strongly related to leakage and urinary retention, but not to the length of time the catheter had been in situ, fluid intake or the type of drainage bag employed. The 18 patients for whom blockage was a problem had a higher urinary pH than others in the sample and showed a higher concentration of ammonium ions. These characteristics could be used to identify patients more likely to develop a blocked catheter, thus enabling nurses to plan care rather than resorting to crisis management, as so often happens (Getliffe, 1994).

Activity

➤ Access the article by Getliffe (2003a) cited above. Consider the proactive approaches suggested by the author.

➤ Search the literature for research on catheter maintenance solutions and discuss the findings with your mentor or lecturer.

Leakage

Leakage around the outside of the catheter follows blockage.

Pain and discomfort

Pain and discomfort are experienced if rigid or irritant catheters remain in the bladder. If a leaking catheter is replaced with a larger one, the problem is exacerbated and discomfort increases.

The closed urinary drainage system

The earliest indwelling catheters emptied into glass-stoppered bottles. Dukes introduced the closed system of drainage in 1928, but its value in preventing infection was not appreciated until the 1960s, when two independent teams established that it could reduce the development of sepsis from 80 per cent to 10 per cent (Gillespie, 1960; Sandford, 1964).

Portals of entry

The term 'closed drainage' is, however, not strictly accurate as there are numerous portals of entry for pathogens (Figure 7.1) and the system must be opened to allow emptying and be disconnected when the drainage bag is changed.

There is some debate concerning the source of pathogens responsible for CAUTI. Possible routes are indicated below, but there is disagreement over the most important. According to one school of thought, migration from the contaminated bag constitutes a major factor (Maizels and Shaeffer, 1980), contamination of the catheter from the drainage bag occurring within 24 hours (Rogers et al., 1996). Another view holds that access via the periurethral space (that between the walls of the catheter and the urethra) is of greater importance (Garibaldi et al., 1980). A resolution of this debate would be welcome in view of the associated clinical implications. Endemic and epidemic infections have been associated with contamination of the environment and nurses' hands

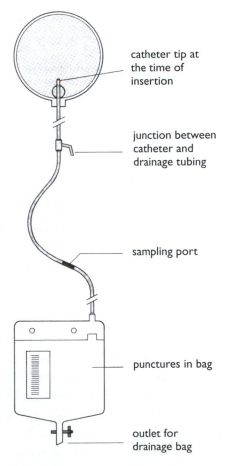

catheter tip at the time of insertion

junction between catheter and drainage tubing

sampling port

punctures in bag

outlet for drainage bag

Figure 7.1 The 'closed system' of catheter drainage: portals of entry

by bacteria of the same strain (Sanderson and Weissler, 1992). This does not, however, prove that they are exogenously (from outside) acquired: organisms from the perianal (around the anus) region may first contaminate the immediate patient/ resident environment, colonize the hands of patients/residents and healthcare workers, and then gain access to the bladder when the catheter is manipulated. Whatever the source, a strict regimen of hand hygiene on the part of both patient/ resident and healthcare workers is necessary before and after the system is handled.

INFORMATION BOX 7.2

Access of pathogens to the 'closed system' of drainage

Pathogens can gain access to the closed system of drainage by the following routes:

➤ On the catheter tip during insertion

➤ During disconnection of drainage bag and tubing (accidental or planned change)

➤ By migrating along the lumen of the catheter from a contaminated drainage system

➤ By migration via the periurethral space in the film of moisture between the outside of the catheter and the urethra

---

Recommendations for clinical practice: reducing the problems of catheterization

Recommendations for clinical practice are possible, although some questions remain unanswered and more research is needed (Getliffe, 2003b). Avoiding the use of catheters, considering the aspects outlined below and removing a catheter as soon as it is no longer necessary are vital in maintaining patient/resident safety and reducing the risk of CAUTI.

▬ PRACTICE APPLICATION 7.2 ▬

Summary Checklist for Safer Catheterization

The decisions taken by healthcare staff prior to inserting a urinary catheter can have far-reaching consequences for the patient/resident. Making the correct choices can reduce the incidence of catheter-related complications, especially infection.

Checklist

➤ Does the person really need a urinary catheter or is there a viable alternative?

➤ Does the person possess sufficient information to understand the need for urinary catheterization and give valid consent (see below)?

➤ Do I need to consult another professional?

➤ Choose a catheter of the correct gauge.

➤ Choose a catheter of the correct length for gender and age.

➤ Choose the most appropriate catheter material for the length of time the person is likely to be catheterized and for particular personal characteristics.

➤ For adults, choose an indwelling catheter with a 10 ml balloon for routine use.

➤ Choose the most appropriate bag and drainage system.

➤ Use aseptic technique with sterile gloves for catheter insertion.

➤ Instill anaesthetic lubricating gel into the urethra prior to catheterization.

➤ Choose non-irritant solutions, for example sterile normal saline, for cleansing around the urinary meatus.

➤ Ask again whether catheterization is the only option for this person.

➤ Ensure that a record of catheterization is made, the reason for its insertion and include a reminder for staff to review the continuing need for a urinary catheter; thus avoiding the unnecessary use of a catheter (Saint et al., 2005).

Patient/resident education

It is important that patients/residents and carers understand why catheterization is needed and are provided with sufficient knowledge about catheter care (see below).

INFORMATION BOX 7.3

Providing education for catheter care

Patient education in relation to catheter care has traditionally been poor (Roe and Brocklehurst, 1987). In an experimental study, subjects receiving an educational intervention and an information booklet proved more knowledgeable about the function of the catheter and its associated risks as well as demonstrating better handwashing performance, although this was not sustained over time (Roe, 1989). The author concluded that it is worth educating patients about their catheters, teaching should begin as soon as the need for catheterization is apparent and it should be reinforced at regular intervals.

Choice of catheter material

Many catheters are made of plastic or latex. These substances are inexpensive but not suitable for long-term indwelling catheters because they are particularly irritant (Belfield, 1988). In addition, latex allergy is an increasing problem in both staff and patients/residents (Chapter 2).

Teflon, silicone, silicone–Teflon combinations, elastomers and hydrogels are newer, more suitable materials, their smooth finish being less likely to result in encrustation or irritation (Cox et al., 1988). Catheters with novel coatings such as silver alloy or antibiotics are also available (see Further Reading). Long-term catheterization is common in community settings and making the correct choice about the type of catheter is important. However, a recent Cochrane Review concluded that the evidence was not sufficient because few trials existed and these were small, and that better quality trials are required to provide evidence about which catheters were best for particular patients (Jahn et al., 2007).

Some people are more likely to develop encrustations than others, suggesting that the formation of deposits is not simply a reaction between alkaline urine and the catheter. It is possible to identify patients particularly at risk of developing encrustations (Kunin et al., 1987) and to plan their care accordingly. There is a difference in infection rates associated between silicone and latex catheters (Pellowe and Pratt, 2004).

Catheter length

The length of the urethra should determine catheter length. The standard catheter length for males is 40 cm. For females, in whom the urethra is shorter, the standard catheter length is 25 cm. Women should not be given male-length catheters because this increases the risk of kinking and dragging, leading to accidental disconnection. An excessively long catheter is also more difficult to conceal beneath clothing if the individual is mobile. Infants and small children need smaller catheters depending on their age and size.

Catheter gauge

Catheter gauge is measured using a unit called a Charrière (Ch), 1 Ch measuring 0.33 mm. The optimal gauge is 12–14 Ch for males and 10–12 Ch for females. Larger gauges are not usually justified because a 12 Ch catheter is capable of draining 100 l of fluid over 24 hours, a capacity far greater than the actual requirement. Larger dimensions are necessary only when problems are anticipated. For example, experience may show that particular patients produce urine containing considerable amounts of debris, and these may fare better with a larger catheter. Following prostate surgery, an irrigation catheter or a larger gauge catheter (18–30 Ch) is essential to drain blood clots. There is no justification for fitting a larger gauge catheter than that required: it will irritate the urethral mucosa, promoting bypassing and leakage, and will be painful (Crow et al., 1986).

Balloon size

Balloons on self-retaining catheters are available in two standard sizes, 10 ml and 30 ml, with smaller (for example for infants and children) and larger ones intended for special purposes. A larger size might be required for a woman with weak pelvic muscles catheterized in the long term, or to prevent bleeding from the prostate bed following surgery. The 10 ml size is recommended for routine use. The catheterized bladder is always fully drained and thus permanently collapsed. A larger balloon would be in greater contact with the bladder wall and would therefore be more likely to cause irritation. Larger balloons induce leakage (Kennedy et al., 1983) and can damage the bladder neck (Steggall, 2007). Balloons should be filled with sterile water because saline may crystallize, blocking the inflation channel. Deflation and removal are then difficult.

Catheter insertion

Insertion should be performed with an aseptic technique using sterile gloves and equipment, sterile local anaesthetic or lubricating gel being used before the catheter is inserted. Recent guidelines recommend the use of sterile normal saline for cleansing the urethral meatus before catheter insertion (Pratt et al., 2007).

Meatal hygiene care

The results of trials involving the use of disinfectants such as chlorhexidine and povidone iodine have produced mixed results (Falkiner, 1993). Meatal hygiene should be daily washing with soap and water (National Institute for Health and Clinical Excellence, 2003). The epic 2: national evidence-based guidelines confirm that routine daily personal hygiene such as showering or bathing is sufficient for meatal care (Pratt et al., 2007).

Management and choice of drainage system

Management and choice of drainage system also merit consideration in view of their possible contribution to infection.

Choice of bag

The following features for the bag are highly desirable:

- A sampling port in the bag tubing to allow the aspiration of specimens without breaking the system. This should be disinfected with an alcohol-impregnated swab before a sample is collected (Nicol et al., 2008).
- The system should have non-return valves and a sufficient length of tubing for the bag to hang free.
- The outlet should never touch the floor and the bag should always be positioned lower than the bladder so that the urine drains under gravity.
- The bag must be supported in order to prevent dragging, which could damage the urethra or bladder.
- A leg bag of the appropriate capacity should be selected if the person is mobile.
- Some people may be able to use a catheter valve in place of drainage bag (National Institute for Health and Clinical Evidence, 2003).

Emptying

Emptying disrupts the closed system of drainage. Frequent emptying is sometimes avoided because it may increase risk of contamination (Crow et al., 1986). A full bag looks unsightly and the contents develop an odour. The decision of when to empty is thus a judgement made according to individual circumstance. Hands and the environment can become contaminated during emptying, so non-sterile gloves and a plastic apron should be worn and the hands should be decontaminated before and afterwards. Cross-infection can be avoided by using a sterile receptacle that is only used once. This may not be possible on the grounds of expense, but disposables provide an acceptable alternative (Roe, 1993).

Bag changes

Bag changes involve disconnection of the closed system and may be avoided to reduce this situation. The Department of Health recommends a change after 5–7 days, a figure supported by research findings (Rogers et al., 1996). Prompt disposal is essential in hospital to prevent cross-infection. Suggestions that bags could be reused in the community may be impractical as people at home may lack the facilities to decontaminate bags adequately, or may be unable to do so through lack of manual dexterity if they are disabled or infirm (Roe, 1993).

Additives to the drainage system

Additives to the drainage system are no longer thought to offer any advantage in preventing infection and are ineffective once infection has become established (Stickler et al., 1987).

Irrigation

Irrigation is essential after a transurethral resection of the prostate (TURP) to relieve physical blockage by blood clots and may be necessary for patients catheterized in the long term if encrustations form. It is possible to anticipate problems and employ catheters with three-way taps so that irrigation can be performed without disconnecting the drainage system. Proprietary solutions intended for instillation in order to reduce encrustation are available. Most are weakly acidic and may help by reducing pH, thus decreasing urease activity as well as exerting mechanical action, but their value in controlled trials has yet to be established.

Auditing the use of urinary catheters

Urinary infections were the most common nosocomial infection reported during the second national prevalence survey, occurring in 23 per cent of patients, mainly those with catheters. They were especially common in urosurgical and gynaecology patients over 75 years of age (Emmerson et al., 1996). Urinary infections still account for nearly 20 per cent of HCAIs (Hospital Infection Society/Infection Control Nurses Association, 2007). A study by Crow et al. (1986) revealed that 44 per cent of patients developed significant bacteriuria within 72 hours, this figure rising to 90 per cent 17 days later. Preventing CAUTI is vitally important, and an audit of guidelines has been suggested as one of the ways forward (French, 1993). Process and outcome measures are available (Curran, 1993; see below).

INFORMATION BOX 7.4

Auditing the use of urinary catheters

Process

➤   To determine the incidence of CAUTI

➤   To assess whether the use of indwelling urethral catheters is appropriate

➤ To determine whether the choice of catheter is appropriate (according to research findings)

➤ To determine whether catheter care is appropriate (according to research findings)

➤ To identify catheter-associated procedures that could be avoided if their use were abandoned

➤ To target infection control and other resources to clinical settings with a high incidence of catheter-associated problems

➤ To ensure that healthcare professionals have the knowledge and resources to select, insert and maintain catheters and give appropriate care to patients/residents

Outcome

➤ To reduce the incidence of CAUTI

➤ To reduce patients/residents' discomfort and inconvenience

➤ To reduce costs through the appropriate use of resources

SELF-ASSESSMENT

1. Bacteriuria indicating infection is defined as the presence of 100,000 or more pathogens per ml of urine. True? or False?

2. What is biofilm?

3. Which of the following are true?

   (a) Urinary tract infections are mainly due to Gram-negative organisms
   (b) Both Gram-negative and Gram-positive organisms cause urinary infection
   (c) The bacterium *Escherichia coli* is a common cause of urinary infection
   (d) All of these

4. Catheter blockage commonly affects 40–50 per cent of people who are catheterized long term. True? or False?

5. List the portals of entry for pathogens in the 'closed' urinary drainage system.

6. What are the standard length catheters for men and for women?

REFERENCES

Beachy EH (1981) Bacterial adherence: adhesion receptor interactions mediating the attachment of bacteria to mucosal surfaces. *Journal of Infectious Diseases* **143**: 325–45.

Belfield PW (1988) Urinary catheters. *British Medical Journal* **296**: 836–7.

Cox AJ, Hukins DW and Sutton TM (1988) Comparison of in vitro encrustation on silicone and hydrogel coated latex catheters. *British Journal of Urology* **61**: 156–61.

Crouzet J, Bertrand X, Venier AG et al. (2007) Control of the duration of urinary catheterization: impact on catheter-associated urinary tract infection. *Journal of Hospital Infection* **67**: 253–7.

Crow R, Chapman R, Roe B et al. (1986) *Study of Patients with an Indwelling Urinary Catheter and Related Nursing Practice*. Nursing Practice Research Unit, University of Surrey.

Curran E (1993) A programme to audit the use of urinary catheters. *Journal of Clinical Nursing* **1**: 329–34.

Emmerson AM, Enstone JE, Griffin M et al. (1996) The Second National Prevalence Survey of Infection in Hospitals – overview of the results. *Journal of Hospital Infection* **32**: 175–90.

Falkiner FR (1993) The insertion and management of indwelling urethral catheters – minimising the risk of infection. *Journal of Hospital Infection* **25**: 79–90.

French GL (1993) Closing the loop: audit in infection control. *Journal of Hospital Infection* **24**: 301–8.

Garibaldi RA, Burke JP, Britt A et al. (1980) Meatal colonisation and catheter-associated bacteriuria. *New England Journal of Medicine* **303**: 316–18.

Getliffe K (1994) The characteristics and management of patients with recurrent blockage of long-term urinary catheters. *Journal of Advanced Nursing* **20**: 140–9.

Getliffe K (2003a) Managing recurrent urinary catheter blockage: problems, promises, and practicalities. *Journal of Wound, Ostomy and Continence Nursing* **30**(3): 146–51.

Getliffe K (2003b) How to manage encrustation and blockage of Foley catheters. *Nursing Times* **99**(29): 59–61.

Gillespie WA (1960) The diagnosis, epidemiology and control of urinary tract infection in urology and gynaecology. *Journal of Clinical Pathology* **13**: 187–94.

Health Protection Agency (HPA) (2007) Press Statement *Infections caused by ESBL-producing E. coli*. Available www.hpa.org.uk/.

Hospital Infection Society/Infection Control Nurses Association (HIS/ICNA) (2007) *Summary of Preliminary Results of The Third Prevalence Survey of Healthcare Associated Infections in Acute Hospitals* (for England) (2006). Available www.his.org.uk/.

Jahn P, Preuss M, Kernig A et al. (2007) Types of indwelling urinary catheters for long-term bladder drainage in adults. *Cochrane Database Systematic Review*, CD004997. Available www.cochrane.org/reviews/.

Kennedy AP, Brocklehurst JC and Lye M (1983) Factors related to the problems of long-term catheterisation. *Journal of Advanced Nursing* **8**: 207–12.

Kunin CM, Chin QF and Chambers A (1987) Formation of encrustations on indwelling urinary catheters in the elderly. *Journal of Urology* **138**: 899–902.

Maizels M and Schaeffer AJ (1980) Decreased incidence of bacteriuria associated with instillation of hydrogen peroxide into the urethra catheter drainage bag. *Journal of Urology* **123**: 841–5.

Montgomerie JZ and Morrow JW (1978) Pseudomonas colonisation in patients with spinal cord injury. *American Journal of Epidemiology* **108**: 328–36.

Mulhall A (1991) Biofilms and urethral catheter infections. *Nursing Standard* **5**(18): 26–8.

Mulhall A, King S, Lee K et al. (1993) Maintenance of closed urinary drainage systems: are practitioners more aware of the dangers? *Journal of Clinical Nursing* **2**: 135–40.

National Institute for Health and Clinical Excellence (NICE) (2003) *Infection Control, Prevention of Healthcare-associated Infection in Primary and Community Care*. Clinical guideline 2. NICE, London. Available www.nice.org.uk/.

Nicol M, Bavin C, Cronin P and Rawlings-Anderson K (2008) *Essential Nursing Skills*, 3rd edn. Mosby, Edinburgh.

Pascual A, Ramirez de Arellano E, Martinez-Martinez L et al. (1993) Effect of polyurethane catheters and bacterial biofilms on the in vitro activity of antimicrobials against *Staphylococcus epidermidis. Journal of Hospital Infection* **24**: 211–18.

Pellowe C and Pratt R (2004) Catheter-associated urinary tract infections: primary care. *Nursing Times* **100**(2): 53–4.

Pratt RJ, Pellowe CM, Wilson JA et al. (2007) epic2: National evidence-based guidelines for preventing healthcare-associated infections in NHS hospitals in England. *Journal of Hospital Infection* **65** (Supplement 1): S1–S64. Available www.epic.tvu.ac.uk.

Roe B (1989) Long-term catheter care in the community. *Nursing Times* **85**(36): 43–4.

Roe B (1993) Catheter-associated urinary tract infection: a review. *Journal of Clinical Nursing* **2**: 197–203.

Roe B and Brocklehurst JC (1987) Study of patients with indwelling catheters. *Journal of Advanced Nursing* **12**: 713–18.

Rogers J, Norkett DI, Bracegirdle P et al. (1996) Examination of biofilm formation and risk of infection associated with the use of urinary catheters with leg bags. *Journal of Hospital Infection* **32**: 105–15.

Saint S, Kaufman SR, Thompson M et al. (2005) A reminder reduces urinary catheterization in hospitalized patients. *Joint Commission Journal on Quality and Patient Safety* **31**(8): 455–62.

Sanderson PJ and Weissler S (1992) Recovery of coliforms from the hands of nurses and patients: activities leading to contamination. *Journal of Hospital Infection* **21**: 85–94.

Sandford JP (1964) Hospital acquired urinary tract infection. *Annals of Internal Medicine* **60**: 903–14.

Sobota AE (1984) Inhibition of bacterial adherence by cranberry juice: potential use for urinary tract infections. *Journal of Urology* **131**: 1013–16.

Steggall M (2007) Elimination – urine. In C Brooker and A Waugh (eds) *Foundations of Nursing Practice: Fundamentals of Holistic Care*. Mosby, Edinburgh.

Stickler DJ and Chawla JC (1987) The role of antiseptics in the management of patients with long term indwelling bladder catheters. *Journal of Hospital Infection* **10**: 219–28.

Stickler DJ, Clayton CL and Chawla JC (1987) The resistance of urinary tract pathogens to chlorhexidine bladder washouts. *Journal of Hospital Infection* **10**: 28–39.

Trilla A, Gatell M, Mensa J et al. (1991) Risk factors for nosocomial bacteraemia in a large Spanish teaching hospital: a case control study. *Infection Control and Hospital Epidemiology* **12**: 150–6.

FURTHER READING AND INFORMATION SOURCES

Ha US and Cho YH (2006) Catheter-associated urinary tract infections: new aspects of novel urinary catheters. *International Journal of Antimicrobial Agents* **28**(6): 485–90.

Lindsay D and von Holy A (2006) Bacterial biofilms within the clinical setting: what healthcare professionals should know. *Journal of Hospital Infection* **64**: 313–25.

Robinson J (2004) A practical approach to catheter-associated problems. *Nursing Standard* **18**(3): 38–42.

Tew L, Pomfret I and King D (2005) Infection risks associated with urinary catheters. *Nursing Standard* **20**(7): 55–62.

CHAPTER 8

Wound infections

CHAPTER OUTCOMES

After reading this chapter, you should be able to:

➤ Name the four categories of wound described by the National Research Council (1964) and state their significance when calculating wound infection rates

➤ Describe each of the stages of wound healing/tissue repair

➤ Explain the terms 'collagen', 'fibroblast', 'connective tissue', 'angiogenesis', 'epithelialization' and 'granulation'

➤ Explain what is meant by healing by first (primary) and secondary intention, and primary and secondary wound closure

➤ Discuss the criteria used to determine wound infection

➤ State the factors that contribute to the development of wound infection

➤ Describe the ideal wound healing environment

➤ Debate the role of the aseptic dressing techniques in the treatment of surgical and chronic wounds

Introduction to wounds, healing and wound infection

The ability of tissues to undergo repair depends on the condition of the wound and the general health of the person.

The wound condition (the specific microenvironment), which is influenced by the wound-dressing product, is important. Healing proceeds better in a wound that has been covered as a moist environment encourages cells to multiply and migrate more easily across the wound surface (Winter, 1962) (Figure 8.1). A moist environment promotes healing and, today, it is accepted that dressing products that create this environment should be used. A second important function of the dressing is occlusion: extraneous pathogens are prevented from contaminating the wound while organisms already present are unable to escape, preventing cross-infection. The basic characteristics of the 'ideal' wound dressing are outlined below but it is important to remember that there are many different dressing products that have specific functions depending on the particular wound, for example a specific dressing designed for the stage of wound healing or the amount of exudate produced from the wound and so on.

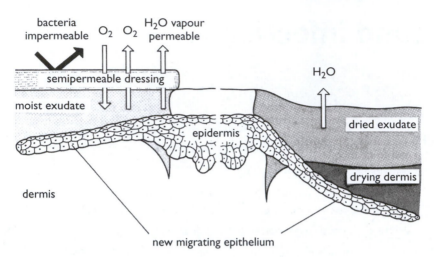

WOUND COVERED   WOUND EXPOSED

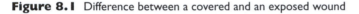

Figure 8.1 Difference between a covered and an exposed wound

INFORMATION BOX 8.1

Basic characteristics of the 'ideal' wound dressing

➤   Absorbs excess exudate and toxins

➤   Maintains a moist environment over the wound surface

➤   Permits gaseous exchange

➤   Presents an occlusive barrier to microorganisms

➤   Provides thermal insulation

➤   Does not contain particulate contaminants

➤   Is non-adherent

The skin is the body's major barrier against invading pathogens; when it is no longer intact, infection becomes a major risk. In the case of surgical wounds, infection usually originates in theatre (Pollock and Evans, 1983). The surfaces of chronic wounds (pressure ulcers and leg ulcers, for example) are frequently covered in microorganisms, some of which are capable of operating as pathogens (Leaper, 1995), but there is no evidence that they interfere with healing in normal circumstances (Brennan et al., 1985). The presence of foreign material is, however, known to slow healing and increase the risk of infection in all types of wound.

The person's general health will influence healing, this includes nutritional status, metabolic disturbance and genetically inherited traits (for example a bleeding disorder). A holistic approach is therefore appropriate in order to promote healing and prevent infection, taking both the above factors into consideration.

Historical aspects of wound care

In the past, the development of sepsis with the formation of pus was considered not only normal, but also desirable. Many different substances were applied to secure it. One of the earliest records from a Mesopotamian clay tablet from 2500 BC advocated the use of honey and resin, which have antiseptic properties. Some people remain enthusiastic about these 'natural' remedies, but the modern approach to wound healing, with its emphasis on occlusion and providing a moist environment, is more effective than folk cures.

During the 16th century, air was considered particularly injurious to healing tissues, so wounds were kept warm, dark and moist until the 1860s, when Lister discovered that applying carbolic spray to surgical dressings reduced infection. His discovery was possible because major advances were made in chemistry throughout the 1800s, notably the isolation of chlorine and iodine, which have disinfectant properties. Through Lister's work and the increasing sophistication of anaesthesia, longer operations became possible, and a higher proportion of patients survived. Today, the care of patients undergoing surgery remains an important nursing responsibility. However, the prevention of surgical sepsis also depends on the patient's general health and the surgeon's skill. The care of patients/residents with chronic wounds such as pressure ulcers and leg ulcers remains a major nursing challenge.

Classifying wounds

Numerous categories of wound classification exist. The amount of tissue lost and the extent of contamination are among those most commonly employed. Both influence the risk of infection.

Amount of tissue lost

There are two categories here:

- A wound in which there is minimal tissue loss (a cut with a knife or a surgical incision) and healing occurs by first or primary intention (see below).
- A wound where extensive tissue is lost and healing is by secondary intention (see below), with more extensive tissue replacement and regeneration (as seen, for example, with pressure ulcers, venous leg ulcers and burns). This type of wound is more often contaminated and heals more slowly so there is greater scope for infection to supervene. In the case of non-surgical wounds, the patient's underlying poor health may have contributed to the development of the lesion in the first place. Poor nutrition and a poorly controlled underlying disease such as diabetes mellitus contribute to poor wound healing (Murphy, 2006). The choice of an appropriate dressing plays a key role in the healing of wounds in this category (Westaby, 1985).

Extent of wound contamination

The system of wound classification was developed by the National Research Council (1964) to allow a direct comparison of infection rates between wounds likely to share similar degrees of contamination (see below). Operations performed at anatomical locations that are normally sterile and those in parts of the body where bacteria are present clearly cannot be expected to show a similar rate of sepsis.

INFORMATION BOX 8.2

Wound classification

➤ **Clean wounds**: no inflammation, no lapse in aseptic technique during surgery and no entry into the respiratory and gastrointestinal tracts. Cholecystectomy, hysterectomy and appendicectomy without evidence of inflammation are placed in the clean category

➤ **Clean contaminated wounds**: those generated by surgical procedures that involve entry into the respiratory or gastrointestinal tract, but where no significant spillage has occurred

➤ **Contaminated wounds**: evidence of acute inflammation without the formation of pus, or where gross spillage has occurred from a hollow internal organ. An otherwise clean operation in which there has been a major breach of aseptic technique and recent traumatic wounds are considered to be contaminated

➤ **Dirty wounds**: pus or a perforated internal organ is encountered. Traumatic wounds not of recent origin are also placed in this category

Source: Adapted from the National Research Council system of wound classification, 1964

Wound healing

The stages of wound healing are outlined below, drawing attention to factors that may influence the development of sepsis. The process of healing is divided into numerous stages for convenience, but in reality they overlap and the process is continuous.

There are two main phases:

■ The **proliferative** phase, when most tissue regeneration takes place
■ The **maturation** phase, when the new tissues become stronger.

A number of proteins called 'growth factors' are important throughout both stages. They enhance wound healing by promoting the development of new blood vessels, attract cells to the wound bed, stimulate cell division and help to regulate the synthesis and breakdown of the extracellular matrix. Wound bed preparation is important to enhance the healing of chronic wounds (Collier, 2003; see below).

■ **PRACTICE APPLICATION 8.1** ■

Wound Bed Preparation
Access the article by Collier (2003).

Activity

➤ Which five factors are important in wound bed preparation?

➤ List the methods of debridement.

➤ Read the section entitled 'Decrease bacterial burden' and then find out which methods are employed in your workplace/placement.

➤ Investigate the effectiveness of topical antimicrobial drugs.

Proliferative phase of wound healing

The proliferative phase (Figures 8.2 and 8.3) encompasses:

■ The inflammatory response

■ Collagen synthesis: tissue regeneration and the replacement of cells lost through trauma

■ Angiogenesis: the formation of new blood vessels

■ Epithelialization: the growth of epithelium over the raw, wounded surface.

Healing by first or primary intention

This type of healing occurs in wounds in which tissue loss is minimal and the wound edges can be brought together, for example with sutures.

The inflammatory response

The inflammatory response continues for approximately three days (see Chapter 2). Heavy contamination (with bacteria or cellular debris) prolongs inflammation and interferes with healing and the cosmetic result. Surgical debridement may be necessary to prevent complications.

Collagen synthesis

Collagen synthesis commences as inflammation subsides and the macrophages responsible for ingesting debris in the wound attract fibroblast cells to the local area. Fibroblasts are connective tissue cells producing collagen, a tough protein that gives strength to skin, bone and tendons. Collagen forms a meshwork to support the granulation tissue that will eventually fill the cleft of the wound. Collagen synthesis reaches a peak between the fifth and seventh postoperative day and proceeds more effectively in moist, occluded wounds. Infection disrupts healing; many pathogens release an enzyme called 'collagenase', which digests collagen fibres, reducing the strength of the new tissue. Collagen synthesis is promoted at low pH in an environment where high concentrations of lactate ions and vitamin C are present. These conditions are most prevalent deep within the tissues, where cells that are still viable undergo metabolism to release lactate. Thus, collagen formation begins deep within the undamaged areas and works outwards.

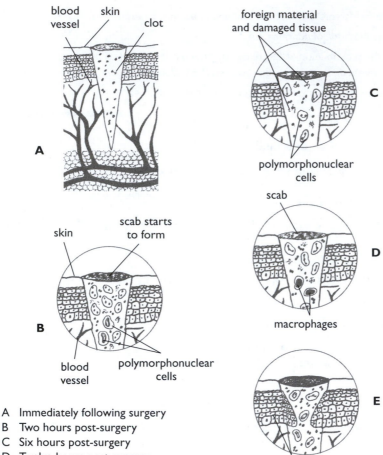

A   Immediately following surgery
B   Two hours post-surgery
C   Six hours post-surgery
D   Twelve hours post-surgery
E   Twenty-four hours post-surgery

Figure 8.2 Hour-by-hour view of the wound healing process I

Source: Adapted from Westaby, 1985

Angiogenesis

Angiogenesis commences deep in the tissues, just as collagen formation is occurring. New capillaries are stimulated by low oxygen tension to grow from the healthy margins of the wound and invade the area of regeneration.

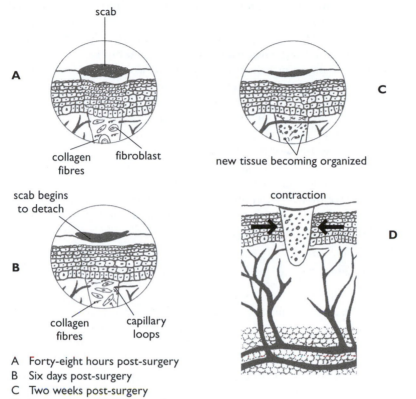

A Forty-eight hours post-surgery
B Six days post-surgery
C Two weeks post-surgery
D Later, contraction reduces the
   area of the wound, with tissue loss

Figure 8.3 Hour-by-hour view of the wound healing process II
Source: Adapted from Westaby, 1985

Epithelialization

Epithelialization commences within 24 hours in a clean wound with minimal tissue loss. Healthy epidermal cells at the edges of the wound multiply and then move in a sheet across the surface until the raw area is completely covered by a new, intact layer, several cells thick (Figure 8.3). In dry wounds, new epithelial cells cannot migrate as effectively as they would in a moist environment because their progress is impeded by collagen fibres attaching the hard scab to the underlying dermis. Where the cells meet at the middle of the damaged area, further movement is inhibited. Once epithelialization is complete, a protein called 'keratin' is deposited in skin cells, making them tough and waterproof. Cells lining the sebaceous glands and hair follicles present in the skin also multiply and migrate first upwards and then over the wound surface, contributing to epithelialization. Severely damaged tissues (such as full-thickness burns) take longer to undergo epithelialization because the sebaceous glands and hair follicles are lost: skin grafting may be necessary.

Epithelial cells retain the ability to multiply throughout the life of the individual because they are undifferentiated (that is, they have not undergone specialization). Highly differentiated tissues (for example neurones and muscle cells) are unable to multiply after embryonic life, and when irrevocably damaged can be replaced only by non-functional scar tissue. Epithelialization seals the wound from pathogenic invasion, but the new cells are delicate so the tissue must be handled gently. The epithelialization of a clean surgical wound is generally complete by the third post-operative day; this is why dressings applied in the operating theatre are usually kept intact until this time. Once an intact layer of cells has formed, the protective scab from the blood clot previously covering the damaged area is able to slough away. At one time, it was common to swab clean wounds with normal saline or other solutions. This practice is now discouraged, being a waste of time and resources. Unnecessary interference may also traumatize the fragile new tissue and increases the possibility of contamination. A scab visible over a wound is indicative of under-lying repair and should not be removed.

Healing by secondary intention

Healing by secondary intention occurs when there has been greater tissue loss and more granulation tissue is needed to occupy the resulting space. Wounds that heal by secondary intention include pressure ulcers and some traumatic wounds where it is neither desirable nor possible to bring the wound edges together. Healthy granulation tissue, which is moist and red, forms in the wound bed. Healing occurs mainly by contraction effected by specialized cells in the granulation tissue called 'myofibroblasts'; epithelialization is of less importance than in lesions where tissue loss has been slight (Leaper, 1995). Tissue repair is often prolonged, with repeated episodes of inflammation, fibroblast activity, excessive formation of collagen and renewed damage. Scarring can be pronounced because of the formation of excess granulation tissue. However, scarring from exuberant granulation can occur in poorly managed surgical wounds, and there may be hypertrophy in chronic or surgical wounds that have become infected: the inflammatory response is prolonged and necrotic tissue, foreign bodies or excess suture material may be retained.

Phase of maturation of wound healing

The signs and symptoms of inflammation gradually subside during the proliferative phase of healing in surgical and properly managed non-surgical lesions, but the wound retains its red, raised appearance and may feel itchy for several months. The collagen fibres are haphazardly arranged. Throughout the phase of maturation, which may take up to a year, they realign at right angles to the direction of wound-ing. This laces the edges together in a tight three-dimensional weave. As maturation progresses, the wound becomes less vascular, the fibroblasts shrink and the tissue becomes stronger, although this varies between tissues of different types. Intestinal anastomoses may regain the strength of the original tissue within seven days. Skin and fascia slowly regain strength.

Surgical intervention and approaches to wound repair

Minor wounds heal spontaneously. When damage is more extensive, surgical intervention is required to speed tissue repair, avoid infection and help to reduce deformity. The approach chosen will depend on the amount of tissue lost. The edges of a clean wound can be sutured together if there has been minimal tissue loss. When extensive areas of tissue have been removed, plastic surgery is necessary, employing flaps or skin grafts. The method of closure is dictated by the estimated risk of infection. Experience with traumatic wounds sustained during warfare has illustrated the dangers associated with the immediate closure of heavily contaminated wounds: abscess formation, septicaemia and dehiscence (bursting or splitting open). Three approaches to wound repair are possible (Figure 8.4):

- Primary closure
- Delayed primary closure
- Secondary intention.

Primary closure

Primary closure is appropriate for clean wounds, clean contaminated wounds and traumatic wounds where thorough debridement has been possible.

Delayed primary closure

Delayed primary closure is the method of choice for large, heavily contaminated wounds, usually traumatic in origin (Whiteside and Moorhead, 1994). The wound is left open or loosely packed and covered with a sterile, non-adherent dressing. Suturing or grafting is not undertaken until 4–5 days after injury, when the development of infection appears to be reduced. By this stage, the inflammatory response is well developed and may boost the immune reaction.

Mechanical cleansing is necessary to remove debris from heavily contaminated wounds (for example traumatic wounds or infected joints after orthopaedic surgery) and helps to reduce the risks of infection in acute wounds (Towler, 2001). It may be undertaken in theatre before the tissues are closed or be performed in conjunction with delayed wound closure. A stream of sterile irrigating fluid is driven across the surface by hydrostatic pressure to remove contaminants physically. The high pressure of the fluid required to maintain continuous irrigation may be damaging, so intermittent irrigation via a syringe, with frequent dressing changes, may be used instead.

Secondary intention approach

In the secondary intention approach, the wound is allowed to close through contraction, granulation and epithelialization. Granulation occurs upwards from the base until the cavity is filled. It is appropriate to allow healing by secondary intention when there has been considerable tissue loss. It is also appropriate for superficial burns and donor sites where skin has been lost over a wide surface area but the wound is not deep. Disadvantages of this method include scarring, contracture and distortion. These effects are most marked around bones and joints where the tissues become constricted during movement.

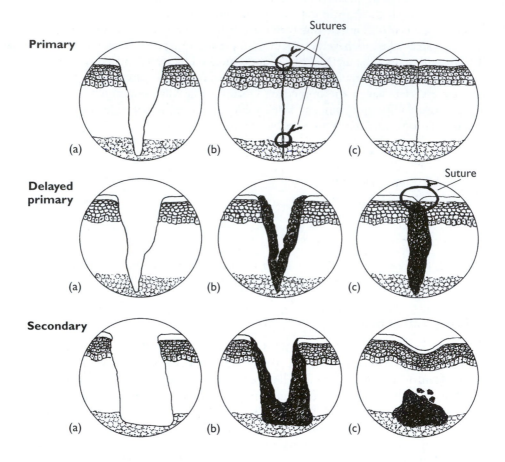

Figure 8.4 Approaches to wound repair

Source: Adapted from Westaby, 1985

Wound (surgical site) infection

Wound infection occurs when the number and activity of bacteria present in the wound overwhelm the immune system. This results in wound breakdown and delayed healing (Murphy, 2006). As with any healthcare-associated infection, wound infection adds to the cost of personal and health care, interferes with recovery, detracts from quality of life and in severe cases contributes to mortality. In the past, surgical wound infection contributed directly to the length of hospitalization (Coello et al., 1993), but this is becoming less likely as people are discharged into the care of community nurses. The effect may be to reduce the hotel costs associated with hospital stay, but it will not diminish the expense of staff time, dressings or antibiotics.

The first major research study to examine the surgical wound infection rate was carried out by Cruse and Foord (1973) in Canada. The incidence of surgical wound sepsis was determined prospectively in an 850-bed hospital over a period of five years. A follow-up study has since been published (Cruse and Foord, 1980). All wounds were examined daily until the twenty-eighth postoperative day, excluding patients with burns and those who had undergone gynaecological, rectal and oral procedures. Initially, 23,649 wounds were examined, of which 1,124 became infected, which gave an overall sepsis rate of 4.8 per cent. However, rates differed according to wound category, dirty wounds being over 20 times more likely to become infected (Table 8.1).

Table 8.1 Infection rates for different wound categories

Type of wound	Percentage
Clean	1.8
Clean contaminated	8.9
Contaminated	21.5
Dirty	28.3

Source: Cruse and Foord, 1973

Overall, the results suggest that surgical wound infection is most closely associated with the type of procedure undertaken. This is substantiated by more recent research (Coello et al., 2005). Standards are best judged according to the rates obtained for clean wounds, the development of sepsis then being independent of extraneous factors such as the degree of contamination and the presence of necrotic tissue. Most hospital infection prevention and control teams today would consider a clean wound infection rate of 1 per cent to be exemplary, 1–2 per cent to be acceptable and a higher level to be indicative that investigation should be undertaken to review and improve current practice. Surgery is increasingly being performed on a daycare basis, and unless special provision is made to follow up patients in the community, infection may not be reported. In areas where purchasers demand this type of information before placing contracts, initiatives to follow patients up at home are being instituted (Holmes and Readman, 1994).

In the 1993–94 second national prevalence survey, wound infections accounted for 10.7 per cent of all nosocomial (hospital-acquired) infections. They were less common than urinary or lower respiratory tract infections (Emmerson et al., 1996). The organisms responsible are shown in Table 8.2. The third national prevalence survey conducted in 2006 found that surgical site infection accounted for 13.8 per cent of HCAIs in acute hospitals (Hospital Infection Society/Infection Control Nurses Association, 2007).

Table 8.2 Bacteria associated with surgical wound infection

Bacteria	Postoperative day of onset
Staphylococcus	3–5 days
Gram-negative rods	5 days
Streptococcus	2–3 days
Clostridium perfringens (very rare, causes gas gangrene)	1–3 days

Auditing wound infection

Surgical wound infection is a key area for clinical audit because the information yielded (Glenister, 1993):

- Can be used to help to evaluate changes in practice
- Is useful in studying the epidemiology of wound infection
- Provides data on the quality of healthcare required by commissioners of healthcare.

During the audit cycle, the level of surgical infection can be taken as the standard. The collection, analysis and interpretation of data are used to obtain and measure this agreed standard. Data collection is the most time-consuming and difficult part of the exercise. It requires careful planning, tight criteria for the inclusion of subjects and a clear definition of the criteria used to determine the existence of infection if the results are to be considered reliable and the resulting decisions are to be sound. The best use of surgical wound audit involves a re-examination of the same clinical area on repeated occasions, especially after the implementation of change, rather than the production of league tables (Humphreys and Emmerson, 1993). The findings must be interpreted with caution, as comparisons are only meaningful between areas with similar patient profiles and if valid definitions of wound infection are used (Bruce et al., 2001).

Shorter hospital stays and day surgery mean that, for certain procedures, most infections occur after discharge, for example appendicectomy and prosthetic knee surgery; post-discharge surveillance for surgical site infection is needed to avoid an underestimation of surgical site infection (Manniën et al., 2006).

Identifying wound infection

The inflammatory response to infection and tissue damage is similar, so confusion inevitably arises when identifying wounds that are clinically infected and those which are merely colonized with commensal flora not invading the tissues (Hutchinson and Lawrence, 1991). Some authors suggest that clinical infection should be diagnosed in the presence of bacterial counts greater than 10^5 colony-forming units per gram of tissue (Borneside and Borneside, 1979). There is, however, evidence that burns continue to heal in the presence of higher bacterial counts, although the risks of graft rejection are increased (Pruitt, 1984). Microorganisms present in wound exudate may not necessarily be invading the tissues, and their presence should thus be regarded as indicative but not diagnostic of infection. The results of microbiological examination must therefore be evaluated in conjunction with other factors, which have been identified by Cutting and Harding (1994):

- Abscess formation
- Cellulitis
- Discharge
- Delayed healing
- Discoloration

- Friable granulation tissue
- Pockets of infection
- Throbbing pain
- Odour
- Dehiscence.

Abscess formation

Abscesses are localized collections of necrotic tissue, bacteria and phagocytic leuco-cytes (purulent material) contained within a fibrin network. They may exert consider-able pressure, forcing bacteria into the surrounding tissues or the blood and lymphatic vessels, resulting in septicaemia. Wherever possible, an abscess should be incised and drained. Antibiotics cannot penetrate a mass of purulent tissue and will be ineffective. Staphylococci are the pyogenic bacteria most likely to cause abscesses.

Cellulitis

Cellulitis is diffuse inflammation of the connective tissue, usually occurring subcutane-ously. The causative organism in most cases is the haemolytic streptococcus. The pres-ence of cellulitis is indicated by the classic hallmarks of inflammation: erythema and local heat with accompanying pain and oedema. Vesicles may develop in severe cases, leading to ulceration and necrosis. The rare condition of necrotizing fasciitis is caused by strep-tococci, although other bacteria may become involved as the condition progresses.

Abnormal discharge

Exudate (protein-rich serous fluid, leucocytes and debris) from a freshly created wound is normal but should diminish as healing occurs in acute wounds. In chronic wounds, however, exudate may continue for longer periods and may increase. The normal exudate contains substances that include growth factors, enzymes and nutrients, and promotes tissue repair (Fletcher and Anderson, 2007). A healthy wound is moist rather than wet. Excessive exudates can result in maceration (Murphy, 2006). It can be managed by selecting the most appropriate dressing product for the level of exudate. The amount of exudate to be expected and therefore judged as 'normal' depends on the nature and extent of the wounding (see below): considerable quantities of protein-rich serum may escape from burns, necessitating fluid replacement therapy.

INFORMATION BOX 8.3

Abnormal wound discharge

The following types of wound discharge should not be considered normal and suggest that infection has occurred:

➤ Serous exudate – where there is evidence of severe inflammation

➤ Serosanguinous (serous fluid and blood) – may occur before wound dehiscence

> ➤ Seropurulent (serous fluid and pus)
>
> ➤ Haemopurulent (blood and pus)
>
> ➤ Purulent (thick pus) – this must be distinguished from slough (moist, devitalized – dead – tissue), which may be present without infection

Delayed healing

The length of time that a wound of a given type should take to heal is a matter of clinical judgement. Factors other than infection (poor nutrition, pre-existing metabolic disorders, corticosteroid therapy and age, for example) may be operating and must be taken into consideration, especially if there is no other indication of sepsis.

Discoloration

Again, much depends on clinical judgement, especially familiarity with the expected appearance of inflamed tissues responding to trauma in the normal way and the effect of different dressing materials. Sepsis is sometimes mistakenly attributed to the effect of a wound care product (Leaper, 1996). Healthy granulation tissue appears moist (rather than wet) and red or pink, discoloration suggesting infection. A yellow membrane developing over the surface of a wound represents fibrin. If removed, it will return within a few days.

Friable granulation tissue

Friable granulation tissue that bleeds spontaneously or in response to light pressure suggests infection. It looks raw and is tender.

Pockets of infection

'Pockets' of infection may develop in the deepest part of a granulating wound. They must be drained to allow the new, healthy tissue to develop. Specific dressing products that conform to the wound are used when cavities are present.

Throbbing pain

Throbbing pain is an indication of severe inflammation, the resulting oedema exerting pressure on adjacent tissues. Chemicals released as part of the inflammatory response (Chapter 2) further contribute to the pain.

Odour

Odour may be detectable in healthy wounds but should not be pervasive or unpleasant. It is caused by putrefaction of the tissues with the activity of Gram-negative and anaerobic bacteria. Streptococcal and staphylococcal infections do not usually produce a noticeable odour; an offensive putrid smell indicates the presence of anaerobes. Odour is among the most distressing problems experienced by people with wounds such as leg ulcers, severely reducing their quality of life and restricting their social activities (Fletcher and Anderson, 2007).

Dehiscence

Dehiscence occurs in severely infected wounds because the bacteria break down collagen, undermining the strength of the regenerating tissues.

Factors associated with surgical wound infection

Factors influencing the development of surgical sepsis fall into two categories (Cruse and Foord, 1973):

- The dose of contaminating bacteria
- The patient's resistance.

Dose of contaminating bacteria

Many factors affect the dose of contaminating bacteria including conditions in the operating theatre, the length of the operation and theatre attire (Chapter 5). The importance of conditions in theatre warrants further discussion and other factors, such as skin preparation and chemoprophylaxis (Chapter 4), are also addressed in this section.

Conditions in the operating theatre

Postoperative infections in general surgery are mainly endogenous, but airborne organisms cause some cases, especially in orthopaedic patients when prostheses are inserted (Babb et al., 1995).

Exogenous surgical infection is possible via the airborne route or by contact spread from hands or instruments. A single skin scale from a staphylococcal carrier may transport up to a hundred individual bacteria. Skin scales may become airborne, settle onto the hands of staff or the drapes and then become carried into the wound. The number of airborne particles in the operating room is proportional to the number of people present and their level of activity; this is because the friction of clothing against the skin releases skin scales. Special ventilation systems are used to filter out airborne bacteria and to prevent those in the corridors and theatre suite entering the operating room. Further precautions to reduce infection include:

- Restricting the number of people present in theatre during an operation and reducing the levels of activity of those who are present: spectators should use a viewing gallery
- Regularly maintaining the operating environment: dust should not be allowed to settle on any surface, and filters in the ventilation system should be checked (see below).

Considerable research has been undertaken with orthopaedic patients because infection is so damaging and will ultimately reduce mobility to less than that present before surgery. Treatment with antibiotics is not always successful, and the removal of the prosthesis is in some cases inevitable.

INFORMATION BOX 8.4

Theatre ventilation systems

Ventilation systems in operating theatres are designed to filter airborne bacteria and to prevent the spread of bacteria from the theatre suite and corridors to the operating theatre.

Several points should be noted:

➤ Ventilation systems must undergo regular and properly planned maintenance.

➤ Airborne bacteria are removed by forcing air through filters before it enters the operating theatre.

➤ The higher air pressure in operating theatres prevents unfiltered air moving into the theatres from other areas of the theatre suite.

➤ Filtered air is continually being renewed in the operating theatre, most systems renewing the air about 20 times every hour.

➤ Specialized ventilation systems may be installed in some high-risk situations, for example orthopaedic surgery involving the use of prostheses.

Preoperative hair removal

The evidence that hair removal from the site prior to surgery leads to a reduction in surgical site infection is insufficient and inconclusive (see below).

■ PRACTICE APPLICATION 8.2 ■

Preoperative Hair Removal

The practice of removing hair from the operation site, by shaving, clipping or use of depilatory creams, varies across specialties and the wishes of particular surgeons.

Activity

➤ Is hair removal prior to surgery routine in your placement?

➤ If so, which method is used?

➤ When is it undertaken – the day of surgery or before?

➤ Access the articles below and discuss their findings with your mentor.

Resources

Cruse PJE and Foord R (1980) The epidemiology of wound infection: a 10-year prospective study of 62,939 wounds. *Surgical Clinics of North America* **60**: 27–40.

Hallstrom R and Beck SL (1993) Implementation of the AORN skin standard. *Association of Operating Room Nurses' Journal* **583**: 498–506.

Seropian R and Reynolds BM (1971) Wound infection after pre-operative depilatory versus razor preparation. *American Journal of Surgery* 121: 251–5.

Tanner J, Moncaster K and Woodings D (2007) Preoperative hair removal: a systematic review. *Journal of Perioperative Practice*. 17(3): 118–21, 124–32.

Preoperative skin hygiene

Preoperative showering with antiseptics reduced the rate of infection in the study by Cruse and Foord (1973). This finding has been highly publicized by pharmaceutical companies, but the results have not been supported by other large-scale, well-planned epidemiological studies (Byrne et al., 1990; Lynch et al., 1992). There is no evidence that one antiseptic might be of more benefit than another (Lipp, 2005).

Bowel preparation

Bowel preparation is essential to reduce the risk of endogenous infection with Gram-negative bacilli in patients undergoing procedures involving the gastrointestinal tract. This preparation usually involves measures to empty the bowel and chemo-prophylaxis.

Chemoprophylaxis

Chemoprophylaxis given systemically to surgical patients has dramatically reduced the incidence of surgical wound infection. Nevertheless, antibiotics are not 'wonder drugs'. It is good practice to prescribe them only to protect a particular patient from bacteria known to represent a specific threat according to the type of procedure undertaken, and not as part of a blanket policy intended to 'destroy all known germs' (Chapter 4). For example, the patient undergoing abdominal or gynaecological surgery will benefit from prophylactic metronidazole because anaerobes in the gut or vagina may cause infection; the drug is of no value to the patient with a traumatic wound restricted to the surface tissues where anaerobes do not survive.

Duration of operative procedures

The duration of the operation is related to the development of surgical sepsis as the exposure of the tissues is increased during longer procedures. Tissues are also likely to be manipulated more during long, complicated operations, introducing more opportunities for operator error and contamination by contact. After the first hour, the infection rate tends to double for every additional hour that the operation is prolonged. However, the use of minimally invasive techniques for many surgical procedures including some joint surgery is increasing.

Reducing the number of people present and the amount of movement in theatre helps to reduce the risk of infection – movement increases the number of airborne particles so that more are available to settle into the wound.

Wound site

The wound site appears to be a major factor influencing the development of sepsis. Wounds in well-vascularized regions fare better, as discussed below. Moist areas are difficult to manage, especially if dressings are difficult to apply and retain in position, for example over incisions in the inguinal (groin), perianal (around the anus) and vulval areas. Tissue at other, unexpected anatomical locations may also be susceptible to contamination and infection. A high incidence of infection has been associated with coronary artery bypass graft operations when the veins have been harvested from the legs (Wells, 1983). The bacteria responsible were mainly faecal in origin, suggesting contamination from the perineum. The health professional who harvests the veins should scrub again and put on a new gown and gloves before undertaking further clean activities.

Vascularization

Vascularization influences infection and tissue necrosis. The beneficial effects of inflammation depend on an adequate blood supply; thus poor vascularization and/ or excessive blood loss delays healing. Non-surgical wounds tend to develop at anatomical locations where vascularization is poor, for example minor trauma may trigger the formation of ulcers on the front of the leg, especially in older adults and others with impaired circulation.

Poor surgical technique

Delayed healing and sepsis are the products of poor surgical technique. Roughly handling the tissues, the excessive use of diathermy and tight suturing impair healing and promote infection (Leaper, 1995).

Length of pre- and postoperative stay

The longer the period spent in hospital before surgery, the higher the wound infection rate: Cruse and Foord (1973) reported a rate of 1.1 per cent for those admitted one day before surgery compared with 2 per cent for those present in hospital for a week before their operation. The present trend towards day-case surgery and the move towards GPs performing minor procedures are therefore to be welcomed. However, more work is required to detect possible differences between the infection rate for day-case and outpatient surgery.

Presence of foreign bodies

Foreign bodies promote the development of infection. Sutures, especially multi-braided types, trap bacteria (Gristina et al., 1985). If a wound has resulted through cardiac or orthopaedic surgery, underlying bone or the presence of a prosthesis will increase the potential for infection (Murphy, 2006). For the normal, healthy adult patient, it has been estimated that 10^6 bacteria must be present for every gram of tissue to result in clinical infection: local and humoral immunological defence mechanisms are usually able to cope with a smaller number of bacteria but are more easily overwhelmed in the presence of foreign material: one silk suture dramatically reduces the threshold for clinical infection. Resistance to invading pathogens develops more rapidly in wounds held together with sterile skin-closure strips than in those which have been conventionally sutured. Particles from gauze and cotton dressings may leave contaminants in a wound and should not be used. Capillary loops may grow up into the weave, leading to trauma when they are removed (Wood, 1976).

Wound drainage

Wound drainage is intended to prevent the accumulation of body fluids (blood, serous exudates, bile and so on) within the tissues, which will operate as a nidus (focus) for infection and promote abscess formation. Closed suction drainage significantly reduces the incidence of postoperative sepsis. In the study by Cruse and Foord (1973), the infection rate for clean contaminated wounds without drainage was 2.2 per cent compared with 1.8 per cent for those treated by drainage without suction through a separate stab wound. With closed suction drains, the infection rate was 0.6 per cent. The rate of infection was substantially higher when the drain was inserted via the wound itself. When drains are manipulated, an aseptic technique must be adopted; skin bacteria have been isolated from the lumen of drains, indicating that they may move from the exterior towards the internal tissues as well as in the reverse direction. The presence of a haematoma also increases the risk of infection.

Patient's resistance

For people admitted from a waiting list to undergo elective operations, it is possible to enhance resistance to infection through careful nursing and medical assessment and intervention. The following measures place the individual in a better position to withstand the challenge of surgery:

- Optimal fluid and electrolyte balance
- Optimal nutritional status, with the correction of any negative nitrogen balance
- The correction of a low haemoglobin level
- The control of any underlying metabolic disorder, for example diabetes mellitus
- The opportunity to learn and practise deep breathing and leg exercises
- The opportunity to discuss the operation, to anticipate what will happen in hospital and during the longer term recovery at home, and to plan for any resulting change, for example stoma formation or mastectomy.

In emergency situations where this is not feasible, physical and psychological recovery may be slower.

The factors outlined below influence the development of postoperative wound infection.

Age

People between the ages of 20 and 40 years have a lower infection rate, probably because their immune system is functioning optimally (Ayliffe et al., 1977). This has major clinical implications as a high proportion of surgical patients fall into the older age group.

Gender

Gender also influenced the ability to withstand infection in the study undertaken by Ayliffe et al. (1977). After general surgical procedures (stripping varicose veins, hernia repairs and gut operations), males were more likely to develop infection, especially staphylococcal infection, than females. Males carry staphylococci more often than females and disseminate them more easily, especially from the perineal area (Hare and Thomas, 1956).

Nutritional status

Cruse and Foord (1973) detected a significant association between post-surgical sepsis and obesity: for clean wounds, overweight people had an infection rate of 13 per cent compared with 1.8 per cent for those of ideal body weight. Subcutaneous adipose tissue is poorly vascularized, and it may be difficult to secure haemostasis during closure. Secondary Gram-negative infection is probably also more common in this group. Moist skin folds may harbour sufficient bacteria to form a reservoir, the bacteria reaching the wound by contact spread.

Undernourishment is also important. The rate of post-surgical sepsis for people significantly below their ideal body weight was 16.6 per cent in the study by Cruse and Foord (1973). The inflammatory response, the immunological response and tissue repair all depend on adequate supplies of protein. A negative nitrogen balance impedes healing and increases the opportunity for infection to supervene.

Metabolic disorders

Metabolic disorders are believed to alter the ability of the tissues to withstand pathogenic invasion, but the mechanism is obscure and may vary between one type of patient and another. Diabetes mellitus is one of the most common metabolic disorders and therefore among the easiest to establish. The clean wound infection rate for diabetic patients was 10.7 per cent in the study by Cruse and Foord (1973). The physiological mechanism remains to be clarified, but there are suggestions that neutrophil migration may occur more slowly than in people without diabetes.

Temperature

Maintaining the patient's normal body temperature around the time of surgery appears to decrease infection and promote healing (Kurz et al., 1996).

Corticosteroids

The association between a depressed inflammatory response and corticosteroid therapy has been well established. Physical and psychological stress may, by increasing the release of corticosteroid hormones from the adrenal cortex, suppress healing, increase the rate of surgical wound infection and delay recovery (Boore, 1978).

Malignancy

Malignancy is often cited as a risk factor for post-surgical sepsis. In a study by Bucknall (1982), conducted on over a thousand patients undergoing a laparotomy, malignancy and its associated problems of anaemia and malnutrition resulted in a significantly higher infection rate.

Aseptic dressing technique

The purpose of the aseptic (non-touch) dressing technique is to avoid contact between open tissue, the fingers and any other potentially contaminated item that could lead to cross-infection. Dressing procedures frequently take the form of time-consuming rituals that are not evidence based (Bree-Williams and Waterman, 1996). In the absence of supporting research, the following are offered as a means by which to save time, resources and patient discomfort:

- Question the need to change the dressing at all. A larger, more absorbent dressing may be applied to deal with seeping exudate ('strike-through') in order to avoid discomfort, environmental contamination and cross-infection. Daily changes are usually unnecessary and may be painful. Transparent polyurethane dressings permit inspection without removal.

- Cleanse the hands with an alcoholic handrub at the bedside immediately before handling the dressing. Time walking to a sink is saved, especially if the hands have to be decontaminated more than once during the procedure.

- Avoid the application of solutions to wounds that are already clean. This increases the risk of contamination and cools the wound, slowing cell division and the action of phagocytic cells.

- Research with occlusive and semi-permeable dressings such as hydrocolloids suggests that the surfaces of healthy granulating wounds may be colonized by, rather than infected with, saprophytic organisms, even though these are capable of pathogenic activity (Brennan et al., 1985). A clean rather than a complicated aseptic procedure may be more appropriate for this type of wound. Microorganisms can never be completely removed from the wound surface; they may even be beneficial.

- Use of strongly acidic or alkaline solutions (such as hydrogen peroxide) is not recommended. They damage new tissue, destroy the delicately balanced microflora (microorganisms present in a specific area) of the wound and soon lose their antiseptic properties (Leaper, 1996).

With chronic wounds, it is vital that the healthcare professional responsible for providing treatment understands the aetiology of the wound, otherwise an inappropriate regimen may be selected and tissue repair will not be promoted. Occlusive, semi-permeable dressings are more appropriate than cheaper cotton wool or gauze. They provide a more effective physiological environment for healing, are less likely to traumatize the tissues and do not disseminate bacteria into the air when removed (Lawrence et al., 1992). It is helpful to anticipate the way in which the wound is likely to respond to treatment. Occlusive, semi-permeable dressings promote auto-debridement so the wound may appear to become larger before the formation of granulation tissue (Melhuish et al., 1994), contraction eventually indicating that progress is occurring. The use of some hydrocolloids is associated with odour, which, although it may be unpleasant, is not an indication of infection or necrosis.

■ SELF-ASSESSMENT ■

1. Wounds heal best under moist conditions. True? or False?

2. Which processes occur during the proliferative phase of wound healing?

3. Give an example of a wound that heals by first (primary) intention and one that heals by secondary intention.

4. How does the application of cold solutions to already clean wounds slow healing?

5. Give two examples of wound discharges that suggest infection.

6. Preoperative shaving reduces the risk of surgical wound infection. True? or False?

■ REFERENCES ■

Ayliffe GAJ, Brightwell KM, Babb BJ et al. (1977) Surveys of hospital infection in the Birmingham region. *Journal of Hygiene* **79**: 299–313.

Babb JR, Lynam P and Ayliffe GAJ (1995) Risk of airborne transmission in an operating theatre containing four ultra clean air units. *Journal of Hospital Infection* **31**: 159–68.

Boore J (1978) *Prescription for Recovery.* RCN, London.

Borneside GH and Borneside BB (1979) Comparison between moist swab and tissue biopsy methods for quantitation of bacteria in experimental incision wounds. *Journal of Trauma* **19**: 103–5.

Bree-Williams FJ and Waterman H (1996) An examination of nurses' practices when performing aseptic technique for wound dressings. *Journal of Advanced Nursing* **23**: 48–54.

Brennan SS, Foster M and Leaper DJ (1985) Antiseptic toxicity in wounds healing by secondary intention. *Journal of Hospital Infection* **8**: 263–7.

Bruce J, Russell EM, Mollison J et al. (2001) The quality of measurement of surgical wound infection as the basis for monitoring: a systematic review. *Journal of Hospital Infection* **49**: 99–108.

Bucknall TE (1982) Burst abdomen and the incisional hernia – a prospective study of 1129 major laparotomies. *British Medical Journal* **184**: 931–3.

Byrne DJ, Napier A and Cuschieri A (1990) Rationalising whole body disinfection. *Journal of Hospital Infection* **15**: 183–7.

Coello R, Glenister H, Ferres J et al. (1993) The cost of infection in surgical patients: a case control study. *Journal of Hospital Infection* **25**: 239–50.

Coello R, Charlett A, Wilson J et al. (2005) Adverse impact of surgical site infections in English hospitals. *Journal of Hospital Infection* **60:** 93–103.

Collier M (2003) Wound bed preparation: theory to practice. *Nursing Standard* **17**(36): 45–52.

Cruse PJ and Foord R (1973) A five year prospective study of 23,649 surgical wounds. *Archives of Surgery* **107**: 206–10.

Cruse PJ and Foord R (1980) The epidemiology of wound infection: a 10-year prospective study of 62,939 wounds. *Surgical Clinics of North America* **60**: 27–40.

Cutting KF and Harding KG (1994) Criteria for identifying wound infection. *Journal of Wound Care* **3**: 198–201.

Emmerson AM, Enstone JE, Griffin M et al. (1996) The Second National Prevalence Survey of Infection in Hospitals – overview of the results. *Journal of Hospital Infection* **32**: 175–90.

Fletcher J and Anderson I (2007) Wound management. In Brooker C and Waugh A (eds) *Foundations of Nursing Practice: Fundamentals of Holistic Care*. Mosby, Edinburgh.

Glenister H (1993) How do we collect data for surveillance of wound infection? *Journal of Hospital Infection* **24**: 283–9.

Gristina AG, Price JL, Hobgood CD et al. (1985) Bacterial colonisation of percutaneous sutures. *Surgery* **98**: 12–19.

Hare R and Thomas CG (1956) The transmission of *Staphylococcus aureus*. *British Medical Journal* **2**: 840–4.

Holmes J and Readman R (1994) A study of wound infections following inguinal hernia repair. *Journal of Hospital Infection* **28**: 153–6.

Hospital Infection Society/Infection Control Nurses Association (2007) *Summary of Preliminary Results of The Third Prevalence Survey of Healthcare Associated Infections in Acute Hospitals* (for England) (2006). Available www.his.org.uk/.

Humphreys H and Emmerson AM (1993) Control of hospital-acquired infection: accurate data and more resources, not league tables. *Journal of Hospital Infection* **25**: 75–8.

Hutchinson JJ and Lawrence JC (1991) Wound infection under occlusive dressings. *Journal of Hospital Infection* **17**: 83–94.

Kurz A, Sessler DI, Lenhardt R et al. (1996) Perioperative normothermia to reduce the incidence of surgical wound infection and shorten hospitalisation. *New England Journal of Medicine* **312**: 1195–9.

Lawrence JC, Lilly HA and Kidson A (1992) Wound dressings and airborne dispersal of bacteria. *Lancet* **339**: 807.

Leaper D (1995) Risk factors for surgical infection. *Journal of Hospital Infection* (Supplement) **30**: 127–39.

Leaper D (1996) Antiseptics in wound healing. *Nursing Times* **92**(39): 63–8.

Lipp A (2005) The evidence base for using preoperative antiseptics. *Nursing Times* **101**(50): 26–8.

Lynch W, Davey PG, Malek M et al. (1992) Cost-effectiveness of the use of chlorhexidine detergent in pre-operative whole-body disinfection in wound prophylaxis. *Journal of Hospital Infection* **21**: 179–91.

Manniën J, Wille J, Snoeren R, van den Hof S (2006) Impact of postdischarge surveillance on surgical site infection rates for several surgical procedures: results from the nosocomial surveillance network in the Netherlands. *Infection Control and Hospital Epidemiology* **27**(8): 809–16.

Melhuish JM, Plassman P and Harding KG (1994) Circumference, area and volume of the healing wound. *Journal of Wound Care* **3**: 380–4.

Murphy F (2006) Assessment and management of patients with surgical cavity wounds. *Nursing Standard* **20**(45): 57–66.

National Research Council (1964) Post-operative wound infection. *Annals of Surgery* (Supplement) **160**(2): 1–192.

Pollock AV and Evans M (1983) Microbiological prediction of abdominal surgical wound infection. *Archives of Surgery* **122**: 33–7.

Pruitt BZ (1984) The diagnosis and treatment of infection in the burned patient. *Burns* **11**: 79–81.

Towler J (2001) Cleansing traumatic wounds with swabs, water or saline. *Journal of Wound Care* **10**: 231–4.

Wells FC (1983) Wound infection in cardiothoracic surgery. *Lancet* **1**: 1209–10.

Westaby S (1985) *Wound Care.* Heinemann, London.

Whiteside MC and Moorhead RJ (1994) Traumatic wound management. A guide to treatment of gunshot and bomb injuries. *Journal of Wound Care* **3**: 183–6.

Winter GD (1962) Formation of the scab and the rate of epithelialisation of superficial wounds in the skin of the young domestic pig. *Nature* **193**: 293–4.

Wood RA (1976) Disintegration of cellulose dressings in open granulating wounds. *British Medical Journal* **1**: 1444–5.

FURTHER READING AND INFORMATION SOURCES

Bale S and Jones V (2006) *Wound Care Nursing*, 2nd edn. Mosby, Edinburgh.

Cole E (2003) Wound management in the A&E department. *Nursing Standard* **17**(46): 45–54.

Enoch S, Grey JE and Harding KG (2006) ABC of wound healing. Recent advances and emerging treatments. *British Medical Journal* **332:** 962–5.

European Wound Management Association (2005) *Position Document Identifying Criteria for Wound Infection*. Medical Education Partnership, London.

Haley RW, Culver DH, Morgan WM et al. (1985) Identifying patients at high risk of surgical wound infection. A simple multivariate index of patient susceptibility and wound contamination. *American Journal of Epidemiology* **121**(2): 206–15.

Health Protection Agency – www.hpa.org.uk/.

Hess CT (2005) *Wound Care*. Lippincott Williams & Wilkins, London.

Johnstone CC, Farley A and Hendry C (2005) The physiological basis of wound management. *Nursing Standard* **19**(43): 59–66.

Morgan D (2004) *Formulary of Wound Management Products*. Euromed Communications, Haslemere.

Nicol M, Bavin C, Cronin P and Rawlings-Anderson K (2008) *Essential Nursing Skills*, 3rd edn. Mosby, Edinburgh.

Webster J and Osborne S (2007) Preoperative bathing or showering with skin antiseptics to prevent surgical site infection. *Cochrane Database Systematic Review* **12**(2): CD004985.

CHAPTER 9

Respiratory infections

CHAPTER OUTCOMES

After reading this chapter, you should be able to:

➤ State the prevalence of lower respiratory tract infection and pneumonia in hospital inpatients

➤ Discuss the increasing importance of community-acquired pneumonia

➤ List the organisms responsible for lower respiratory tract infection

➤ Explain why postoperative and ventilated patients are at particular risk of developing lower respiratory tract infection and suggest strategies to help to reduce these risks

➤ List the organisms responsible for upper respiratory tract infection and suggest preventive strategies in each case

Introduction: the importance of respiratory infections

Respiratory infections are common in both hospital and community settings. The third national prevalence survey conducted in 2006 found that infections of the lower respiratory tract (not pneumonia) and pneumonia together accounted for 19.9 per cent of HCAIs in acute hospitals (Hospital Infection Society/Infection Control Nurses Association, 2007). Hospital-acquired infections affecting the respiratory tract cause considerable morbidity and mortality. This type of respiratory infection generally affects those who are critically ill.

Other respiratory infections and those arising from pathogens in the respiratory tract – pulmonary tuberculosis, severe acute respiratory syndrome (SARS), Legionnaire's disease and meningococcal meningitis – are covered in Chapter 14. Drugs used to treat tuberculosis are outlined in Chapter 4.

Lower respiratory tract infections

Lower respiratory tract infections (LRTIs) involve the bronchi and alveoli (Figure 9.1). They include two serious conditions – acute bronchitis and pneumonia:

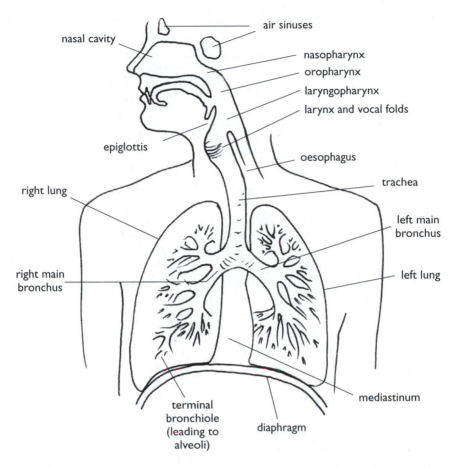

Figure 9.1 The respiratory tract

- **Acute bronchitis** (inflammation of the bronchi) is an acute respiratory infection in which the dominant symptom is coughing without localized infection. This should not be confused with chronic bronchitis, which is a type of chronic obstructive pulmonary disease (COPD). Acute bronchitis is usually a community-acquired infection and typically arises as a complication of upper respiratory tract infection (URTI) caused by a virus, when bacterial infection supervenes. Some children seem prone to bronchitis. It appears to be related to poor living conditions (overcrowding, poor hygiene and poor nutrition) and is exacerbated by maternal smoking, especially during pregnancy. Individuals who have experienced childhood bronchitis are at risk of developing further symptoms during their teenage years if they then smoke.

- **Pneumonia** (inflammation of the lung) is a serious condition, responsible for most deaths caused by infection of the respiratory tract, especially in older adults and infants. It may be acquired in hospital or the community. The alveoli become filled with pus, air is excluded, and the lung is said to be 'consolidated'. In bronchopneumonia, consolidation is widely distributed; in lobar pneumonia, it is localized.

Hospital admission is arranged to:

- Administer antibiotics – although many cases are viral, this may be difficult to determine, and no time must be lost in instituting treatment
- Provide physiotherapy – percussion, breathing exercises and postural drainage.

Community-acquired pneumonia

In the community, bacterial pneumonia is most frequently caused by *Streptococcus pneumoniae* (Riley and Riley, 2003). Infection is most common in people with pre-existing health problems, frequently developing as a complication of some other respiratory infection (for example influenza or measles). Treatment is complicated because some strains of *Streptococcus pneumoniae* are now resistant to penicillin. Vaccination has been recommended in the UK since 2003 (Bedford and Lane, 2006). The pneumococcal vaccine is part of the childhood immunization programme (Chapter 2) and it is also offered to people over 65 years of age. It is also recommended for people following splenectomy and those with dysfunction of the spleen, sickle cell disease, coeliac disease, chronic renal disease, chronic respiratory disease, chronic heart conditions, liver disease, diabetes mellitus, immunosuppression and HIV. Following vaccination, about 80 per cent of healthy adults develop a good antibody response within three weeks. Practice nurses working in primary care settings usually offer immunization.

Other bacteria responsible for community-acquired pneumonia include *Mycoplasma pneumoniae*, *Haemophilus influenzae*, *Legionella pneumophila* (Chapter 14) and *Staphylococcus aureus*, including the strain that produces the Panton–Valentine leukocidin toxin (see below).

INFORMATION BOX 9.1

Panton–Valentine leukocidin

Some strains of the bacterium *Staphylococcus aureus* produce a virulent toxin known as 'Panton–Valentine leukocidin' (PVL), which damages white blood cells. This strain of *S. aureus* is responsible for several infections including a life-threatening, community-acquired pneumonia in previously fit and healthy children and young adults.

Resource

Health Protection Agency – www.hpa.org.uk.

Hospital-acquired pneumonia

In the third national prevalence survey of infection in hospitals, pneumonia was the third most common (13.9 per cent) HCAI in acute hospitals (Hospital Infection Society/Infection Control Nurses Association, 2007). It mainly affects critically ill and postoperative patients. Risk factors include obesity, impaired consciousness, a history of smoking and underlying respiratory disease. In hospital, bacteria, viruses or fungi can cause pneumonia, but most hospital-acquired pneumonia is caused by *S. aureus* and Gram-negative opportunists (Inglis et al., 1993).

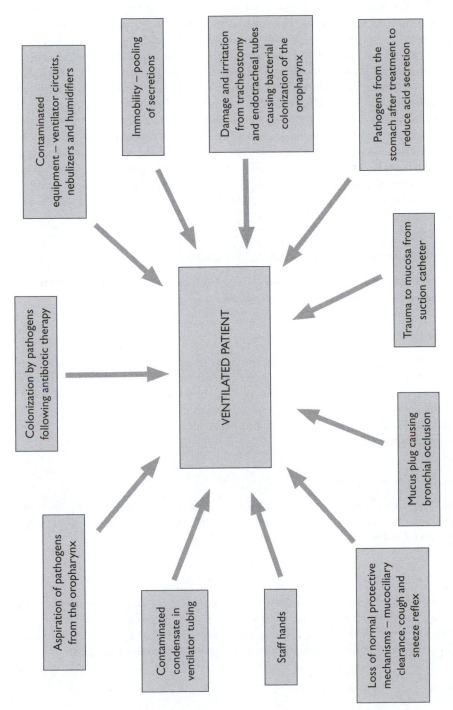

Figure 9.2 Infection risks in ventilated patients

Infection can arise from other people by cross-infection or from an environmental source (as, for example, with *Legionella pneumophila*). The bacteria responsible are frequently resistant to antibiotics (Koeman et al., 2001). Airborne transmission is not a major route in hospital except for *L. pneumophila*. Instead, most cases of hospital-acquired pneumonia develop in patients who require mechanical ventilation (Figure 9.2). Ventilator-associated pneumonia (VAP) is diagnosed if infection arises more than 48 hours after endotracheal intubation and mechanical ventilation. These patients are at particular risk because they have lost the protective coughing and sneezing reflexes, their risk being increased further by antibiotic therapy and other invasive procedures.

VAP occurs when the bronchioles and alveoli become contaminated with pathogens. In health, they are kept free of microorganisms by the mucociliary escalator: foreign particles become trapped in the mucus, are wafted upwards by ciliary action and are eventually swallowed. However, the upper respiratory passages harbour bacteria, including potential pathogens, and these may be transferred to the lower airways during invasive procedures.

Sources of pathogens for hospital-acquired pneumonia

There are a variety of sources of pathogens, such as those from the oropharynx, which can cause hospital-acquired pneumonia.

Aspiration of pathogens from the oropharynx

The aspiration of pathogens colonizing the oropharynx is the most important source of bacterial pneumonia in hospital inpatients. Although many healthy people aspirate their secretions during sleep, the body's immunological defences deal with these. In ventilated patients, the risk of aspiration is increased by the presence of endotracheal and tracheostomy tubes, and because the patients are sedated or have been anaesthetized.

Colonization of the oropharynx

Colonization of the oropharynx increases the risk of developing pneumonia and complicates its treatment. Gram-negative bacilli replace the normal flora if the patient receives antibiotics (Johanson et al., 1972).

Colonization of the stomach

Colonization of the stomach results if the patient receives drugs to neutralize (for example antacids) or suppress (H_2-receptor antagonists, for example cimetidine) the secretion of gastric acid. These are commonly prescribed for the critically ill patient to reduce the risk of peptic ulceration caused by stress (Craven et al., 1986).

Endotracheal and tracheostomy tubes

Endotracheal and tracheostomy tubes irritate the respiratory mucosa and promote Gram-negative colonization of the oropharynx. Contaminated secretions enter the trachea from the mouth and pharynx, secretions then seeping down through the space between the outer wall of the endotracheal tube and the tracheal wall. The endotracheal tube should provide an airtight seal sufficient to occlude this space, but leakage is possible during the periodic deflation of the cuff. Bacteria of the same strain have been isolated from the mouth and trachea of ventilated patients (Sanderson, 1983).

Contaminated ventilator circuits

Contaminated ventilator circuits may lead to cross-infection by delivering bacteria-laden air directly to the lower airways (Phillips, 1967).

Nebulizers

Nebulizers create aerosols of minute droplets that penetrate deeply into the narrowest airways and thus present a significant problem. This is especially so for small-volume medication nebulizers (Botman and de Krieger, 1987).

Humidification

Humidification of the circuit is essential to prevent dehydration of the airways. Humidifiers do not produce aerosols so if the water in the reservoir becomes contaminated, the bacteria are less likely to be inhaled. However, water vapour tends to condense in the tubing (Stucke and Thompson, 1980). The condensate may become heavily contaminated and can drain into the trachea, increasing the risk of infection (Craven et al., 1984).

Tracheobronchial suction

Tracheobronchial suction, intended to reduce the risk of infection in pooled secretions, may contribute to its development if poor technique results in the transfer of bacteria (Fiorentini, 1992). Mucous membranes are more easily damaged by trauma than skin, and abrasions from the suction catheter further increase the risk of infection (see below).

PRACTICE APPLICATION 9.1

Reducing Infection Risks Associated with Tracheobronchial Suctioning

Patients who require suctioning of their respiratory secretions have a high risk of developing healthcare-associated pneumonia. This risk is increased for patients with a tracheostomy and those being ventilated.

Activity

➤ Access the article by Moore (2003) and read the list in Box 4 (p. 50). Identify the points that directly relate to reducing infection risks and discuss them with your mentor.

➤ Find out how often the suction container and tubing are changed in your placement or workplace.

Resource

Moore T (2003) Suctioning techniques for the removal of respiratory secretions. *Nursing Standard* 18(9): 47–53.

Bronchial occlusion with mucus plug

Postoperative respiratory infection arises when a bronchus becomes occluded with a plug of tenacious mucus. The patient may be frightened to move after surgery and reluctant to expectorate, especially if pain is poorly controlled. After some major surgery, immobility is complete because the patient is sedated and ventilated. Occlusion results in the pooling of secretions in the air passages distal to the obstruction, which then collapse when the air within the alveoli is absorbed but not replaced. Gaseous exchange in that area ceases. The tissue is still perfused, but the blood reaching it no longer receives oxygen and cannot be relieved of carbon dioxide. There is a change in the normal ventilation/perfusion ratio, which produces a right-to-left shunt. The bigger the mucus plug, the greater the problem, because a larger airway is obstructed. An extensive area of the lung will thus be affected, leading to collapse (atelectasis). Conditions are now favourable for bacterial growth and multiplication.

Prevention of hospital-acquired pneumonia

The risk of developing hospital-acquired pneumonia can be reduced by early ambulation and physiotherapy to improve lung expansion in postoperative patients (see below).

PRACTICE APPLICATION 9.2

Preventing Postoperative Chest Infection

Postoperative chest infections can be prevented by early ambulation and by teaching deep breathing exercises during the preoperative period, either individually or to groups of people (Lindeman and Van Aernan, 1971). As more operations are performed on a day-case basis with only a few hours before surgery, there will be an increasing need to organize pre-assessment clinics to provide information and teaching for the postoperative period. Written, audio or web-based information may also be provided. The importance of reducing smoking before surgery can be emphasized at the same time if necessary. Other actions include:

➤ Anaesthetic equipment should be disinfected between patients, taking care to avoid recontamination during its assembly so that spread by contact is avoided

➤ Effective pain control should be ensured in order to allow physiotherapy and early ambulation

➤ Patients with abdominal or chest incisions can be taught how to support the wound during deep breathing and coughing

> An upright position allows chest expansion and prevents the stasis of respiratory secretions

> Postoperatively, physiotherapy is important to encourage coughing and expectoration. If infection occurs, the mucus plug may have to be removed by bronchoscopy and aspiration if physiotherapy is insufficient to dislodge it. Antibiotics are of secondary importance to mechanical clearing

> Maintain hydration, as dehydration increases the viscosity of respiratory secretions (sputum), which then become difficult to dislodge

For critically ill patients, hospital-acquired pneumonia remains difficult to prevent and expensive to treat (Kelleghan et al., 1993). Some general ways of preventing pneumonia in intubated patients having mechanical ventilation are outlined below.

INFORMATION BOX 9.2

Preventing pneumonia in ventilated patients

> Wash the hands before and after every contact with an intubated patient

> Use clean gloves for all routine contact with respiratory equipment and wash the hands afterwards

> Use heat–moisture exchange (HME) filters with microbial filtration where possible; otherwise, date and change the ventilator circuits every 48 hours (Craven et al., 1982)

> Date and change the connector tubing every 24 hours (Craven et al., 1982)

> Remove condensation from the ventilator tubing if humidification is being used: it may support the growth of Gram-negative bacteria, leading to colonization and infection (Stucke and Thompson, 1980)

> Change oxygen masks and tubing between patients

> Store all respiratory equipment clean and dry

> Provide oral care at an appropriate frequency, as the mouth can operate as a source of respiratory pathogens. The use of an oral antiseptic, such as chlorhexidine 2 per cent, during oral hygiene for intubated patients having mechanical ventilation is provisionally recommended in draft guidance from the National Institute for Health and Clinical Excellence (NICE) (2007) in collaboration with the National Patient Safety Agency

> Position the patient to prevent the stagnation of respiratory secretions. The draft guidance from NICE (2007) recommends that intubated patients having mechanical ventilation be positioned in a sitting or semi-recumbent position unless this is inappropriate, such as patients with spinal injuries

> Provide physiotherapy

> Ensure effective pain relief to permit movement and physiotherapy

NB The NICE guidance *Technical Patient Safety Solutions for Prevention of Ventilator-associated Pneumonia in Adults* is expected to be issued August 2008.

Contaminated equipment has been incriminated in outbreaks (Gorman et al., 1993), but risks can be reduced by autoclaving any equipment used in respiratory therapy. This includes the ventilator and its circuits, nebulizers, humidifiers and non-disposable equipment used during endotracheal suction. If autoclaving is not possible, equipment can be decontaminated in an automated washing machine or with chemical disinfectants followed by rinsing with tap water.

Ventilators

Ventilators need not be routinely decontaminated if filters are used to protect the inspiratory and expiratory circuits. The routine use of heat–moisture exchange (HME) filters and closed suction systems in ventilators has reduced the risk of VAP. HME filters cut down the need to humidify the gases being administered to ventilated patients.

The routine disinfection of equipment is no longer necessary, the HME filter alone being changed every 24–48 hours. Where HME filters are not used, changing the circuits is recommended every 48 hours (Craven et al., 1982). Condensate collecting in ventilator tubing should be regularly drained.

Humidifiers

Humidifiers should always be used during oxygen therapy to prevent dehydration of the respiratory mucosae. They should be filled with sterile water and decontaminated every 48 hours (Craven et al., 1982).

Nebulizers

Nebulizers used to deliver medication easily become contaminated. They should be washed with detergent and dried every time they are used. Mouthpieces should be changed every 24 hours (Cobben et al., 1996).

Upper respiratory tract infections

Upper respiratory tract infections (URTIs) involve the nasal passages, pharynx, tonsils and epiglottis (see Figure 9.1 above). Most are minor infections acquired in the community and are caused by viruses. URTIs can, however, have serious consequences for the very young and older adults. They also account for a high proportion of days lost from work and school in the UK, so their impact on the health of individuals and their social and economic consequences should not be dismissed.

Coughs and colds

Coughs and colds (the common cold is also known as 'coryza') are mainly caused by rhinoviruses, members of the picornavirus group. There are about 200 different types so somebody who has just recovered from one cold may succumb to another caused by a different rhinovirus. It was traditionally believed that transmission occurred by inhaling virus particles contained in airborne droplets, but there is evidence that it also takes place by contact, especially via the hands. In laboratory simulations, Gwaltney et al. (1978) showed that volunteers' hands became contaminated after shaking hands with infected subjects; they were more likely to develop colds than individuals exposed to viral aerosols released by sneezing. Rhinoviruses survive in the inanimate environment if they are protected by mucus. Objects that are handled frequently (door knobs, light switches and crockery, for example) thus become contaminated, and the viruses are passed to a new host, reaching the eyes or nose when the face is touched. General hygiene and handwashing are especially important in schools to prevent infection by rhinoviruses. Self-inoculation is the most common form of transmission (Hendley et al., 1973).

Colds are a nuisance and can cause problems in people with pre-existing respiratory difficulties, especially older adults (Nicholson et al., 1996). There is no evidence that developing an URTI is related to becoming wet or 'chilled'. Colds are common in the UK, which has been attributed to the damp climate, but they also develop in hot, dry countries. In babies and young children, URTI is usually harmless, as it is in adulthood, but it can interfere with feeding and may be associated with acute otitis media (see below) or involvement of the lower airways. The community nurse's advice is helpful, reassuring parents and determining whether medical intervention is necessary for colds (Taylor, 1988). Medical treatment is seldom necessary (see below). The nasal discharge associated with colds contains virus particles, dead cells from the nasal mucosa and bacteria, but these are of the same type as are present in health. Bacterial invasion of the damaged epithelium is rare, and antibiotics are seldom required (see Chapters 1 and 4).

Other viruses responsible for 'colds' include:

- Parainfluenza virus
- Reoviruses
- Coxsackie viruses
- Adenoviruses
- Respiratory syncytial virus (RSV) (see below)
- Coronaviruses (NB a specific coronavirus causes SARS; Chapter 14)
- Echoviruses.

PRACTICE APPLICATION 9.3

Managing URTIs in Babies and Children

> **Antipyretics** reduce an elevated temperature. Paracetamol dose calculated on body weight is safe and has valuable analgesic properties. Aspirin and aspirin-containing preparations should not be given to children under the age of 16 years, as it has been associated with the development of encephalopathy (brain disease) and hepatitis (inflammation of the liver – Reye's syndrome)

> **Decongestant drops** may be helpful before a feed to allow an infant to breathe as well as to swallow

> ➤ **Antihistamines** may be useful in cases of allergy when the nasal mucosa is swollen, but they do not speed recovery. They cause drowsiness, which may be annoying in older children

> ➤ **Antitussive medicines** to suppress coughing are of possible value if the household has been disturbed all night or the child is distressed

> ➤ **Antibiotics** are not usually necessary as most infections are viral. They are of value only when there is evidence of bacterial infection, such as streptococcal throat infection or in some cases of associated acute otitis media

Activity

➤ Investigate the advice available to parents or carers of a child with an URTI.

Resources

British National Formulary – www.bnf.org/.

NHS Direct – www.nhsdirect.nhs.uk/.

Acute otitis media and otitis media with effusion

Acute otitis media (AOM) is inflammation of the middle ear; it is a common childhood complaint. It typically leads to pain, raised temperature and discharge from the ear (otorrhoea); the child rubs the ear and is fretful and irritable. The middle ear is lined with respiratory mucosa and often becomes inflamed during an URTI. Purulent fluid collects in the middle ear causing the tympanic membrane (ear drum) to bulge and change in appearance. This increases pressure and causes pain. The tympanic membrane may perforate under pressure to release bloodstained mucopurulent discharge, which relieves pain and other symptoms.

Antibiotics should not be routinely prescribed for the initial treatment of AOM, although delayed treatment after 72 hours if the child's condition has not improved is another approach (Scottish Intercollegiate Guidelines Network, 2003). A short initial course of antibiotics, such as amoxicillin, may be beneficial for some groups of children, such as those under two years of age with severe disease. Pain-relieving drugs (paracetamol), which also reduce temperature, are useful. When frequent attacks of AOM occur, the child should be referred to an otolaryngologist (ear and throat specialist) (Scottish Intercollegiate Guidelines Network, 2003).

Otitis media with effusion (OME), often known as 'glue ear', is the term used to describe inflammation accompanied by the collection of viscous fluid within the middle ear. OME, which usually resolves spontaneously, should not be treated with antibiotics (Scottish Intercollegiate Guidelines Network, 2003). Some groups of children with OME should be carefully monitored so that hearing loss and problems with speech and language developmental delay, behavioural problems and difficulties at school can be detected. Referral to an otolaryngologist is required if problems occur. In some cases, the fluid is aspirated from the middle ear and grommets (plastic aeration tubes) inserted through the tympanic membrane into the middle ear.

Croup

Croup (laryngeal spasm) is a feature of viral infection involving the larynx and trachea. The child initially develops a snuffly nose, inspiration then becoming noisy and sounding harsh (stridor). This is distressing for the child and frightening for the parents/carers. Treatment traditionally involved the use of steam to liquefy secretions and relieve obstruction, the modern alternative being a steamy bathroom. Most children recover without treatment, but croup remains a worrying condition because:

- Children occasionally develop airway obstruction and exhaustion, and thus require emergency admission to ensure that the airway remains patent
- Rarely, acute epiglottitis supervenes, emergency treatment being essential. This is usually caused by bacteria such as *Haemophilus influenzae*
- Children occasionally experience repeated attacks of croup, suggesting allergy.

Respiratory syncytial virus

Respiratory syncytial virus (RSV) is a virus responsible for acute respiratory infection in infants and young children, often severe in babies under the age of six months. Bronchiolitis (inflammation of the bronchioles) and pneumonia may result, and death is not uncommon. In older children, RSV infection is usually milder. By the age of four years, most children show serological evidence of previous infection, but this does not necessarily result in lasting immunity. Outbreaks of RSV have been documented in the community and may occur in hospital, especially among very sick children, contributing to morbidity and mortality. Virus particles are present in nasal secretions, nosocomial spread being via the hands. This is supported by the results of a study in which the incidence of RSV declined after a strict handwashing regimen was introduced among staff and parents (Isaacs et al., 1991).

Pertussis

Pertussis (whooping cough) is caused by a small Gram-negative bacterium called *Bordetella pertussis*. Following exposure to a source of infection, the bacteria become attached to ciliated cells lining the respiratory mucosa. Nonspecific symptoms without the typical cough develop within 5–7 days. The child appears to have a cold but is highly infectious, releasing a large number of bacteria from the nasopharynx. Finally, the infection enters the paroxysmal phase, characterized by coughing that ends in 'whoop' and/or vomiting. However, the presentation varies and may be a persistent cough alone. Pertussis is particularly severe in infants under six months of age (Bedford and Elliman, 2006). Vaccination is an important public health measure in the control of this frightening and unpleasant infection, which can in severe cases be life-threatening. The bacteria are never carried in a healthy throat (Weiss and Hewlett, 1986).

Diphtheria

Diphtheria is caused by the Gram-positive bacillus *Corynebacterium diphtheriae*. It is a very rare infection in the UK, but travellers to Eastern Europe, countries of the former Soviet Union and areas in the developing world may be exposed to the organism. The disease results in an acute respiratory illness characterized by the formation of a tenacious 'membrane' (consisting of white blood cells, bacteria and respiratory epithelium) within the upper respiratory tract. This membrane can cause laryngeal obstruction, leading to death without emergency treatment, such as a tracheostomy, to maintain a patent airway. *Corynebacterium diphtheriae* also produces an exotoxin that circulates in the blood to cause complications such as myocarditis and peripheral neuropathy.

The management of patients and contacts with diphtheria includes:

- Informing the proper officer of the relevant public health authority, as diphtheria is a notifiable disease
- Case isolation
- PPE – gloves, aprons and masks – for staff and visitors
- Treating the patient with penicillin and diphtheria antitoxin
- Treating contacts with erythromycin and immunizing them with diphtheria toxoid
- Meticulous attention to oral hygiene and pain relief
- Monitoring vital signs, especially respiration. Cardiac monitoring should be undertaken if myocardial involvement is suspected.

It is important to stress that active immunization against diphtheria, administered during childhood, is very effective. Others who may need immunization include contacts of a case of diphtheria, healthcare workers, laboratory staff and those who travel to countries where the disease is endemic.

Influenza

RNA viruses belonging to the family of orthomyxoviruses, which have an affinity for mucoproteins present on the surface of human and other mammalian cells, cause influenza. There are three types of influenza virus: A, B and C. The surface of each type is coated with a number of specific antigens (V, H and N) to which the host responds by secreting the corresponding antibody. Standard nomenclature is employed to classify the different strains according to their surface antigens.

Influenza is transmitted via infected nasopharyngeal secretions, resulting in an acute illness with fever, headache, anorexia, myalgia and profound malaise, although (contrary to popular belief) relatively minor respiratory symptoms. The antiviral drugs oseltamivir and zanamivir are used within 48 hours of the onset of symptoms to shorten the duration of symptoms for specified groups. For post-exposure prophylaxis in specified groups and for use in influenza epidemics (see Further Reading). Severe colds are sometimes erroneously labelled 'flu' by sufferers. In young people, influenza is an unpleasant, debilitating illness, disrupting work or school. The consequences can be grave for older adults or those in poor health (Riley and Riley, 2003). Pneumonia may supervene. This is usually attributed to colonization of the traumatized respiratory epithelium by potential pathogens (*Staphylococcus aureus* and *Haemophilus influenzae*), but in some cases the virus itself may be responsible.

Influenza viruses are widespread throughout the world, producing epidemics every few years. Spread across the community is most common for type A, which is the most virulent (Grist, 1989), type C being least likely to cause epidemics. World-wide pandemics have been recorded but are difficult to predict. In 1918, 20 million people – including young adults – died from influenza. More recently, the pandemic of Asian flu resulted in a high incidence of infection but a lower rate of mortality. Most major outbreaks represent the emergence of new variants of influenza virus with different surface antigens (antigenic drift). This is most marked with type A. The population has no immunity against the new antigens so infection becomes rife. The existence of the three different strains of the virus (A, B and C), the differences in the surface antigens displayed by members of the same strain and the phenomenon of antigenic drift contribute to the difficulties of controlling influenza. No single vaccine will give lasting immunity. Instead, annual vaccination is necessary as each new strain emerges. Immunizing those over 65 reduces the rate of influenza-related hospital admissions (Riley and Riley, 2003). At-risk groups benefiting from immunization include all those over 65 years of age and those:

- Over six months of age who have:
  - chronic respiratory disease including asthma who require use of a nebulizers
  - chronic heart disease
  - chronic renal disease
  - diabetes requiring insulin or hypoglycaemic drugs
  - immunosuppressive conditions
- Living in long-stay facilities (see below)
- NHS staff who deal with or support patients/clients and social service care staff (Department of Health, 2007).

PRACTICE APPLICATION 9.4

Protecting Care Home Residents against Flu

Residents in care homes and other long-stay facilities benefit from an annual influenza vaccination. Hayward et al. (2006) conducted a study to determine whether or not the vaccination of staff is also beneficial for residents.

Activity

➤ Access the article by Hayward et al. (2006). Consider their findings and discuss them with your mentor.

➤ If you work in a care home:
  ➤ are carers and other staff offered flu vaccination?
  ➤ are residents routinely vaccinated against flu?

Uptake of the vaccine is usually high (Health Protection Agency, 2006). The influenza vaccine, prepared from inactivated, highly purified viruses, is cheap and safe with few side-effects (Govaert and Dinant, 1993).

Most offers of immunization are made within the primary care setting, and most people who accept request it the following year. Practice nurses are in a key position to run immunization clinics, maintain registers of people at risk and liaise with practice managers so that reminders and repeat prescriptions are issued. The failure of susceptible people to accept vaccination is serious because it leads to increased mortality, although many deaths will not be directly attributed to the influenza itself. Outbreaks are expensive because a large number of patients are admitted to hospital over a short period of time and normal services are disrupted (Grist, 1989).

Avian influenza

Avian influenza ('bird flu') is a highly contagious disease of birds caused by influenza A viruses (Campbell, 2006). In birds it can present as a mild illness with low mortality to a highly contagious disease with nearly 100 per cent mortality rate. The bird flu that has recently affected wild birds, poultry and some people is the highly pathogenic strain H5N1. It is a threat because the virus can remain viable in bird droppings for long periods and is able to spread among birds and from birds to other animals through ingestion and inhalation. Migratory birds often carry H5N1 without symptoms but domestic flocks of poultry appear especially susceptible to rapid, fatal epidemics. The widespread occurrence of H5N1 has prompted concern that it might give rise to a new human influenza illness with pandemic potential, although so far it appears to have infected only people having close contact with birds. However, once established in a human population, the virus could spread rapidly and there is at present little available to prevent this because effective vaccines and antiviral drugs are presently in low supply. A global strategy for tackling avian flu has been recommended because it is a highly pathogenic condition that has the potential to spread rapidly across countries and continents, disrupting the lives of millions of people, threatening regional and international trade depending on the poultry industry and outstripping the health resources of any individual country. As well as a global strategy, the World Health Organization (2005) has recommended that all countries develop a national strategy to control avian influenza. In the UK, the Department of Health (2005) has responded by developing a contingency plan to minimize the spread of the new virus, provide treatment, cope with the eventuality of large numbers of people falling ill and dying and reduce its impact on the health and social services and its economic consequences. Drugs having the greatest potential for treatment are oseltamivir and zanamivir.

SELF-ASSESSMENT

I. Which of the following operate as respiratory pathogens?

(a) staphylococci
(b) rhinoviruses
(c) Gram-negative bacteria
(d) all of these

2. Bacterial community-acquired pneumonia is most frequently caused by *Streptococcus pneumoniae*. True? or False?

3. Pneumonia accounts for 13.9 per cent of HCAIs in acute hospitals. True? or False?

4. Which groups of patients in hospital are most likely to develop pneumonia?

5. Name five sources of pathogens for hospital-acquired pneumonia.

6. A pyrexial child with an upper respiratory tract infection may benefit from which of the following?

   (a) two paracetamol tablets
   (b) an antitussive
   (c) aspirin
   (d) paracetamol dose calculated on body weight

7. The pathogen responsible for whooping cough is *Haemophilus influenzae*? True? or False?

8. Which groups of people should be offered an annual influenza vaccination?

REFERENCES

Bedford H and Elliman D (2006) Prevention, diagnosis and management of pertussis. *Nursing Times* 102(46): 42–4.

Bedford H and Lane L (2006) Pneumococcal vaccination and the new child vaccination schedule. *Nursing Times* 102(39): 44–5.

Botman A and de Krieger RA (1987) Contamination of small volume medication nebulisers and its association with oropharyngeal colonisation. *Journal of Hospital Infection* 10: 204–8.

Campbell S (2006) Avian influenza. Are you prepared? *Nursing Standard* 21(5): 51–6.

Cobben NA, Drent M, Jonkers EF et al. (1996) Outbreak of severe *Pseudomonas aeruginosa* respiratory infections due to contaminated nebulisers. *Journal of Hospital Infection* 33: 63–70.

Craven DE, Connolly M, Lichtenberg G et al. (1982) Contamination of mechanical ventilator tubing changes every 24 or 48 hours. *New England Journal of Medicine* 306: 1505–8.

Craven DE, Goularte TA and Make BJ (1984) Contaminated condensate in mechanical ventilator circuits: a risk factor for nosocomial pneumonia? *American Review of Respiratory Diseases* 129: 625–8.

Craven DE, Kunches LM, Kilinsky V et al. (1986) Risk factors for pneumonia and fatality for patients receiving continuous mechanical ventilation. *American Review of Respiratory Diseases* 133: 792–6.

Department of Health (DH) (2005) *Pandemic Flu. Key Facts*. Available www.dh.gov.uk.

Department of Health (DH) (2007) *Summary of Flu Immunisation Policy.* Available www. dh.gov.uk.

Fiorentini A (1992) Potential hazards of tracheobronchial suctioning. *Intensive Critical Care Nursing* **8**: 217–26.

Gorman LJ, Sanai L, Notman W et al. (1993) Cross-infection in an intensive care unit by *Klebsiella pneumoniae* from ventilator condensate. *Journal of Hospital Infection* **23**: 17–26.

Govaert TM and Dinant GJ (1993) Adverse reactions to influenza vaccine in elderly people: randomised double blind placebo trial. *British Medical Journal* **307**: 988–99.

Grist N (1989) Influenza update. *Practitioner* **233**: 56–9.

Gwaltney JM, Moskalski PB and Hendley JO (1978) Hand to hand transmission of rhinovirus colds. *Annals of Internal Medicine* **88**: 463–7.

Hayward A, Harling R, Wetten S et al. (2006) Effectiveness of an influenza vaccine programme for care home staff to prevent death, morbidity, and health service use among residents: cluster randomised controlled trial. *British Medical Journal* **333**: 1241.

Health Protection Agency (HPA) (2006) *Seasonal Influenza.* Available www.hpa.org.uk.

Hendley JO, Wenzel RP and Gwaltney JM (1973) Transmission of rhinovirus colds by self-inoculation. *New England Journal of Medicine* **291**: 1361–4.

Hospital Infection Society/Infection Control Nurses Association (2007) *Summary of Preliminary Results of The Third Prevalence Survey of Healthcare Associated Infections in Acute Hospitals* (for England) (2006). Available www.his.org.uk/.

Inglis TJ, Sproat LJ, Hawkey PM et al. (1993) Staphylococcal pneumonia in ventilated patients: a twelve month review of cases in an intensive care unit. *Journal of Hospital Infection* **25**: 207–10.

Isaacs D, Dickson H, O'Callaghan C et al. (1991) Handwashing and cohorting in prevention of hospital acquired respiratory syncitial virus. *Archives of Disease in Childhood* **66**: 227–31.

Johanson WG, Pierce AK and Sandford JP (1972) Nosocomial respiratory tract infections with Gram-negative bacilli. *Annals of Internal Medicine* **77**: 701–14.

Kelleghan SI, Salemi C, Padilla S et al. (1993) An effective continuous quality improvement approach to the prevention of ventilator-associated pneumonia. *American Journal of Infection Control* **21**: 322–30.

Koeman M, van der Ven AJ, Ramsay G et al. (2001) Ventilator-associated pneumonia: recent issues on pathogenesis, prevention and diagnosis. *Journal of Hospital Infection* **49**: 155–62.

Lindeman CA and Van Aernan B (1971) Effects of structured and unstructured pre-operative teaching. *Nursing Research* **20**: 319–32.

National Institute for Health and Clinical Excellence (NICE) in collaboration with the National Patient Safety Agency (NPSA) (2007) *Prevention of Ventilator-associated Pneumonia: Consultation.* Available www.nice.org.uk.

Nicholson KG, Kent J, Hammersley V et al. (1996) Risk factors for lower respiratory complications of rhinovirus infections in elderly people living in the community. *British Medical Journal* **313**: 119–23.

Phillips I (1967) *Pseudomonas aeruginosa* respiratory tract infections in patients receiving mechanical ventilation. *Journal of Hygiene* **65**: 229–35.

Riley C and Riley S (2003) Influenza and pneumococcal disease in the community. *Nursing Standard* **18**(4): 45–51.

Sanderson PJ (1983) Colonisation of the trachea in ventilated patients: what is the bacterial pathway? *Journal of Hospital Infection* **4**: 15–18.

Scottish Intercollegiate Guidelines Network (SIGN) (2003) *Diagnosis and Management of Childhood Otitis Media in Primary Care.* Available www.sign.ac.uk/pdf/sign66.pdf.

Stucke VA and Thompson REM (1980) Infection transfer by respiratory condensate during positive pressure respiration. *Nursing Times* (Infection Control Supplement) **76**(7): s3–s7.

Taylor B (1988) Coughs and colds in children. *Health Visitor* **612**: 313–15.

Weiss AA and Hewlett EL (1986) Virulence factors of *Bordetella pertussis*. *Annual Review of Microbiology* **40**: 661–86.

World Health Organization (WHO) (2005) *WHO Checklist: Influenza Pandemic Preparedness Planning.* WHO, Geneva.

FURTHER READING AND INFORMATION SOURCES

Department of Health (DH) (2007) *Bird Flu and Pandemic Influenza: What are the Risks?* Available www.dh.gov.uk.

Jefferson T, Foxlee R, Del Mar C et al. (2008) Physical interventions to interrupt or reduce the spread of respiratory viruses: systematic review. *British Medical Journal* **336**: 77–80.

National Institute for Health and Clinical Excellence (NICE) (2003) *Flu Prevention – Amantadine and Oseltamivir.* Technical appraisal TA67. Available www.nice.org.uk.

CHAPTER 10

Infections associated with intravascular devices

CHAPTER OUTCOMES

After reading this chapter, you should be able to:

➤ Identify and discuss the portals of entry and sources of infection associated with intravascular devices

➤ Define the terms 'bacteraemia', 'phlebitis', 'septicaemia' and 'systemic inflammatory response syndrome'

➤ List the factors that place patients/residents at risk of developing sepsis related to the presence of an intravascular device

➤ Explain how the risk of infection may be reduced for patients/residents with intravascular devices

Introduction

Intravascular devices are used extensively in hospital and increasingly in community settings. In hospital, 60 per cent of patients require cannulation (Lavery and Ingram, 2006). Intravenous lines are inserted to:

- provide intravenous access
- deliver medication, fluids, blood or nutrients
- enable haemodynamic monitoring including central venous pressure and other measurements
- allow frequent blood sampling.

Their insertion is an invasive procedure, breaching the skin, which is the body's primary defence against infection. Pathogenic invasion is possible from a number of sites and sources (Figure 10.1). Many infections result from microorganisms on the person's skin gaining access extraluminally (between the vein and the cannula) from the insertion point, or intraluminally (within the lumen of the cannula) following contamination of the hubs or stopcock (Elliott et al., 1995).

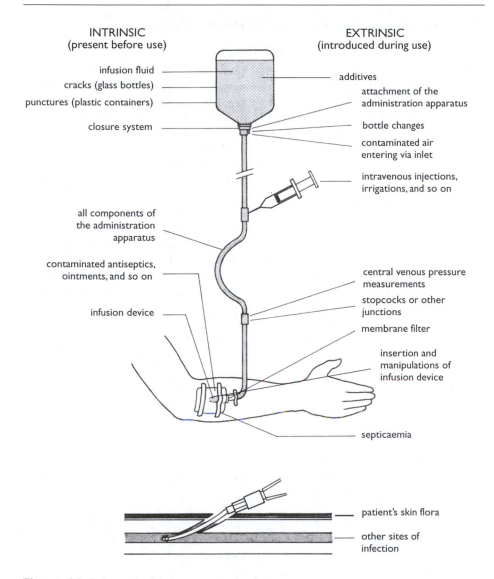

INTRINSIC
(present before use)

EXTRINSIC
(introduced during use)

infusion fluid

cracks (glass bottles)

punctures (plastic containers)

closure system

all components of
the administration
apparatus

contaminated antiseptics,
ointments, and so on

infusion device

additives

attachment of the
administration apparatus

bottle changes

contaminated air
entering via inlet

intravenous injections,
irrigations, and so on

central venous pressure
measurements

stopcocks or other
junctions

membrane filter

insertion and
manipulations of
infusion device

septicaemia

patient's skin flora

other sites of
infection

Figure 10.1 Intravascular therapy: portals of entry

Voluntary surveillance of morbidity and mortality from sepsis arising as a complication of intravascular devices by the Public Health Laboratory Service (now Health Protection Agency) indicated an increase of 39 per cent between 1989 and 1991 (Elliott, 1993). Waghorn (1994), recording data collected in a district general hospital, listed 39 episodes of sepsis associated with intravascular devices over a two-year period, including six fatalities. The rapid increase in the number of bacteraemias due to meticillin-resistant *Staphylococcus aureus* (MRSA) throughout the 1990s led to the introduction of mandatory surveillance in 2001 (Duerden, 2007).

Infections associated with intravascular devices

Infection may be associated with peripherally sited intravenous cannulae and with central venous access devices (CVADs). The risk of sepsis is increased when new techniques are introduced and the experience of staff is limited, particularly when infection prevention and control protocols are being developed. The introduction of intravascular volume control sets was initially associated with a poor level of maintenance, evidence being seen of leakage, dirty injection ports and breaches in asepsis during handling (Dumas et al., 1971). A later study recorded lower infection rates explained through the introduction of newer, less easily contaminated equipment and strict protocols for asepsis (Leroy et al., 1989). Infection showed a definite association with breaches in asepsis in all these studies, with clear links to poor hand hygiene. Protocols for managing intravascular devices differ between centres, contributing to the variation in infection rate that has been recorded (Nyström et al., 1983). There are guidelines for the insertion and care of some types of intravascular devices in the UK (Pratt et al., 2007), but auditing to identify problems remains important (Elliot, 1993; Elliot et al., 1995). Another factor contributing to the disparity in sepsis rate is the lack of consensus regarding the criteria accepted as evidence of infection. Authors employ different definitions so comparisons between findings are not meaningful (see below). Clinically suspected intravascular catheter-related sepsis is defined as persistent pyrexia (of more than 38.5 °C) returning to normal when the device is removed (Haddock et al., 1983). Most authorities believe that the device should only be considered responsible for the infection in the absence of any other explanation for the patient's symptoms.

INFORMATION BOX 10.1

Definitions of intravascular-associated infection

➤   Colonization of the catheter (Maki and Ringer, 1987)

➤   Phlebitis (Tager et al., 1983)

➤   Septicaemia (Ricard et al., 1985)

➤   Culture of a newly withdrawn intravascular line (Maki et al., 1977). Infection is considered to be present if 15 or more bacteria are isolated, allowing for accidental contamination during removal

---

Bacterial colonization and infection of intravascular devices

The first step towards infection is colonization of the catheter (Cercenado et al., 1990). The organisms responsible are often those growing at the site of insertion. Bacteria and proteins adhere to the surface of the catheter, forming a biofilm (Chapter 7). As the biofilm develops, the organisms become incorporated into it and are protected. They multiply, eventually reaching a sufficient number to cause infection. The biofilm further protects the bacteria by offering mechanical protection from antibiotics so infection (once established) is more difficult to treat unless the device is removed.

Bacteria forming part of the normal skin flora, especially the coagulase-negative *Staphylococcus epidermidis*, cause most colonization and infection associated with intravascular devices. This originates from the patient's skin or from staff handling the device (Maki and Ringer, 1987). It colonizes plastic more easily than other bacteria through its ability to adhere to plastic surfaces (Pascual et al., 1993). However, Gram-negative opportunists cause a significant number of intravascular infections (Vázquez et al., 1994). Other microorganisms, including *Staphylococcus aureus* and the fungus *Candida albicans*, are also important causes of intravascular catheter-associated infection.

Presentation of infection associated with intravascular cannulation

Infection associated with intravascular cannulation may present in a variety of forms:

- localized cutaneous infection
- phlebitis
- bacteraemia and septicaemia.

Localized cutaneous infection

Localized cutaneous infection may develop at the point where the cannula enters the skin. It is characterized by the signs of inflammation, which include localized erythema (redness) and heat.

Phlebitis

Phlebitis (inflammation of the vein), the most common complication associated with intravascular therapy, usually results from chemical or mechanical irritation. The main predisposing factors are the infusion of hypertonic (higher osmotic pressure than body fluids) solutions and the presence of particulate matter derived from incompletely reconstituted drugs, fragments of rubber or glass from vials and plastic from the cannula. Erythema develops proximal to the site of venepuncture, with pain. Bacteria are seldom responsible for phlebitis, but septicaemia is more common in patients who have developed it (Francombe, 1988).

Bacteraemia and septicaemia

Bacteraemia (the presence of bacteria in the blood, also called bloodstream infection) may be transient or may lead to septicaemia and overwhelming sepsis. Bacteraemia caused by MRSA is most commonly linked with the presence of invasive devices such as peripherally sited intravenous cannulae and CVADs (Health Protection Agency, 2007).

Septicaemia (multiplication of bacteria in the blood) produces the signs and symptoms of infection – fever and rigors. Intravascular devices are not the only cause of bacteraemia and septicaemia, but in hospital they are the most common source. Bacteraemia and septicaemia are very serious and can lead to overwhelming sepsis and life-threatening systemic inflammatory response syndrome (SIRS) (see below).

INFORMATION BOX 10.2

Systemic inflammatory response syndrome

SIRS describes a condition characterized by:

➤ abnormal white blood cell count ($< 4.0 \times 10^9/l$ or $> 12 \times 10^9/l$ or 10 per cent immature neutrophils)

➤ abnormal body temperature

➤ increased heart rate (tachycardia)

➤ increased respiratory rate (tachypnoea).

Overwhelming sepsis is one trigger for SIRS, as are major trauma, severe haemorrhage, acute pancreatitis (inflammation of the pancreas), conditions that result in poor tissue perfusion and so on (Adams, 2003).

SIRS occurs when inflammatory mediators are released into the blood leading to an abnormal response with widespread effects and damage. It occurs in critically ill patients and is associated with multiple organ dysfunction syndrome (MODS) including kidney failure, abnormal blood coagulation (disseminated intravascular coagulation – DIC), acute respiratory distress syndrome (ARDS) and gastrointestinal failure.

Risk factors associated with intravascular infection

The risk factors include:

■ the patient's condition
■ the length of time the device is in situ
■ the presence of phlebitis
■ the material and type of device.

Patient's condition

The risk of infection is highest among immunocompromised individuals, the group most likely to require intravascular therapy for parenteral nutrition and to administer drugs (such as antibiotics and cytotoxic therapy).

Length of time the device remains in situ

The longer the device (cannula or catheter) remains in place, the greater the risk of biofilm formation, colonization and infection (Clarke and Raffin, 1990).

Presence of phlebitis

Phlebitis, whether from chemical or mechanical irritation of the blood vessel, predisposes to infection. Measures aimed at reducing the incidence of phlebitis are outlined below.

PRACTICE APPLICATION 10.1

Reducing the Incidence of Phlebitis

Staff education

➤ Increase staff awareness of infection prevention and control protocols in relation to intravascular devices and provide regular updates.

➤ Include education about intravascular devices in pre-registration courses.

Duration of intravascular cannulation

➤ Keep an accurate record of the date of cannula insertion in the nursing notes. The Nursing and Midwifery Council (2007) guidelines stress the importance of good record keeping in protecting the welfare of patients/clients.

➤ Many studies and most specialists advocate the routine rotation of the cannula site every 48–72 hours, although an audit study by Stonehouse and Butcher (1996) found no correlation between the length of time the cannula remained in situ and phlebitis.

➤ Cannulae should be replaced whenever signs of phlebitis are observed.

Recognizing the problem

➤ Observe the site for signs of phlebitis at least once a day, and check the site prior to nursing interventions involving the cannula or intravenous infusion, for example intravenous injection.

➤ Grade signs of phlebitis using a recognized scale.

➤ Audit the incidence of phlebitis.

Expert teams

➤ Where one exists, use the specialist cannulation team.

➤ Consult the infection prevention and control team.

Mechanical problems: trauma and irritation

➤ Use the smallest cannula appropriate for the situation.

➤ Secure the cannula properly to avoid movement.

➤ Select the insertion site carefully: some sites may cause discomfort or be inconvenient.

➤ Select cannulae made from material least likely to cause trauma.

Chemical problems

➤ Ensure that no hypertonic fluids are infused via a peripheral vein.

➤ Make sure that drugs for intravenous injection are prepared and administered correctly to avoid the possibility of problems caused by undissolved residues and changes in pH.

Filtration of particulate material

➤ Consider the use of filters to minimize the effects of particulate matter such as drug residues, rubber, plastic, glass and microorganisms.

Problems of infection

➤ Use an aseptic technique during insertion of the cannula and any other dealings with the cannula or infusion.

➤ Clean the site prior to insertion of the cannula.

➤ Cover the insertion site with a well-secured dressing.

➤ Decontaminate or wash the hands before and after dealing with the cannula or infusion.

➤ Check the infusion fluid for signs of contamination, for example deterioration, colour change or damage to the container.

➤ Check the expiry date of the infusion fluid.

➤ Flush the cannula with heparin or sodium chloride (according to local protocols) to help to prevent blockage and subsequent bacterial colonization of the device.

The material and type of device

The material used in the manufacture of the device influences the incidence of infection. Teflon and Silastic catheters resist bacterial adherence and colonization better than other plastics (Toltzis and Goldmann, 1990). Various different types of intravascular device carry different levels of risk (see below).

Trials are taking place to establish whether new types of intravenous devices made of new materials can help to reduce the rates of colonization and bacteraemia. However, the most important factors appear to be the way the insertion site is managed, including dressing changes and adherence to infection prevention protocols, rather than the type of device (Moretti et al., 2005).

Types of intravascular device

The earliest single-use peripheral intravascular devices, introduced in 1945, were made of plastic. They were superseded in 1950 by newer designs in which a plastic catheter covered a steel needle. In a modified form, these models are still used to establish short-term venous access, but single and multilumen catheters are now available. These have revolutionized the care of patients/clients undergoing long-term nutritional and intravascular therapy, improving treatment prospects and quality of life by removing the need for difficult and repeated venepuncture. The most familiar examples include:

■ **Broviac catheters** (Broviac et al., 1973) – these consist of a narrow silicone rubber catheter 'tunnelled' subcutaneously between the point of insertion into the skin and entry into a central vein via a Dacron cuff. Tissue grows up into the cuff, securing the catheter into position. This helps to prevent bacterial invasion. The site heals within approximately 10 days of insertion. Dressings are no longer necessary.

■ **Hickman catheters** (Hickman et al., 1979) – the catheter bore is wider, as this model is intended for the administration of blood products and can be used for patients undergoing bone marrow transplantation (Figure 10.2).

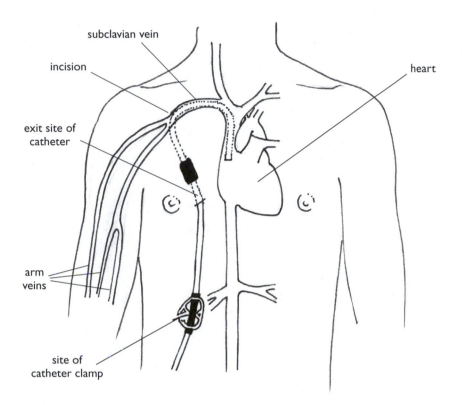

Figure 10.2 A Hickman catheter: position and insertion

CVADs and arterial catheters have been associated with a higher rate of sepsis than peripheral lines (Nyström et al., 1983; Waghorn, 1994). However, complications appear to be less problematic when allowance is made for the extended time they remain in situ compared with peripheral lines, and the high risk of infection seen in immunocompromised patients, who are most likely to use them (Decker and Edwards, 1988). There is no evidence that subcutaneously 'tunnelled' subclavian catheters reduce the incidence of sepsis arising through contamination of the skin–catheter junction, especially when highly trained staff are responsible for care (Keohane et al., 1983).

Prevention of infection associated with intravascular devices

Infection prevention and control protocols should include guidelines for insertion and subsequent management of intravascular devices. An opportunity to consider the recent guidelines for preventing infections associated with CVADs is provided below.

┌───┐

━━ PRACTICE APPLICATION 10.2 ━━

CVADs: Preventing Associated Infection

Access the evidence-based guidelines by Pratt et al. (2007) and locate the section dealing with CVADs (pp. 33–49).

Activity

➤ Select one of the nine intervention categories, for example 'General asepsis', and discuss the guidelines and the strength of evidence with your mentor, or a member of the infection prevention and control team.

➤ Compare the guideline for the intervention category chosen with the protocol in your placement/workplace.

└───┘

Insertion of the intravascular catheter

A strict aseptic technique is required to reduce the risk of transferring bacteria from the skin of the patient or health professional into the blood vessel. Pratt et al. (2007) stress the importance of skin cleansing/antisepsis before the intravascular catheter is inserted; the guideline recommends the use of alcoholic chlorhexidine solution (2 per cent chlorhexidine in 70 per cent alcohol). The hands should be decontaminated immediately before the catheter is introduced. Sterile gloves, gowns and drapes should be used during the insertion of CVADs as this has been shown to reduce the infection rate (Raad et al., 1993); this is easier to ensure if the insertion is performed in theatre. Once in situ, the catheter should be secured with sterile tape rather than sutured, in order to avoid traction. Traction could carry any bacteria present deeper into the wound or result in mechanical trauma, increasing the risk of non-bacterial phlebitis (Maki et al., 1973). The insertion site should be covered with an appropriate water vapour-permeable dressing (Pratt et al., 2007).

Shaving the site should be avoided if possible. It causes skin damage, increasing the number of microorganisms present and therefore the risk of infection (Cruse and Foord, 1980).

Maintaining the intravascular system

Proper maintenance of the intravascular system is vital in preventing infection. This includes:

- hand hygiene
- skin cleansing at dressing change
- dressing selection
- checks for contamination of the infusion fluid
- use of filters
- access to an intravascular therapy team.

Readers are directed to Pratt et al. (2007) for comprehensive guidelines covering all aspects of maintaining CVADs.

Hand hygiene

Hand hygiene is essential to reduce cross-infection. The hands should be decontaminated before intravascular lines are accessed and connections should only be manipulated with gloved hands.

Skin cleansing at dressing change

Skin cleansing with 2 per cent chlorhexidine in 70 per cent alcohol solution around the insertion site at each dressing change is recommended (Pratt et al., 2007). An aqueous (water-based) solution of chlorhexidine may be necessary if the device could be damaged by alcohol. The use of chlorhexidine reduces infection more effectively than cleansing with povidone iodine or 70 per cent alcohol (Maki et al., 1991). This is not surprising as the bacteria responsible for the infections associated with intravascular devices are often those normally present on the skin, especially *Staphylococcus epidermidis,* a Gram-positive coccus that chlorhexidine continues to destroy some time after its application.

Dressing selection

A sterile dressing that is permeable to water vapour while preventing the passage of microorganisms is commonly used to protect the insertion site. The use of a transparent dressing permits inspection of the insertion site and the early detection of infection or other problems. Occlusive dressings that trap moisture on the skin should not be used as this encourages the growth of skin commensals, thus increasing the risk of infection. Sterile gauze and tape dressings will be appropriate in some situations, such as when blood is seeping from the site. There is some evidence that transparent dressings have no advantage over sterile gauze changed at regular intervals (Ricard et al., 1985; Maki and Ringer, 1987). Gauze dressings do have disadvantages, however; patients cannot shower/bathe, site observation is only possible at dressing change and the dressing must be changed more frequently.

Checks for contamination of infusion fluids

The contamination of intravascular infusion fluids, although responsible for a number of outbreaks during the 1970s, is now a rare cause of sepsis because of the introduction of strict quality control during commercial preparation. Problems may still arise when fluids intended for parenteral administration are prepared on hospital premises without these high standards (Frean et al., 1994). Before the bag is changed, the healthcare practitioner should check that it has not reached the expiry date, the bag is patent and the fluid is clear. With contamination, the contents appear cloudy.

Use of filters

Filters positioned intraluminally between the intravenous cannula and fluid adminis-tration set reduce the risk of phlebitis and prevent bacteria gaining access to the vein (Francombe, 1988). They are particularly valuable when the administration set will be manipulated frequently but are not suitable for use with blood, blood products, lipid (fat) emulsions or with catheters used for haemodynamic monitoring.

Access to an intravascular therapy team

Access to the services of a multidisciplinary intravascular therapy team is considered to be of key importance, especially in conjunction with CVADs. Keohane et al. (1983) reported a reduction in phlebitis from 25 per cent to 4 per cent when the team incorporated a specialist nutrition nurse attending to patients undergoing parenteral therapy.

▮ SELF-ASSESSMENT ▮

1. List four intrinsic and four extrinsic sites and sources of pathogenic invasion causing intravascular infection.

2. Phlebitis is usually a complication of bacterial infection. True? or False?

3. Define bacteraemia.

4. Research evidence suggests that the infection rate is invariably higher when a CVAD is used. True? or False?

5. Which antiseptic is recommended for skin cleansing/antisepsis prior to the insertion of a CVAD?

▮ REFERENCES ▮

Adams S (2003) Shock, systemic inflammatory response and multiple organ dysfunction. In C Brooker and M Nicol (eds) *Nursing Adults: The Practice of Caring.* Mosby, Edinburgh.

Broviac JW, Cole JJ and Scribner BH (1973) A silicone rubber atrial catheter for prolonged parenteral alimentation. *Surgery, Gynecology and Obstetrics* **136**: 602–6.

Cercenado E, Javier E and Rodriguez M (1990) A conservative procedure for the diagnosis of catheter-related infections. *Archives of Internal Medicine* **150**: 1417–20.

Clarke DE and Raffin TA (1990) Infectious complications of indwelling long-term central venous catheters. *Chest* **97**: 966–72.

Cruse PJ and Foord R (1980) The epidemiology of wound infection: a 10 year prospective study of 62,939 wounds. *Surgical Clinics of North America* **60**: 27–40.

Decker MD and Edwards KM (1988) Central venous catheter infectious. *Paediatric Nursing Clinics of North America* **14**: 503–9.

Duerden B (2007) Bloodstream infections and their control. *Nursing Times* **103**(46): supplement Clean, Safe Care. Reducing Healthcare-associated infection, pp 6–7.

Dumas RJ, Warner JF and Dalton MP (1971) Septicaemia from intravascular infusions. *New England Journal of Medicine* **284**: 257–60.

Elliott TS (1993) Line-associated bacteraemias. *Public Health Laboratory Service CDR* 3 R: 91–6.

Elliott TS, Faroqui MH, Tebbs SE et al. (1995) An audit programme for central venous catheter-associated infections. *Journal of Hospital Infection* **30**: 181–91.

Francombe P (1988) Intravascular filters and phlebitis. *Nursing Times* **29**(84): 34–5.

Frean JA, Arntzen L, Rosekilly I et al. (1994) Investigation of parenteral nutrition fluids associated with an outbreak of *Serratia odorifera* septicaemia. *Journal of Hospital Infection* **27**: 263–73.

Haddock G, Barr J, Burns HJ et al. (1983) Reduction of central venous catheter complications. *British Journal of Parenteral Therapy* **3**: 124–8.

Health Protection Agency (HPA) with National Statistics (2007) *National Confidential Study of Deaths Following Meticillin Resistant Staphylococcus aureus (MRSA) Infection.* Available www.hpa.org.uk/.

Hickman RO, Bruckner CD, Clift RA et al. (1979) A modified right atrial catheter for access to the venous system on marrow transplant recipients. *Surgery, Gynecology and Obstetrics* **148**: 871–5.

Keohane PP, Jones BJ, Attrill H et al. (1983) Effect of catheter tunnelling and a nutrition nurse on catheter sepsis during parenteral nutrition. *Lancet* **2**: 1388–90.

Lavery I and Ingram P (2006) Prevention of infection in peripheral intravenous devices. *Nursing Standard* **20**(49): 49–56.

Leroy O, Billiau V, Beussart C et al. (1989) Nosocomial infection associated with long-term arterial cannulation. *Intensive Care Medicine* **15**: 241–5.

Maki DG and Ringer M (1987) Evaluation of dressing regimens for prevention of infection with peripheral intravenous catheters. Gauze, a transparent polyurethane dressing and an iodophor-transparent dressing. *Journal of the American Medical Association* **258**(17): 2396–403.

Maki DG, Goldman D and Rhame FS (1973) Infection control in intravascular therapy. *Annals of Internal Medicine* **79**: 867–87.

Maki DG, Ringer M and Alvardo CJ (1991) Prospective randomised trial of povidone, iodine, alcohol and chlorhexidine for prevention of infection associated with central venous and arterial catheters. *Lancet* **338**: 339–43.

Maki DG, Weise CE and Sarafin H (1977) A semi-quantitative culture method for identifying intravascular catheter-related infection. *New England Journal of Medicine* **296**: 1305–9.

Moretti EW, Ofstead CL, Kristy RM et al. (2005) Impact of central venous catheter type and methods on catheter-related colonization and bacteraemia. *Journal of Hospital Infection* **61**: 139–45.

Nursing and Midwifery Council (NMC) (2007) *A-Z Advice Sheet: NMC Record Keeping Guidance.* NMC, London. Available www.nmc-uk.org.

Nyström B, Larson OS, Dankert J et al. (1983) Bacteraemia in surgical patients with intravascular devices: a European multicentre incidence study. *Journal of Hospital Infection* **4**: 338–49.

Pascual A, Ramirez de Arellano E, Martinez-Martinez L et al. (1993) Effect of polyurethane catheters and bacterial biofilms on the *in vitro* activity of antimicrobials against *Staphylococcus epidermidis*. *Journal of Hospital Infection* **24**: 211–18.

Pratt RJ, Pellowe CM, Wilson JA et al. (2007) epic2: National evidence-based guidelines for preventing healthcare-associated infections in NHS hospitals in England. *Journal of Hospital Infection* **65** (Supplement 1): S1–S64. Available www.epic.tvu.ac.uk.

Raad II, Hohn DC and Gilbreath BJ (1993) Prevention of central catheter-related infections by using maximal sterile barrier precautions during insertion. *Infection Control and Hospital Epidemiology* **15**: 231–8.

Ricard P, Martin R and Marcoux A (1985) Protection of indwelling vascular catheters; incidence of bacterial contamination and catheter-related sepsis. *Critical Care Medicine* **13**: 542–3.

Stonehouse J and Butcher J (1996) Phlebitis associated with peripheral cannulae. *Professional Nurse* **12**(1): 51–4.

Tager IB, Ginsberg M, Ellis S et al. (1983) An epidemiological study of the risks associated with peripheral intravascular catheters. *American Journal of Epidemiology* **118**: 839–51.

Toltzis P and Goldmann DA (1990) Current issues in central venous catheter infection. *Annual Review of Medicine* **41**: 169–76.

Vázquez F, Mendoza MC, Villar MH et al. (1994) Survey of bacteraemia in a Spanish hospital over a decade. *Journal of Hospital Infection* **26**: 111–21.

Waghorn DJ (1994) Intravascular device-associated systemic infections: a 2 year analysis of cases in a district general hospital. *Journal of Hospital Infection* **28**: 91–102.

FURTHER READING AND INFORMATION SOURCES

Casey A and Elliott TS (2007) Infection risks associated with needleless intravenous devices. *Nursing Standard* **22**(11): 38–44.

Department of Health (DH) (2001) Guidelines for preventing infections associated with the insertion and maintenance of central venous catheters. *Journal of Hospital Infection* **47**: Supplement S47–S67.

Ingram P and Lavery I (2005) Peripheral intravenous therapy: key risks and implications for practice. *Nursing Standard* **19**(46): 55–64.

Lavery I and Ingram P (2005) Venepuncture: best practice. *Nursing Standard* **19**(49): 55–65.

Mermel LA, Farr BM, Sherertz RJ et al. (2001) (Infectious Diseases Society of America, American College of Critical Care Medicine, Society for Healthcare Epidemiology of America) Guidelines for the management of intravascular catheter-related infections. *Journal of Intravenous Nursing* **24**(3): 180–205.

Royal College of Nursing (RCN) (2005) *Standards for Infusion Therapy*. RCN, London.

CHAPTER 11

Enteric infection

CHAPTER OUTCOMES

After reading this chapter, you should be able to:

➤ Differentiate between food-borne infections and intoxications

➤ List the main organisms responsible for food-borne infection

➤ List the main organisms responsible for food-borne intoxication

➤ Explain to a member of the public effective strategies for preventing food-borne illness at home

➤ Explain why food-borne disease is a problem in hospitals, care homes, prisons and so on and identify the main steps taken to prevent and control it

Introduction

All food contains microorganisms. Some cause spoilage by altering the appearance, taste or smell, but food that has 'gone bad' is unlikely to be consumed and therefore does not cause a threat to health. Items contaminated by enteric bacteria or their toxins, however, can give rise to unpleasant illness even though their appearance, smell and taste are unchanged. The illnesses caused by contaminated food can range from very mild to serious illness, which may lead to death in vulnerable people.

This chapter provides information about the common bacteria, viruses and protozoa that cause enteric infections. *Clostridium difficile* is dealt with in Chapters 4 and 6 and *Vibrio cholerae*, the bacterium that causes cholera, is discussed in Chapter 14.

Incidence of enteric infection

Enteric infection is a major health problem. Every year 1.3 million people in England and Wales develop food-borne diseases. The number of cases reported to the Health Protection Agency is increasing (O'Brien, 2006). This is, however, only the tip of the iceberg, as isolated cases are not reported, whereas large outbreaks, when several people have eaten the same food, are more likely to be investigated (Tranter, 1990). A recent audit and re-audit of statutory notifications of suspected gastroenteritis or food poisoning by general practitioners (GPs) in an area of Yorkshire highlighted considerable differences in reporting activity and the timing of notifications (Day and Sutton, 2007).

The main contributory factors in enteric infection are:

- The advance preparation of food
- Inadequate cooking
- Inadequate cooling
- Improper storage
- Reheating.

Faults during food production and processing, transport and storage before reaching the consumer also contribute.

Risk factors

Risk factors are related to the immune status of the individual (intrinsic) and factors associated with modern lifestyle affecting food choice and preparation (extrinsic).

Intrinsic factors

The following groups are at particular risk:

- **The very young** – The immune system in the very young is not mature so susceptibility to infection is high. Traditionally, specialist community public health nurses (health visitors) have played a major role in educating the public about the importance of hygiene, especially when infant feeds are prepared. The incidence of gastroenteritis is higher for bottle-fed babies, vomiting and diarrhoea developing either because feeds are too concentrated or because of infective gastroenteritis. Sick children are at greatest risk. The trend towards early discharge means that these infants are now likely to be cared for in the community. They often require special feeds administered enterally, and these feeds may become contaminated, especially if they are prepared by parents/carers at home (Anderton et al., 1993).
- **Older adults** – Fewer organisms are required to produce an infective dose, while diarrhoea and vomiting are more likely to result in dehydration and electrolyte imbalance.
- **People with severe illnesses,** especially those who are immunocompromised – This group includes those with cancer and those with HIV/AIDS.

Extrinsic factors

Those most at risk are:

- **Frail people** (including older adults) – Frail people may not be able to get out to buy fresh food.
- **People with limited financial means** – Individuals in this group may be unable to afford good-quality produce. Lacking transport, they may rely on local shops where turnover is slower and perishable items may remain longer on the shelves. They are

also less likely to throw away suspect items because they cannot afford waste. Lack of refrigeration can be a problem, especially in bed and breakfast accommodation where families with young children are housed by the social services.

- **People who frequently eat out** or rely on a high proportion of pre-prepared food – Mass production and pre-prepared meals or snacks are associated with an increased risk.
- **People travelling overseas** – The number has increased dramatically over the past 20 years, exposing people to potentially lower standards of hygiene than in developed countries.
- **People living or eating meals in establishments** – This includes residents of schools, prisons, care and nursing homes and hospitals, where mass catering is inevitable.

Food-borne illness is usually mild, resolving spontaneously within a few days, but the consequences can occasionally be more serious. Fluid and electrolyte imbalance can be severe, dangerous and expensive. It can also be difficult to treat in infants, older adults and people with some pre-existing chronic conditions.

Food infection and intoxication

The term 'food poisoning' is used to describe vomiting or diarrhoea following the consumption of food contaminated with bacteria or their toxins. As it also encompasses illnesses resulting from the ingestion of natural poisons (berries or toadstools, for example), 'food-borne illness' is a more accurate term. There are two types of food-borne illness:

- invasive gastrointestinal infection (gastroenteritis)
- intoxication (Table 11.1).

Table 11.1 Food infections and intoxications

Infections	Intoxications
Salmonella	Bacillus cereus
Shigella	Staphylococcus aureus
Campylobacter	Clostridium perfringens*
Listeria	Clostridium botulinum

*Toxins are released after ingestion and not into the food

Infection (invasive gastrointestinal infection) results when bacteria are ingested in contaminated food. They multiply within the gut, giving rise to a systemic, infectious illness characterized by malaise, pyrexia and cramping abdominal pain in addition to nausea, vomiting and diarrhoea. Symptoms generally develop and resolve more slowly than in cases of intoxication because there is an incubation period in which the bacteria establish themselves within the host and multiply before causing symptoms. The victim is infectious, and precautions must be taken when excreta and vomitus are handled. Heating the food to 60 °C kills most bacteria, but the temperature must be high enough and applied for long enough to destroy sufficient bacteria to result in a level below the infective dose. This may be impossible for some dishes likely to deteriorate with heat (such as custards or lightly boiled eggs) or when the food is heavily contaminated. It is not always possible to detect the presence of bacteria by odour.

Intoxication develops when food containing bacterial toxins is consumed. Vomiting, sometimes with diarrhoea, develops within a few hours. The person is not infectious. Toxins are heat stable so contaminated food is not rendered safe by normal cooking, pasteurization (Chapter 5) and other heat treatments.

Invasive gastrointestinal infection

Some important bacteria that cause invasive gastrointestinal infection – *Salmonella, Campylobacter, Shigella* and *Escherichia coli* – are outlined below.

Salmonella

Salmonella is a Gram-negative, motile bacillus able to grow under aerobic and anaerobic conditions. There are over 2,500 different serotypes, including *Salmonella enteritidis* and *Salmonella typhimurium*, which commonly cause enteric infection in the UK. The bacteria *Salmonella enterica* serovar Typhi and *Salmonella enterica* serovar Paratyphi are responsible for the enteric fevers typhoid and paratyphoid respectively (Chapter 14). The optimum temperature for growth is 37 °C, but it can multiply anywhere between 7 °C and 48 °C. It is readily destroyed by sufficient heat but can survive freezing and drying, especially if protected by protein in food. Bacteria have been isolated from the fingers even after the hands have been washed and dried (Pether and Gilbert, 1971). Worldwide, *Salmonella* is a major cause of foodborne illness. There has been a sharp increase in the number of reported cases in the UK in recent years, mainly due to *Salmonella enteritidis* (Baird-Parker, 1990). According to Gillespie et al. (2005), outbreaks of *Salmonella enteritidis* (phage type 4) during 1992–2002 were seasonal (increased likelihood in spring and summer), associated with residential institutions, schools and domestic settings and were related to the use of raw shell eggs and egg products.

The increase in *Salmonella* infection is related to the overcrowding of livestock on farms, mass production and poor hygiene in premises where food is prepared, stored and sold. Contamination during transport has been documented (Hennessy et al., 1996), and cross-contamination can occur to any food in contact with it (see below).

PRACTICE APPLICATION 11.1

Salmonella and Eggs

Salmonella can survive light cooking, raw and undercooked eggs having been widely implicated as the cause of *Salmonella* food-borne illness in traditionally prepared and cook–chill dishes (Lacey and Buckingham, 1993). Several theories have been put forward to suggest the source of contamination:

➤ **Faecal contamination** – via cracks in the shell. Bacteria lodged in the crack may reach the yolk when the egg is broken, or become sucked inside as it cools in the refrigerator. This is less likely with battery hens, for which there is a 'roll-away' system for newly laid eggs. Eggs produced in this way are, however, increasingly unacceptable to consumers.

➤ **Vertical transmission** – via the oviduct of an infected bird. The bacteria are thought to gain access to the egg before the shell develops.

➤ **Cross-contamination** – via the fingers or other contaminated sources to shelled eggs or their products during food preparation or storage.

Pasteurized eggs should be used to prepare lightly cooked and raw egg dishes (such as ice cream and mayonnaise) in all catering establishments and if possible at home (Department of Health, 1993), the Department of Health repeating this advice in 1998. The same document also advises vulnerable people to avoid foods prepared from raw or lightly cooked eggs. Other hygiene measures recommended include the following:

➤ Wash the hands after handling eggs

➤ Do not use eggs with damaged shells

➤ Store the eggs in the refrigerator if possible, or in a cool, dry place

➤ Store eggs separate from raw meat, other foods and possible contaminants

➤ Use the oldest eggs first

➤ Clean kitchen surfaces and equipment after preparing egg dishes

➤ Eat egg dishes soon after cooking or refrigerate them.

Activity

Access the resource below and use the section about 'Keeping eggs safe' to answer the following questions:

➤ Which groups are advised not to eat raw eggs, or eggs with runny yolks?

➤ Which foods may contain raw egg?

➤ What type of egg can be safely used in foods that need raw egg?

Resource

Food Standards Agency (FSA) *Eat well, be well – Eggs.* Available www.food.gov.uk/.

Salmonella has an incubation period of 12–72 hours in the human host, symptoms appearing up to 7 days after ingestion. The illness lasts 2–5 days and is more severe in older adults and the very young. Although the acute stage of infection is usually over quickly, bacteria can be shed in the faeces of asymptomatic carriers for up to three months. Diagnosis is by stool culture; bacteria are not usually present in blood. Management involves fluid replacement as necessary. Antibiotics prolong carriage, but if infection is severe with complications (for example septicaemia or damage to the intestinal mucosa resulting in malabsorption and nutrient loss), ciprofloxacin is prescribed. This reduces the duration of diarrhoea and vomiting, and eliminates *Salmonella* from the stools (Ahmad et al., 1991). Trimethoprim may be used to treat invasive *Salmonella*.

Nosocomial salmonellosis

Between 1992 and 1994, infectious intestinal disease accounted for 15 per cent of all reported outbreaks (189 out of 1,275) in hospitals; of these, 125 were caused by salmonellae. Transmission was mainly by person-to-person spread rather than by the consumption of contaminated food. Hospital outbreaks lasted on average 16 days, with considerable disruption to hospital services. The cost of outbreaks was high as many staff and patients had to be screened, and infection was considered to have contributed to the deaths of five patients (Wall et al., 1996).

An outbreak of *Salmonella* infection at Stanley Royd Hospital in Wakefield, Yorkshire in 1984 involved over 400 patients and staff receiving food from the same kitchen, and the death of 19 older patients. This prompted a public enquiry, with recommendations for the future investigation, control and prevention of outbreaks. Recommendations centred mainly on the improvement of kitchen facilities and practices. As a result, Crown immunity was lifted from hospital kitchens in 1987. Hospital authorities and NHS Trusts whose catering departments fail to comply with requirements are now liable to prosecution in the same way as commercial premises (Department of Health, 1986).

More healthcare-associated outbreaks occur where there is a high incidence of faecal soiling (for example paediatric and maternity units and units caring for older people), and many have been reported in people with mental health problems (Joseph and Palmer, 1989). The opportunity for infection is increased by poor personal hygiene and by movement between different parts of the hospital. Although person-to-person spread is the most important route, it cannot always be distinguished from transmission via contaminated clinical equipment (such as gastroscopes or faulty bedpan washers) because the bacteria can survive well in moist environments. It is frequently impossible to trace the source of infection. Catering staff carrying *Salmonella* may cause infection in sick and healthy people (Dryden et al., 1994).

Controlling an outbreak of *Salmonella* is outlined below.

PRACTICE APPLICATION 11.2

Controlling an Outbreak of *Salmonella*

Galloway et al. (1987) report the following successful control measures in a long-stay hospital. The outbreak involved 11 patients and 12 members of staff over three weeks. The measures taken were:

➤ Screening stool specimens from all patients on wards where diarrhoea had been reported. Patients with a positive stool result were isolated and looked after by staff not responsible for any of the other patients

➤ Screening staff from affected wards, catering staff and others with gastrointestinal symptoms. This helped to eliminate carriers

➤ Cleaning the central and ward kitchens

➤ Destroying soiled furniture

➤ Curtailing admissions until the outbreak was controlled.

Taking food histories from patients and testing food specimens did not help to identify the source of the infection.

Activity

➤ Discuss these measures with your mentor or a member of the infection
prevention and control team.

➤ How appropriate are these measures to your placement/workplace?

Campylobacter

Campylobacter jejuni and *C. coli* are Gram-negative, highly motile bacteria of the
genus *Campylobacter*. Infection was first reported to the Public Health Laboratory
Service in 1977. The number of reported cases has since increased every year, and
it is now one of the most common causes of food-borne disease. Health professionals are more likely to see patients with *Campylobacter* infection than many
other enteric infections because the symptoms of acute abdominal pain and bloodstained diarrhoea can be so severe and frightening that the victim will seek medical
help. The incubation period is 2–10 days, and the illness lasts 10–14 days.

The bacteria are widespread within the environment and have been isolated from
sewage, untreated water, raw or undercooked poultry and unpasteurized milk. They
do not multiply below 30 °C and are thus unlikely to grow on food at room temperature. Cross-contamination readily occurs between stored items, which can then
operate as vehicles for infection. Death is unusual but morbidity is considerable, and
it has been suggested that *Campylobacter* infection may be linked with the later
development of Guillain–Barré syndrome, an acute demyelinating peripheral neuropathy in which the myelin sheath is lost from peripheral nerves.

Campylobacter appears to be less infectious than many of the other bacteria
causing food-borne illness. Person-to-person spread is rare, with only occasional
reports among members of the same household (usually children during the acute
diarrhoeal phase), and community outbreaks are uncommon. Infection has,
however, resulted from handling family pets carrying the bacteria, and vertical
transmission from mother to fetus has been documented. The illness is usually self-
limiting but can if necessary be treated with erythromycin or aminoglycoside antibiotics (Chapter 4).

Shigella sonnei

Shigella sonnei is a Gram-negative rod causing dysentery. Infection results in acute
inflammation of the large bowel (colon) with the passage of loose stools containing blood, pus and mucus. Four species are responsible for clinical illness (Table
11.2). *Shigella sonnei* is the species encountered most often in the UK. The faecal-
oral route disseminates the microorganism, with outbreaks typically occurring in
institutions among young children, such as nursery schools. Control is by improving standards of personal hygiene. Chronic carriage is rare, although those recov-
ering from acute infection may continue to shed bacteria for a few weeks.

Table 11.2 *Shigella* species responsible for dysentery

Species	Distribution	Presentation
Shigella dysenteriae	Tropical and subtropical	Severe
Shigella flexneri	Tropical and subtropical	Moderate
Shigella boydii	Tropical and subtropical	Moderate
Shigella sonnei	Temperate	Mild

Escherichia coli

Escherichia coli is a commensal in the human bowel. Colonization occurs within a few weeks of birth and is of benefit to the host because it reduces the risk of overgrowth by other potentially pathogenic bacteria. However, some serotypes of *E. coli* can cause food-borne infection. These fall into four groups, depending on factors contributing to their virulence and the way in which they interact with the intestinal mucosa (Gould, 1996).

Enteropathic E. coli

Enteropathic *E. coli* (EPEC) is a major cause of severe diarrhoea in infants in developing countries. Most outbreaks have been reported from hospitals or nurseries and in each case traced to a food-handler or to water contaminated with human sewage (Doyle, 1990). This serotype owes its pathogenicity (ability to cause disease) to its ability to adhere strongly to the intestinal mucosa, destroying the microvilli and disrupting absorption.

Enterovasive E. coli

Enterovasive *E. coli* (EIEC) has been responsible for many outbreaks since its pathogenic activity was first described in the 1940s (Doyle, 1990). Food-handlers and contaminated water are the usual source, but person-to-person spread is also possible. EIEC causes invasive dysentery and bloodstained diarrhoea.

Enterotoxigenic E. coli

Enterotoxigenic *E. coli* (ETEC) is the principal agent implicated in travellers' diarrhoea reported by those visiting countries with poor standards of hygiene. Infection is uncommon in the UK except in those returning from overseas but it is a major cause of gastroenteritis among all age groups in developing countries. Outbreaks are generally traceable to a human source. The bacteria invade the intestinal mucosa but produce watery rather than bloodstained diarrhoea, and recovery is usually complete.

Enterohaemorrhagic E. coli

Enterohaemorrhagic *E. coli* (EHEC) causes a wide range of illnesses, from mild diarrhoea to severe abdominal pain with haemorrhagic colitis (inflammation of the colon with bleeding). Symptoms arise from the production of an enterotoxin called vero cytotoxin, which is produced when the bacteria adhere to the intestinal wall. The bacterium is generally known as vero cytotoxin-producing *E. coli* (VTEC) or *E. coli* 0157. The organism is extremely virulent and relatively few bacteria will cause harm (Williams and Ellison, 1998).

The disease is usually self-limiting, and most people recover within about eight days. However, approximately a third of those infected require hospital admission, and a small number (mainly in infants, children and older people) develop haemolytic uraemic syndrome (HUS), a form of renal failure carrying a mortality rate of 17 per cent. Survivors may have residual renal problems.

E. coli 0157 is now recognized as an important pathogen and has caused outbreaks in the USA, Canada and the UK (see below), in households, nurseries, schools, residential homes and hospitals. Person-to-person spread is possible via the faecal-oral route, and asymptomatic carriage is possible. Outbreaks have been linked to the consumption of many types of meat, especially undercooked beef products, cold cooked meats, meat pies and hamburgers, unpasteurized milk and milk products, faecally contaminated water and vegetables washed in it. Dairy cattle may operate as a reservoir. *E. coli* 0157 is uncommon in the UK, but the number of cases reported annually to the Health Protection Agency is increasing.

During 1996, a serious outbreak of *E. coli* 0157:H7 occurred in Lanarkshire, central Scotland. There have been other outbreaks, both before and after, but this outbreak was very serious, with 20 deaths, all of which occurred in people aged over 65 years. The 1996 outbreak was eventually traced to a specific butcher's shop. Infected meat and meat products were supplied from this shop to various other business outlets, which increased the size of the outbreak (Williams and Ellison, 1998). The widespread distribution of infected foods also made tracing the source more difficult.

Various recommendations on food handling, training, minimizing contamination, regulations and enforcement, and managing outbreaks have been published by the Pennington Group (1997), which was established by the government to investigate all aspects of the *E. coli* 0157:H7 outbreak in central Scotland.

At the time of writing, an outbreak of *E. coli* 0157 linked to cold meat purchased from a supermarket in Scotland is confirmed to have affected at least nine people including the death of an older woman.

There are implications for all health and social care professionals in their role as health educators, and in the training and supervision of all staff, especially those who handle food. As with most aspects of infection prevention and control, the importance of proper handwashing protocols cannot be stressed enough (see below).

PRACTICE APPLICATION 11.3

Reducing the Risk of *E. coli* 0157

Visits to farms for educational or recreational purposes carry a risk of infection with *E. coli* 0157 through contact with animals or faeces. Thus taking children, clients or residents to visit farms has health and safety implications.

Activity

Access the HSE information sheet produced for school visits and consider the advice about the following:

> ➤ Eating and drinking in areas where animals are present

> ➤ Washing facilities

> ➤ Putting pens, crayons or fingers in mouths

> ➤ When to wash hands

Resources

Health and Safety Executive (HSE) (reprinted 2002) Information sheet. *Avoiding ill health at open farms – Advice to farmers (with teachers' supplement)*. Available http://hse. gov.uk/pubns/ais23.pdf.

Department for Environment, Food and Rural Affairs (DEFRA) – www.defra.gov.uk/.

Listeria monocytogenes

Listeria monocytogenes is a facultive Gram-positive, non-sporing bacillus present in soil and water as well as on vegetation. Although *Listeria* was identified as an animal pathogen early in the 20th century, it has only recently been recognized as a cause of human disease. Listeriosis can take the following forms (Levy, 1989):

- Intrauterine or perinatal (the time around birth) infection
- Meningitis (inflammation of the meninges; the membranes that cover the brain and spinal cord)
- Bacteraemia, septicaemia
- Rarely, skin infection arising through contact with animals.

Most people develop immunity through exposure to bacteria in the environment. Some are asymptomatic carriers, and only 10–15 per cent of infections occur in healthy people (Levy, 1989). Infection follows the consumption of contaminated food (Schlech, 1991), the incubation period being 7–70 days. Having contact with sheep at lambing time may also cause infection in pregnant women (Health Protection Agency, 2007a).

Listeria causes severe invasive infection in the immunocompromised host, such as those with AIDS, infants, older people and in pregnant women. Pregnant women may remain asymptomatic after infection or develop flu-like symptoms. *Listeria* crosses the placenta and can cause spontaneous miscarriage, stillbirth or the delivery of an acutely ill baby. Neonatal (during the first 28 days of life) listeriosis is classified as being of early (within 2–3 days of delivery) or late (5 days or more) onset. In early-onset cases, the infant develops septicaemia, the mortality rate being 40–50 per cent. With late-onset listeriosis, meningitis is the most common presentation. Mortality in the neonate is 25 per cent, but maternal recovery occurs spontaneously after delivery without treatment. Diagnosis is by blood or cerebrospinal fluid culture in adults. In cases of suspected neonatal infection, swabs are taken from the eyes, ears and placenta. Adults are treated with high doses of ampicillin. Infants are given gentamicin for at least two weeks, the dose being determined by weight. Meningitis caused by *Listeria* is treated with amoxicillin (or ampicillin), or gentamicin.

Listeria infection has resulted from the consumption of unpasteurized milk (in Brie, Camembert and blue vein cheese), chilled cold meats, pâté, undercooked chicken, prepared salads such as coleslaw and cook–chill products. Hard cheeses (such as Cheddar) and processed and cottage cheese are safe, as are pasteurized milk and milk powder heated during production.

Listeria grows at temperatures as low as 2 °C and multiplies in refrigerated food, although growth in temperatures up to 42 °C is possible. Outbreaks may be seasonal, occurring most often during the autumn, which is in contrast to most other agents responsible for food-borne disease. Food probably becomes contaminated from environmental sources during production, a situation exacerbated by modern methods of raising livestock since feed may be contaminated with *Listeria*.

Food-borne intoxication

Some important bacteria that are responsible for causing food-borne intoxication – *Staphylococcus aureus, Clostridium perfringens, Clostridium botulinum, Bacillus cereus* – are outlined below.

Staphylococcus aureus

Staphylococcus aureus causes gastrointestinal symptoms by producing heat-stable enter-otoxins (toxins acting on the gastrointestinal tract). The amount necessary to cause symptoms is unknown but is thought to be as little as 1 µg/100 g of food. Symptoms usually appear within 2–6 hours of ingestion, depending on the amount consumed. The cause of vomiting and diarrhoea is poorly understood: presumably the toxin irritates receptors in the gut wall, relaying impulses to the vomiting centres in the brain. Staphylococcal disease is not reportable in the UK so its incidence is not established. It is thought to vary between countries, depending on eating habits, and appears to be more common in the USA than in the UK (Tranter, 1990). Typical episodes last 2–3 days, and many people recover without seeking the advice of a health professional.

Staphylococcus aureus is a natural food contaminant, the source always being another person. Unwashed hands are usually to blame, especially if the food-handler has a septic lesion not covered by a waterproof dressing. The bacteria multiply in the warm, damp conditions so often provided by inadequately refrigerated display counters in shops, restaurants and fast-food outlets, so releasing toxins. They survive in a saline environment and are particularly associated with salty foods such as ham, and sugary products. The salt or sugar discourages the growth of other bacteria, so a large number of staphylococci flourish unchecked. Other foods incriminated include fish, poultry, cakes with cream or custard fillings and salads. Cross-contamination between items stored close together is possible.

Clostridia

Clostridia are anaerobic, Gram-positive, spore-forming bacteria. They inhabit soil, playing an important role in the decomposition of dead organisms. Some species are commensals in the human gut but may also operate as human pathogens. The toxins are released after ingestion. *Clostridium difficile* is discussed in Chapters 4 and 6.

Clostridium perfringens

Clostridium perfringens is responsible for many outbreaks of food-borne illness, especially in institutions. The tough spores withstand cooking but germinate when the food, often meat, is inadequately reheated. The organism multiplies best between 37 °C and 41 °C. The source of the outbreak is usually difficult to establish because *Clostridium perfringens* is widespread within the environment and is often present within the human gut, especially among long-stay patients/residents.

In a typical outbreak described by Pollock and Whitty (1991), the source was reheated mince. The outbreak involved 58 out of 647 older people, with two deaths. Cases were restricted to the four wards where the meals arrived earliest. Food destined for the other wards remained in the heated trolley for longer and reached a satisfactory temperature, halting the multiplication of bacteria. Contamination occurred in the hospital kitchen; samples from the remaining raw mince did not contain clostridia.

Clostridium botulinum

Botulism was first described during the early 19th century. It is a paralytic illness resulting from the consumption of food contaminated with neurotoxins released by *Clostridium botulinum*. Symptoms develop within 2–6 hours. The muscles supplied by the cranial nerves are usually affected first, leading to visual disturbance, difficulty with speech and swallowing, and then paralysis. Symptoms are variable. This, coupled with the rarity of the disease, makes diagnosis difficult. It is not always possible to detect the toxin in the faeces, blood or gastric washings.

Most cases have been associated with preserved meat, fish or vegetables because the bacteria and their resistant spores can survive under anaerobic conditions that exclude competing bacteria. The toxin is destroyed by heating at 80 °C for 30 minutes; to eliminate spores, however, heat is necessary at 121 °C for 2.5 minutes. This is possible on a commercial scale but difficult to achieve domestically, with clear implications for those who preserve their own produce. The increased availability of frozen food, vacuum packing and the better distribution of fresh produce have reduced the incidence of botulism, which is a serious illness with a high mortality rate.

Bacillus cereus

Bacillus cereus is a Gram-positive rod contaminating rice. Its tough spores are not destroyed by boiling and germinate if the food is subsequently stored overnight without adequate refrigeration. The bacteria multiply and produce toxins. The bacteria are not destroyed during the gentle reheating used to produce 'special fried rice' the next day.

Investigating outbreaks of enteric infection in hospitals, care and nursing homes

A thorough investigation into the cause of infection is vital, and although individual establishments will have specific requirements, the principles apply to all such outbreaks (see below).

> ### INFORMATION BOX I I.I
>
> **Investigating outbreaks of enteric infection**
>
> ➤ The appearance and pattern of symptoms is an important indicator of the causative organism. A sudden outbreak involving several people is indicative of food intoxication (clostridial or staphylococcal). Cases of salmonellosis appear more sporadically from a common source because of the longer incubation period. Virus infections (see below) spread with no relationship to any food source.
>
> ➤ Samples of food (raw and 'left-overs') are obtained if possible to identify a source. A recent meal involving mince or a meat pie suggests clostridial intoxication, the consumption of salty food implicating staphylococci. The food can be examined microscopically. If staphylococci or clostridia are the cause, they will be present in large numbers.
>
> ➤ Stool specimens are obtained for microscopy and culture. Toxins may be revealed by enzyme-linked immunosorbent assay (ELISA) techniques. Infectious patients/residents, and carriers, must be isolated. Staff with symptoms must remain away from work until they are well and have bacteriological clearance. Staff who are carriers must be identified and should not handle food until they are clear of the organism.
>
> ➤ Practices will be examined in the central and unit kitchens. Investigations should include the examination of trolleys used to transport meals.
>
> ➤ Ward/unit practices and facilities should be examined, especially in relation to handwashing. Person-to-person spread of gastrointestinal pathogens is possible, and clinical equipment may act as fomites.

Enteric infection caused by viruses

Outbreaks of diarrhoea and vomiting caused by viruses are common in hospitals and the community. Diagnosis is by electron microscopy but is not always made as many infections are mild and self-limiting. There are no published guidelines for the management of these infections in hospital, but NHS Trusts are increasingly developing their own (Rao, 1995).

Viruses involved in enteric infections

Viruses that cause enteric infections – hepatitis A virus, hepatitis E virus, norovirus, rotavirus – are outlined.

Hepatitis A virus

Hepatitis A virus (HAV) is an RNA virus, which causes inflammation of the liver. Small outbreaks have been reported from families and institutions, larger epidemics resulting from the consumption of contaminated water, milk and food. Symptoms include malaise, nausea, vomiting, abdominal pain and jaundice. The incubation period is 15–50 days with an average of 28 days. Subclinical infection is common and gives lasting immunity in areas where sanitation is poor. The higher standard of living in the UK results in a reduced exposure and increases the risk of infection in adulthood, especially during foreign travel. A safe and reliable vaccine is available and is recommended for:

- people visiting countries where hepatitis A is common
- injecting drug users
- people whose sexual behaviour puts them at risk (unprotected anal sex)
- those whose work puts them at risk (for example those who come into contact with raw sewage)
- people living and working in homes for people with severe learning disabilities and so on (*British National Formulary*, 2007)
- people with a history of liver disease.

There is no specific treatment.

Hepatitis E virus

Hepatitis E virus (HEV) is a calcivirus disseminated by the faecal-oral route. Carrier status has not been reported and it does not appear to progress to chronic liver disease. It is a major cause of epidemic, waterborne hepatitis in many parts of the world, but not the UK, although travellers may become ill after returning home. The incubation period and clinical features are very similar to hepatitis A, but it can be much more severe.

Norovirus

Norovirus is an RNA virus. It is an important pathogen causing sporadic cases and outbreaks of gastroenteritis ('winter vomiting disease'), which in hospital may affect staff as well as patients (Goller et al., 2004). Transmission is by the faecal-oral route and via aerosols generated when infected people vomit. According to the Health Protection Agency (2008), the norovirus is the commonest cause of infectious gastroenteritis in England and Wales. Outbreaks are very common in the community, especially in closed environments such as schools, hotels, hospitals and cruise ships where they have attracted considerable media attention. Outbreaks are particularly common in older people but can occur in all age groups. Outbreaks in hospital frequently result in ward closures. The infection is usually mild and self-limiting, but early detection is vital for social and economic reasons (that is, to reduce the length of time away from work or school), because norovirus is highly infectious, up to 50 per cent of those exposed succumbing (Little and Jenkins, 1995). The infective dose appears to be very low. Spread is possible via contaminated environmental surfaces (Baker et al., 2004). Norovirus frequently contaminates water. As oysters, mussels and other bivalves feed by filtering particles from seawater, they tend to concentrate the virus and cause gastric illness if consumed.

Rotavirus

Rotavirus is an RNA virus responsible for outbreaks of winter vomiting. Cases sometimes show seasonal clustering, although they can occur at any time of the year. Most cases involve infants and young children. Rotavirus is responsible for significant infant mortality in developing countries. Although the illness is not usually severe in the UK, the Health Protection Agency (2007b) estimates that around 18,000 children require admission to hospital each year in England and Wales. A study in Austria identified rotavirus as an important cause of community-acquired gastroenteritis in children aged four years and under (Frühwirth et al., 2001). For a long time, it was believed that the droplet route spread rotavirus, but, as with many other viruses, dissemination appears to depend more on direct contact between individuals, the hands playing a major role. The mainstay of preventing the spread of rotavirus is good hygiene, with emphasis on handwashing.

Protozoal causes of enteric infection

Several protozoa cause enteric infections, including *Giardia intestinalis* (formerly *lamblia*), *Cryptosporidium* spp. and *Entamoeba histolytica*.

Giardia intestinalis

Giardia intestinalis (formerly *lamblia*) is an obligate protozoal parasite. It forms cysts, infection resulting when these are ingested. *Giardia* cannot multiply in food, but it contaminates water in parts of the world where hygiene is poor. Outbreaks have occasionally been reported in developed countries. For example, a large outbreak of waterborne giardiasis affecting over 1,500 people occurred in Norway in 2004–05 (Robertson et al., 2006). Transmission is by the faecal-oral route when contaminated water is consumed or used to wash food served raw, food-handlers probably playing a part. The incubation period is 1–3 weeks, and unless treated, the infection persists for 4–6 weeks. The protozoa inhabit the small bowel, the main symptom being offensive diarrhoea with cramping abdominal pain, sometimes malabsorption, and weight loss. Asymptomatic carriage is common. Cysts can withstand chlorination at concentrations used to disinfect water and may survive for more than 2 weeks in a damp, cool environment. They are destroyed by heat and prolonged freezing, but ice cubes in drinks have been associated with infection. The infectious dose is possibly no more than 10 cysts. Treatment is with metronidazole.

Cryptosporidium spp.

Cryptosporidium spp. are intestinal parasites not recognized as a human pathogen until 1976, although they were known to cause animal disease before this time. *Cryptosporidium* causes infection in the immunocompromised host but may also infect healthy people. The incubation period is 3–10 days. Symptoms include watery diarrhoea, abdominal pain and vomiting lasting up to 6 days in otherwise healthy people. Symptoms persist in patients with an impaired immune system (for example those with HIV disease) and deaths have occurred. Outbreaks have been reported, mainly from schools and nurseries, and mains water supplies are occasionally contaminated. No drug is currently effective against this infection, but it is usually self-limiting in otherwise healthy people. Chronic cryptosporidiosis is an AIDS-defining condition.

Entamoeba histolytica

Entamoeba histolytica is an anaerobic amoeba causing infection when the cysts are ingested in food as a consequence of poor hygiene. The incubation period ranges from two weeks to much longer periods – sometimes years (Todd et al., 2006). Infection results in bloodstained, mucoid diarrhoea. *Entamoeba* is endemic in poor communities in tropical and temperate countries, but outbreaks in the UK are rare. Treatment is with metronidazole.

Preventing food-borne infection

Food-borne infection is largely preventable (Barrie, 1996). Good practices include:

- Complying with legal requirements for catering
- Protecting food from contamination at all stages from production to consumption
- Providing training in food and personal hygiene for all food-handlers
- Educating the public about food hygiene.

Understanding the circumstances likely to result in food-borne disease is the key to its prevention. Disease can only occur if the following events take place in sequence:

1. The item must be contaminated by microorganisms able to operate as human pathogens.
2. It must stand at a temperature favouring microbial growth and reproduction.
3. Time is needed for microbial multiplication and invasion or toxin release.

Contamination may occur at source or at any stage during food production, transport or storage. Food manufacturers use different strategies to disrupt the chain culminating in food-borne disease. Eliminating contamination before storage is achieved by canning, freezing and the much older method of salting. Freezing holds the bacteria at temperatures too low for them to multiply and is acknowledged as one of the safest methods of preserving food. However, *Salmonella* already present can survive until it is thawed, then multiply. In theory, food can remain frozen safely for years provided the equipment is in good working order, but the colour and texture of some items may deteriorate. Vacuum packing is widely used to prevent botulism.

Legal requirements

Food hygiene legislation is enacted by national governments in England, Wales, Scotland and Northern Ireland, which incorporates several European Regulations.

For example, The Food Hygiene (England) Regulations 2006 are intended to ensure that premises where food is prepared are safe and properly maintained, and that food hygiene regulations are strictly enforced during all processes. The regulations cover all aspects of food hygiene, for example the temperature at which hot and cold food must be stored. All premises used to prepare, store or serve food must be registered with the local authority and may be inspected by their environmental health officers. After an inspection, the officers can issue informal warnings, improvement notices specifying remedial action that should be taken within a given period, or prohibition notices, which result in immediate closure of the premises. Those responsible for breaches of the food hygiene laws are liable to prosecution. Detailed information is available on the Food Standards Agency website (see Further Reading).

Training for food-handlers

Providing training for food-handlers, including food-handlers in health and social care premises, is essential under the food hygiene legislation. Ward/unit kitchens are subject to the Food Hygiene Regulations, and managers are responsible for ensuring that they are adhered to:

- The kitchen should be clean
- Items in the refrigerator should be monitored. They should be labelled with the date and discarded if not used
- The temperature of the refrigerator should be monitored, and the refrigerator should be kept clean
- Staff should wash and dry their hands before handling food
- Paper cloths should be used to dry kitchen equipment
- Staff with gastrointestinal symptoms should be aware that they must report to the occupational health department.

Ward and unit kitchens do vary in function. Some, such as the unit kitchen in a care home, may be involved in serving meals, whereas many ward kitchens are only used to prepare hot drinks and possibly a light snack for day-case patients before discharge. Whatever the function performed, the same stringent hygiene regulations apply.

Safe practice at home: educating the public

Healthcare practitioners (for example community nurses and specialist community public health nurses) and social care practitioners have an important role in helping people to develop safe practices regarding food. A programme to educate the public should cover the buying, storing, preparing and cooking of food. A typical programme to promote awareness is outlined below.

Buying food

- Avoid products that do not look fresh

- Avoid cans that are misshapen or pierced
- Avoid using cracked eggs
- Avoid cartons with bulging lids
- Select raw and cooked items that have been displayed on separate cold counters.

Safe storage

- Discard suspect items. Sell-by dates are a suggestion only, whatever the date on the package
- Place the food in the refrigerator as soon as possible after purchase and not more than one and a half hours later
- Keep it refrigerated at 1–4 °C
- Cover all stored food
- Store raw and cooked items separately
- Place raw food such as meat in the bottom of the refrigerator where it will not drip onto items that will be consumed raw
- Store items intended for human and animal consumption apart.

Preparing food

- Wash and dry the hands before touching food and again after handling raw items
- Keep cuts and sores on the hands covered with a waterproof dressing
- Keep all kitchen surfaces scrupulously clean. Never use a chopping board and utensils for cooked food if they have been used for raw meat, unless the board and all utensils have been thoroughly washed with detergent. Kitchen cloths should be kept clean and dry
- Wash fruit and vegetables thoroughly in cold, running water
- Dismantle blenders and food processors after use, washing and drying all the parts thoroughly.

Cooking and reheating

- Thaw frozen food thoroughly before cooking
- Ensure that ovens reach the required temperature before the cooking time begins
- Stir liquids to avoid 'cold spots' around the sides of the saucepan
- Ensure that meat, poultry and fish are cooked thoroughly
- Cool food rapidly and place it in the refrigerator unless it is to be consumed immediately
- If food is to be kept hot before serving, hold it at 63 °C or above

- Never refreeze food that has thawed unless it has been cooked

- Take special care with microwave ovens. 'Cold spots' can develop where heat has failed to penetrate. Always follow the manufacturer's guidelines for the equipment and the food. Heating time should be adjusted if the machine is at a lower wattage, stirring halfway if there is no turntable.

Using new methods safely

New methods of food preparation are sometimes blamed for cases of food-borne disease, but provided the system is monitored correctly, the risk is no greater than with conventionally prepared meals.

Cook–chill

Cook–chill is a method of precooking food in bulk, followed by its rapid cooling to 0–3 °C. The items are reheated immediately before serving, usually in a microwave oven. Cook–chill is used commercially to prepare convenience foods and has been introduced in many hospitals as well as in community-based meal provision for the housebound and people with a disability. Meals should not be stored for longer than five days and should be reheated at 70 °C (Department of Health, 1989). Cook–chill products are safe in hospital providing that production is operated in conjunction with a system of microbiological monitoring (Shanaghy et al., 1993). In a typical hospital system, food is prepared in a central kitchen, portioned, chilled, held under refrigeration for a maximum of five days, put onto cold plates and distributed to the wards in refrigerated trolleys before reheating. In a traditional system of bacteriological monitoring, audit occurs by taking samples at any stage in this process.

A more comprehensive method of quality control is offered by the Hazard Analysis Critical Control Point (HACCP) system. This is a system of control to assure food safety using a more standardized approach than traditional inspection and sampling. It has been used effectively within the food industry for over 20 years (Richards et al., 1993). A flow chart is constructed to depict all stages in production from the arrival of raw articles to the meal reaching the consumer. A number of critical points are selected at which monitoring is considered vital, and sampling is performed with every batch. HACCP promotes the development and refinement of guidelines to ensure good practice and operates as a continual reminder to staff of the need for vigilance at every stage throughout food handling. Shanaghy et al. (1993) found that its introduction improved the microbiological quality of food from a hospital cook–chill system.

SELF-ASSESSMENT

1. Describe how invasive gastrointestinal infection (gastroenteritis) and food-borne intoxication cause food-borne illness.

2. *Salmonella* is spread:

    (a) via the faecal-oral route

    (b) by person-to-person contact

    (c) on contaminated fingers

    (d) via fomites

3. *Campylobacter* causes invasive gastrointestinal infection (gastroenteritis). True? or False?

4. *Escherichia coli* is:

    (a) a harmless commensal in the human gut

    (b) a cause of travellers' diarrhoea

    (c) spread by food-handlers

    (d) able to produce enterotoxins (some serotypes)

5. Where do outbreaks of the norovirus commonly occur?

6. *Cryptosporidium* spp. may contaminate drinking water supplies. True? or False?

7. Food should be stored in the refrigerator at 10 °C. True? or False?

8. Outline the safe practices in relation to food preparation at home.

REFERENCES

Ahmad F, Bray G, Prescott RW et al. (1991) Use of ciprofloxacin to control a *Salmonella* outbreak in a long-stay psychiatric hospital. *Journal of Hospital Infection* **12**: 171–8.

Anderton A, Nwoguh CE, McCune I et al. (1993) A comparative study of the numbers of bacteria present in enteral feeds prepared and administered in hospital and at home. *Journal of Hospital Infection* **23**: 43–9.

Baird-Parker AC (1990) Food-borne salmonellosis. *Lancet* **336:** 1231–5.

Baker J, Vipond IB and Bloomfield SF (2004) Effects of cleaning and disinfection in reducing the spread of Norovirus contamination via environmental surfaces. *Journal of Hospital Infection* **58:** 42–9.

Barrie D (1996) The provision of food and catering services in hospital. *Journal of Hospital Infection* **33**: 13–31.

British National Formulary No 54 (2007) Section 14 Immunological products and vaccines. British Medical Association and Royal Pharmaceutical Society of Great Britain, London. Available www.bnf.org/.

Day F and Sutton G (2007) General practitioner notifications of gastroenteritis and food poisoning: cause for concern. *Journal of Public Health* **29**(3): 288–91.

Department of Health (DH) (1986) *Report of a Public Enquiry into the Outbreak of Salmonella Food Poisoning at Stanley Royd Hospital*. HMSO, London.

Department of Health (DH) (1989) *Chilled and Frozen: Guidelines on Cook-chill and Cook-freeze Catering Systems*. HMSO, London.

Department of Health, Advisory Committee on the Microbiological Safety of Food (1993) *Report on Salmonella in Eggs*. HMSO, London.

Department of Health (DH) (1998) *Expert Advice Repeated on Salmonella and Raw Eggs.* Press release 98/138. DH, London.

Doyle MP (1990) Pathogenic *Escherichia coli, Yersinia entercolitica* and *Vibrio parahaemolyticus. Lancet* **336**: 1111–15.

Dryden MS, Keyworth N, Gabb R et al. (1994) Asymptomatic foodhandlers as the source of nosocomial salmonellosis. *Journal of Hospital Infection* **28**: 195–207.

Frühwirth M, Karmaus W, Moll-Schüler I et al. (2001) A prospective evaluation of community acquired gastroenteritis in paediatric practices: impact and disease burden of rotavirus infection. *Archives of Disease in Childhood.* **84**(5): 393–7.

Galloway A, Roberts C and Hunt EJ (1987) An outbreak of *Salmonella typhimurium* gastroenteritis in a psychiatric hospital. *Hospital Infection* **10**: 248–54.

Gillespie I, O'Brien S, Adak G et al. (2005) Foodborne general outbreaks of *Salmonella enteritidis* phage type 4 infection, England and Wales, 1992–2002: where are the risks? *Epidemiology and Infection* **133**(5): 795–801.

Goller JL, Dimitriadis A, Tan A et al. (2004) Long-term features of norovirus gastroenteritis in the elderly. *Journal of Hospital Infection* **58**: 286–91.

Gould DJ (1996) Hygienic practices (*E. coli* foodborne illness). *Nursing Times* **92**(36): 77–80.

Health Protection Agency (HPA) (2007a) *Infectious diseases. Infections A–Z. Zoonoses. Listeriosis and Risks in Lambing Season.* Available www.hpa.org.uk.

Health Protection Agency (HPA) (2007b) *Infectious diseases. Infections A–Z. Rotavirus.* Available www.hpa.org.uk.

Health Protection Agency (HPA) (2008) *Norovirus (Norwalk-like virus, Small Round Structured Virus/SRS).* Available www.hpa.org.uk.

Hennessy TW, Hedberg C, Slutsker L et al. (1996) A national outbreak of *Salmonella enteritidis* infections from ice cream. *New England Journal of Medicine* **334**: 1282–6.

Joseph CA and Palmer SR (1989) Outbreaks of *Salmonella* infection in hospitals in England and Wales 1978–87. *British Medical Journal* **298**: 1161–4.

Lacey SL and Buckingham SE (1993) Isolation of *Salmonella enteritidis* from cook-chill food distributed to hospital patients. *Journal of Hospital Infection* **25**: 133–6.

Levy J (1989) *Listeria* and food poisoning – a growing concern. *Maternal and Child Health* **14**: 380–3.

Little K and Jenkins M (1995) When winter makes you sick. *Nursing Times* **91**(46): 55–60.

O'Brien S (2006) Foodborne zoonoses. *Student BMJ* (January) **14:** 1–44. Available www.studentbmj.com.

Pennington Group (1997) *Report on the Circumstances Leading to the 1996 Outbreak of Infection with E. coli 0157 in Central Scotland: the Implications for Food Safety and the Lessons to be Learnt.* TSO, Edinburgh.

Pether JVS and Gilbert RJ (1971) The survival of *Salmonella* on the finger tips and the transfer of organisms to food. *Journal of Hygiene* **69**: 673–81.

Pollock AM and Whitty PM (1991) Outbreak of *Clostridium perfringens* food poisoning. *Journal of Hospital Infection* **17**: 179–86.

Rao GG (1995) Control of outbreaks of viral diarrhoea in hospitals – a practical approach. *Journal of Hospital Infection* **30**: 1–6.

Richards J, Parr E and Riseborough P (1993) Hospital food hygiene: the application of Hazard Analysis Critical Control Points to conventional hospital catering. *Journal of Hospital Infection* **24**: 273–82.

Robertson L, Hermansen L, Gjerde B et al. (2006) Application of genotyping during an extensive outbreak of waterborne giardiasis in Bergen, Norway, during autumn and winter 2004. *Applied and Environmental Microbiology* **72**(3): 2212–17.

Schlech WF (1991) Listeriosis: epidemiology, virulence and the significance of contaminated foodstuffs. *Journal of Hospital Infection* **19**: 211–24.

Shanaghy N, Murphy F and Kennedy K (1993) Improvements in the microbiological quality of food samples from a hospital cook–chill system since the introduction of HACCP. *Journal of Hospital Infection* **23**: 305–14.

Todd W, Lockwood D and Sundar S (2006) Infectious diseases. In N Boon, N Colledge and B Walker (eds) *Davidson's Principles and Practice of Medicine*, 20th edn. Churchill Livingstone, Edinburgh.

Tranter HS (1990) Foodborne staphylococcal illness. *Lancet* **336**: 1044–6.

Wall PG, Ryan MJ, Ward LR et al. (1996) Outbreaks of salmonellosis in hospitals in England and Wales 1992–1994. *Journal of Hospital Infection* **33**: 181–90.

Williams P and Ellison J (1998) Food fears. *Nursing Times* **94**(28): 72–5.

FURTHER READING AND INFORMATION SOURCES

British Liver Trust – www.britishlivertrust.org.uk.

Cowcroft NS, Walsh B, Davison KL and Gungabissoon U on behalf of PHLS Advisory Committee on Vaccination and Immunisation (2001) Guidelines for the control of hepatitis A virus infection. *Communicable Disease and Public Health* **4**: 213–27.

Cliver DO and Riemann HP (2003) *Foodborne Diseases*. Academic Press, London.

Cunliffe N, Allan C, Lowe S et al. (2007) Healthcare-associated rotavirus gastroenteritis in a large paediatric hospital in the UK. *Journal of Hospital Infection* **67**(3): 240–4.

Food Standards Agency (FSA) (2006) *Cadbury Recall update 1 August*. Available www.food.gov.uk.

Food Standards Agency (FSA) (2008) *General information on food hygiene legislation*. Available www.food.gov.uk/foodindustry/regulation/hygleg/hygleginfo/.

Health Protection Agency (HPA) (2007) *Guidance for the Management of Norovirus Infection in Cruise Ships.* Available www.hpa.org.uk/publications.

Pennington Group (1997) *Report on the Circumstances Leading to the 1996 Outbreak of Infection with E. coli 0157 in Central Scotland: the Implications for Food Safety and the Lessons to be Learnt.* TSO, Edinburgh.

Pratt R (2003) Prevention and control of viral hepatitis. *Nursing Standard* 17(3): 43–52.

World Health Organization (WHO) (revised 2005) *Drug-resistant Salmonella.* Fact sheet 139. Available www.who.int.

CHAPTER 12

Infection risks from blood and body fluids

CHAPTER OUTCOMES

After reading this chapter, you should be able to:

➤ Describe how HIV infection is transmitted and diagnosed

➤ Describe how hepatitis B infection is transmitted and diagnosed, and outline its effect on the health of the individual

➤ Outline two other viruses causing hepatitis that are transmitted in the same manner as hepatitis B

➤ Describe the precautions that should be taken when handling blood or body fluids and explain the rationale underpinning your recommendations

➤ Outline the public health measures taken to control the spread of HIV and hepatitis B

Introduction: the risk of infection and health and social care practitioners

Infection is an occupational health risk for health and social care staff (see below). The most serious threat to health is exposure to blood and body fluids, leading to parenteral infection. In the UK, health and social care staff are most likely to have contact with patients, clients or residents carrying the hepatitis viruses B and C and the human immunodeficiency virus (HIV). These viruses are often referred to as 'blood-borne pathogens' (BBPs), or 'blood-borne viruses' (BBVs). Sharps injuries are one of the main types of accident sustained by health workers (Watterson, 2004). Nurses appear to be the group most at risk and most injuries take place when disposable syringes and needles are used. Many of these injuries are related to staff behaviour and could be avoided by training (Castella et al., 2003).

PRACTICE APPLICATION 12.1

Occupational Infection Health Risk

Clinical work places health and social care workers at risk of developing infections from parenterally transmitted viruses, as well as other conditions including chicken-pox and tuberculosis (Moore and Kczmarek, 1990). The prevention of infection is a health and safety issue, falling within the remit of the Health and Safety at Work Act 1974. This applies throughout England, Wales and Scotland but not to Northern Ireland, where the Health and Safety of Work Order 1978 makes similar provisions. Section 2 of the Health and Safety at Work Act lays down the duties of employers to employees, stipulating that arrangements must be made for the safe use, storage and transport of all substances and equipment, and that staff should receive training to ensure that they adhere to agreed protocols. The Act applies to all employers, whether NHS Trusts, private hospitals and clinics, nursing and care homes, GPs employing a practice nurse, or social services. It also details the responsibilities of the employer to persons other than employees. On healthcare premises, these include patients, clients and visitors. There is therefore a duty to protect staff and the public from the risks of cross-infection.

Activity

➤ Find out more about assessing and reducing the risk of infection at work by visiting the Health and Safety Executive website (www.hse.gov.uk) and accessing the two publications below.

➤ Consider the guidance in the two publications and relate it to your own practice.

Resources

Advisory Committee on Dangerous Pathogens (2003) *Infection at Work: Controlling the Risk.* HMSO, Norwich.

Health and Safety Executive (2001) *Blood-borne Viruses in the Workplace: Guidance for Employers and Employees.* HSE, London.

Human immunodeficiency virus

Human immunodeficiency virus (HIV) is an RNA virus containing an enzyme called 'reverse transcriptase'. The virus has a long incubation period. Possessing antibodies to HIV demonstrates a previous exposure to the virus, but seroconversion (the secretion/formation of specific antibodies following exposure to an antigen) can take months, so a test yielding negative results should be repeated – it may have been performed too soon. Several serological tests have been developed. Core antigen p24 levels in the blood are used to indicate an increase in viral replication, progression of the disease and infectivity. Information about HIV tests can be obtained from GPs, sexual health clinics (genitourinary medicine clinics), NHS Direct, helplines and websites (for example Terence Higgins Trust) and, in the case of occupational exposure, the occupational health department. Testing is performed only after counselling and discussion to ensure that the individual understands the significance of a positive result and the need for repeat testing if it is negative.

Further information about HIV/AIDS is provided in Chapter 13, including drug treatments.

Transmission of HIV

The transmission of HIV occurs sexually, perinatally (around the time of birth) and parenterally.

Pratt (2003a) outlines possible situations in which exposure is possible:

- **Transmission to people with haemophilia** (a blood-clotting disorder) – since 1987, blood products in the UK have been heat-treated to destroy the virus so this risk has been eliminated. However, over 1,200 people with haemophilia (about 30 per cent of the total) in the UK are seropositive.
- **Drug misuse through sharing contaminated injection equipment** – the risk of transmission is probably enhanced through the recreational use of other substances, including alcohol: these alter behaviour and lower inhibition.
- **Sexual transmission between adults** – men and women can become infected, the risk being especially high for gay men who are the receptive partner during anal intercourse. The rectal mucosa is much more delicate than the vaginal mucosa, the virus gaining access via tears and abrasions. Nevertheless, in some parts of the world, an equal number of both sexes carry HIV. This is the situation in Africa, where the infection is believed to have originated.
- **Vertical transmission** from infected mothers to infants.
- **Iatrogenic transmission** to healthcare professionals – HIV is more easily destroyed than hepatitis B and is less common, but the consequences of infection are so grave that the risk of occupational exposure should never be overlooked.

Occupational health risks

The nature of the exposure is important. For surveillance purposes, two types are considered:

- **Percutaneous exposure** – the skin is cut or penetrated by a hollow needle or a sharp instrument, such as a scalpel blade
- **Mucocutaneous exposure** – the eyes, the inside of the nose or mouth, or non-intact skin is exposed.

The rate of infection following percutaneous injury, although higher than with mucocutaneous exposure, is still low, varying between 0.18 per cent and 0.56 per cent in large epidemiological studies (Henderson et al., 1990; Leentvaar-Kuijpers et al., 1990). In the UK, there were five cases of documented HIV seroconversions after percutaneous exposure of healthcare staff to HIV-positive patients prior to

2005 (Health Protection Agency, 2006), but no further reported HIV seroconversions during 2005.

The risk of health and social care workers acquiring HIV or any other parenterally transmitted infection from patients, clients or residents also depends on:

- The prevalence of the virus in the hospital or community setting where they are employed.

- Expertise – junior staff sustain needlestick injuries more often than experienced staff (Jagger et al., 1990). Thus, early clinical practice should be carefully supervised.

- The types of procedure performed – those who are routinely exposed to blood and body fluids most often are at greatest risk.

- The risk of transmission associated with each accidental exposure – the risk of seroconversion is about 1 in 300 (0.33 per cent) and varies depending on the injury, for example venepuncture or intramuscular injection (Heponstall et al., 1993). HIV has been isolated from blood, semen, vaginal secretions, breast milk, saliva and tears. The level in saliva and tears is probably too low to result in transmission (Lifson, 1988).

- The individual's immune status – those less fit are likely to develop infection.

Public health: reducing the risks of HIV infection

Public health measures include (see also Chapter 13):

- Promoting the use of barrier precautions during 'sexual activity' (with the correct type of condom) and emphasizing the need for 'safe sex'. Explicit advice can be obtained from organizations such as the Terence Higgins Trust.

- Screening all donated blood and heat-treating blood products.

- Discouraging members of the public likely to be carrying HIV from donating blood, semen or tissues. Organs cannot be used if the donor is known to be antibody positive.

- Informing the public and health and social care practitioners of the risks associated with handling blood and body fluids, and how to deal with these.

- Alerting the public to the dangers of sharing potentially contaminated items (razors, toothbrushes, sewing needles and scissors).

- Supplying needles and syringes to people who use intravenous drugs for recreational purposes. The use of 'needle exchange' is well established but remains controversial.

NB An effective vaccine is not available for HIV, but considerable research is being carried out in this area.

Hepatitis

Hepatitis is a generic term for inflammation of the liver; it may be acute or chronic. It is caused by a number of viruses including several hepatitis viruses, rubella, cytomegalovirus and herpes simplex. This chapter outlines the hepatitis viruses B, C, D and other hepatitis viruses. Hepatitis A and hepatitis E, the viruses that cause enteric infections, are discussed in Chapter 11.

Hepatitis B

The hepatitis B virus (HBV) causes an inflammatory condition affecting the liver that is caused by a DNA virus (Figure 12.1).

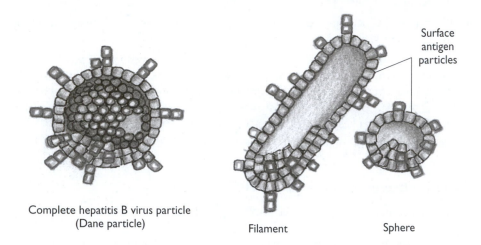

Complete hepatitis B virus particle
(Dane particle)

Filament

Sphere

Surface
antigen
particles

Figure 12.1 The hepatitis B virus

Information concerning its structure has developed through studies of its surface antigens. The terminology in general use is:

- HBV – the entire hepatitis B virus (previously called Dane particle)
- HBsAg – hepatitis B surface antigen
- HBcAg – hepatitis B core antigen
- HBeAg – the e antigen associated with the core of the virus
- Anti-HBs – antibody to hepatitis B surface antigen
- Anti-HBc – antibody to hepatitis B core antigen
- Anti-HBe – antibody to the e antigen.

The virus is detected by testing the blood for surface antigen. It may also cause a change in liver function tests (blood test), for example raised serum aminotransferase, bilirubin and alkaline phosphatase levels.

Infectious particles have been isolated from saliva and semen. Chronic carriers are those remaining HBsAg positive on at least two occasions six months apart. Infectivity is closely associated with the presence of the e antigen, which indicates that active viral replication is occurring.

The incubation period ranges from four weeks to six months. Individuals are probably most highly infectious during the early, acute stages. Most adults (90–95 per cent) recover fully from acute HBV infection (Chapman et al., 2006), but there is a risk of progression to chronic hepatitis. The liver is inflamed and the functional liver cells (hepatocytes) are destroyed in a process known as 'hepatocellular necrosis'.

Only 30–40 per cent of those infected develop symptoms of acute infection, which tend to be nonspecific, fever, malaise and anorexia being most commonly reported. Jaundice does not always develop, or it may be too mild to be noticeable. Between 50 and 60 per cent of patients develop a subclinical infection, remaining asymptomatic despite serological evidence of exposure. These people are most likely to become chronic carriers, at greatest risk of developing liver cirrhosis and hepatocellular cancer, rare but grave complications for which treatment is not always successful (Main, 1991).

Transmission occurs sexually (by vaginal or anal intercourse), through percutaneous sharps injury, by sharing infected needles, via contamination of the mucous membranes and potentially during tattooing/body piercing where equipment is not sterile and standard precautions are not in place. The risk of infection after percutaneous exposure to the blood of a carrier for the e antigen is about 30 per cent (Shaw and Bell, 1993). The risk associated with mucocutaneous exposure does not appear to have been quantified. The hands, however, may carry minute abrasions so the contamination of apparently intact skin may present a significant risk. Many people who develop infection or become carriers cannot recall an injury. As with HIV, the risk of seroconversion depends on the number of people carrying the virus within the local community and the individual's immunological status. In addition, infants whose mothers developed acute HBV infection during the third trimester (the last three months) of pregnancy or who are highly infectious carriers may also become infected by vertical transmission during the perinatal period. Immunization against HBV infection is given to infants born to women who have HBV infection or if a close family member is infected (Department of Health, 2007).

The level of risk depends on how the virus was transmitted; it is highest when transmitted vertically from mother to infant (Chapman et al., 2006).

Groups at high risk of infection

Despite the high rate of asymptomatic carriage, it is possible to identify a number of groups who are at high risk:

- Intravenous drug users
- Men who have sex with men
- Sex workers
- Healthcare professionals
- Immigrants from parts of the world where HBV infection is endemic, for example Africa, Southeast Asia and East Asia
- People in situations in which high standards of hygiene are difficult to maintain.

Reducing the risk of HBV infection

HBV infection is a notifiable disease, the number of cases occurring being recorded by the Health Protection Agency. Prevention involves:

- Effective health promotion regarding unsafe behaviours, such as unsafe sexual practices or the sharing of equipment to inject drugs
- The use of standard precautions in health and social care settings
- The development and implementation of guidelines to prevent spread from contaminated instruments
- Screening all blood for transfusion for HBsAg and excluding carriers from donation
- The use of virus-treated blood and blood products
- Offering vaccine to those at risk in hospital and in community settings.

Immunization has been available against HBV since the early 1980s. Vaccine was originally produced from human plasma, but most is now obtained through a recombinant DNA technique that inserts HBsAg into yeast cells. Both types of vaccine are safe and approximately 90 per cent effective. The duration of immunity has been estimated at between three and five years. The vaccine should be routinely available to health and social care practitioners but uptake is, however, often poor (Spence and Dash, 1990) even though side-effects are minimal. The reasons for low uptake among health professionals include inconvenient appointment times in occupational health departments, pressures of work and misconceptions about the vaccine, especially overlooking the need for boosters (Briggs and Thomas, 1994).

It was initially estimated that only 1–4 per cent of those who had received the standard vaccination consisting of three injections failed to respond (Boxall, 1993), but it has since emerged that a higher proportion may be 'slow responders', requiring up to nine injections to seroconvert (Poole et al., 1994). This suggests that it is not sufficient to evaluate the success of an immunization campaign merely on uptake: serological testing to determine the effectiveness of the vaccine among the recipients is vital. Nevertheless, the number of health professionals becoming infected has declined in recent years. Good record keeping in the occupational health department is essential to manage staff who have been exposed to blood-borne infections (Duthie et al., 1994). Immunization against HBV infection also affords protection against hepatitis D, which depends upon the presence of HBV. The World Health Organization (2004) recommends universal HBV immunization in an attempt to reduce the number of deaths from HBV infection and the number of people who carry HBV. At the time of writing, there are increased calls for immunization against HBV infection to be added to the routine immunization programme in the UK.

Although most cases of HBV infection and HIV passed on within the clinical setting are transmitted from patient to health professional, there have been some instances of members of the public contracting the infection from a healthcare worker (see below).

INFORMATION BOX 12.1

Risk of transmission of blood-borne viruses from healthcare workers to patients

Most cases have occurred when the individual has received treatment from a dentist or surgeon carrying the hepatitis e antigen or HIV. Nosocomial hepatitis B infections between patients have also occurred during the use of medical devices (for example endoscopes, autolets and vials) contaminated with blood and not properly disinfected (Drescher et al., 1994). The first possible case of HIV transmission to six patients was reported in the USA in 1993 (Centers for Disease Control and Prevention, 1993), and further cases have since been investigated.

Resources

Campbell S (2004) Management of HIV/AIDS transmission in health care. *Nursing Standard* 18(27): 33–5.

Department of Health (DH) (2005) *HIV infected health care workers: Guidance on management and patient notification.* Available www.dh.gov.uk.

Department of Health (DH) (2007) *Hepatitis B infected healthcare workers and antiviral treatment.* Available www.dh.gov.uk.

Hepatitis C

Once diagnostic tests had become available for HBV infection, it became apparent that a number of post-viral cases of hepatitis must be associated with infection by another agent. This condition was initially called non-A, non-B hepatitis. It proved to be caused by an RNA flavivirus subsequently named hepatitis C virus (HCV). HCV is endemic worldwide with a high prevalence in East Asia and Eastern Europe (Pratt, 2003b). It is transmitted predominantly via blood and body fluids. Intravenous drug users are most at risk. Risks from blood transfusions have been eliminated by routinely screening donated blood. Donated blood has been screened in the UK for HVC since 1991, but prior to screening, a number of people were infected with HVC, for example people with haemophilia who received infected blood products.

Sexual and mother-to-child HCV transmission occurs and HIV co-infection may increase risk. There is no evidence that HCV is transmitted via breast milk, so breast-feeding is considered safe (Department of Health, 2002). Health and social care workers are at occupational risk through exposure to blood and body fluids. However, for many people, the source of their infection remains a mystery because they do not appear to be in any of the at-risk groups. HCV is more damaging than HBV. So far, 50 per cent of those infected have become chronic carriers, of whom 20 per cent have developed hepatocellular cancer. Seroconversion may not occur until several months after exposure. Many people remain asymptomatic for up to twenty years after infection apart from experiencing occasional nonspecific ill-health and do not realize that anything is wrong (Rogers and Campbell, 2003). The course of the disease is variable and not always easy to predict, but is exacerbated by alcohol consumption. Cirrhosis resulting from hepatitis C is fatal without liver transplantation. An opportunity to investigate the drugs available to manage chronic hepatitis is provided below.

■ PRACTICE APPLICATION 12.2 ■

Drug Treatment for Chronic Hepatitis

The National Institute for Health and Clinical Excellence provides guidance on the drug treatment of people with chronic hepatitis C of varying severity and those with chronic hepatitis B.

Activity

➤ Access the resources below. It might be useful to start with the documents produced for 'Patients, carers and the public'.

➤ Consider the drugs available for different types and stages of chronic hepatitis. Note the doses, duration of treatment, alternatives if treatment is ineffective or people cannot tolerate a drug, and the side-effects.

Resources

British National Formulary – www.bnf.org.

National Institute for Health and Clinical Excellence (NICE) (2004) *Hepatitis C – pegylated interferons, ribavirin and alfa interferon.* TA75. www.nice.org.uk

National Institute for Health and Clinical Excellence (NICE) (2006a) *Hepatitis B (chronic) – adefovir dipivoxil and pegylated interferon alpha-2a.* TA96. www.nice.org.uk

National Institute for Health and Clinical Excellence (NICE) (2006b) *Hepatitis C – peginterferon alfa and ribavirin.* TA106. www.nice.org.uk.

Hepatitis D

Hepatitis D virus (HDV, delta virus) is a defective RNA virus that can cause infection only in the presence of active HBV infection. It is transmitted in the same way as hepatitis B, the same groups being at risk. Injecting drug users are at greatest risk. The incubation period is 30–50 days. Mortality from acute HDV infection is high: 2–20 per cent in those outbreaks so far reported. Infection is diagnosed by finding the antigen (HDAg) in the blood. Routine testing is not undertaken so the prevalence is not known, but it is more common in the countries of the former USSR, the Middle East and Africa than in the UK. Vaccination against HBV infection offers protection against both viruses.

Other hepatitis viruses

An unidentified agent has recently been designated as hepatitis F; this is seen as a possible cause of fulminant hepatitis. A further virus has been identified – hepatitis G – which is transmitted via blood and blood products. Other modes of transmission, for example via sexual intercourse, may occur.

Reducing the risk of exposure to blood-borne viruses

Universal precautions (now generally referred to as standard precautions/principles) for blood and body fluids were developed by the Centers for Disease Control and Prevention in Atlanta during the mid-1980s in response to the emergence of HIV/AIDS as a major health problem (Campbell, 2004). It is not possible to predict whether an individual is carrying a parenterally transmitted viral infection (Havlichek et al., 1991), and as exposure to blood may occur before testing is possible in emergency situations, standard (universal) precautions must be taken whenever blood or body fluids are handled or if contact is possible (Wilson and Breedon, 1990). This means that risk assessment is of the procedure about to be undertaken rather than of the individual patient, client or resident. Guidance from the Department of Health (1998) gives comprehensive information about protecting health-care workers from infection with blood-borne viruses. The document stresses the practical advantages of having common infection control policies for these viruses.

The components of standard precautions required for reducing the risk of exposure to BBVs are handwashing, personal protective equipment (PPE) and dealing with sharps.

Handwashing and decontamination

Appropriate handwashing and decontamination are central to all infection prevention and control (covered in detail in Chapter 5).

Personal protective equipment

The correct and appropriate use of PPE, which includes aprons or gowns, face/eye protection (covered in detail in Chapter 5) and gloves, prevents exposure to BBVs.

Gloves

Gloves are worn to protect the patient/resident during all invasive procedures and to protect the practitioner whenever contact with blood or body fluids takes place or is anticipated. The following points need to be considered when policies for glove use are developed:

- Non-sterile, single-use gloves are adequate when standard (universal) precautions/principles are taken. Sterile gloves are necessary for contact with parts of the body free of microorganisms in health. They should conform to British Standards Institution (BSI) standards.

- Gloves must be changed between patients/residents to prevent cross-infection. Washing is not recommended, as it appears difficult to remove pathogens from the surface of latex and PVC (Dalgleish and Malkovsy, 1988), although this is now contested (Mulhall et al., 1993). Further research is necessary in this area.

- Gloves must be changed between different procedures involving the same patient/resident to prevent endogenous infection (Goldmann, 1991).

- The hands must be washed after gloves have been worn. Virus particles can leak through latex and PVC (Korniewicz, et al., 1989), allergy may develop to the gloves or the lubricating powder they contain (Van Rijwisjk, 1992), and sweating is induced: bacteria are then leached out from beneath the nails and nail beds, increasing the number available for cross-infection (Peireira et al., 1990).

- Gloves must be of sufficient gauge to avoid splitting and tearing, problems reported for numerous brands during tests that simulate clinical procedures (Korniewicz et al., 1989). Double-gloving may be advisable with some brands of PVC glove. Trials have shown that they are more likely to leak than latex varieties, but this risk can be overcome when two pairs are used at once (Korniewicz et al., 1994). Puncture is possible during clinical procedures: electronic testing indicates that, during elective surgical procedures, 24 per cent of gloves become perforated (Green and Grompertz, 1992). They should be removed at once if any defect is observed. Fingernails should be kept short to avoid puncture.

- Gloves must fit well and be available in a range of sizes so that manual dexterity is not compromised. Staff may otherwise be tempted to use expensive, sterile surgeons' gloves when they are unnecessary. Many NHS Trusts now routinely monitor the use of gloves to check expense.

- Some procedures are difficult to perform even with good-quality gloves. For example, needlestick injuries can result when venepuncture is performed clumsily, but this could be reduced by adopting a 'two-tier' system of glove use that would sanction experienced staff undertaking venepuncture without gloves (Jenner, 1990).

Aprons and gowns

Disposable plastic aprons must be worn if clothing is likely to be exposed to blood, body fluids, secretions or excretions. This protection is upgraded to a water-repellent gown where there is a risk of skin being exposed to the above from extensive splashing, such as in the operating theatre or emergency department (Rennie-Meyer, 2007).

Eye protection and face masks

Eye and face protection conforming to BSI standards is required when splashing or aerosols of blood, body fluids, secretions or excretions are possible. This is unusual in ward or care home situations but is a risk in theatre or dentistry when high-speed drills are used. Eye protection (goggles or visors) may not be disposable and must be disinfected after use by washing in a liquid detergent solution, followed by thorough drying.

Other equipment

Equipment such as theatre shoes and phlebotomy cuffs may become splashed with blood and should be decontaminated or discarded (Forseter et al., 1990; Thomas et al., 1993). Hepatitis B virus can survive for at least a week in dry plasma (Bond et al., 1983) and HIV survives for several days if protected by plasma (Hanson et al., 1989).

Dealing with sharps

The handling of sharps should be performed with care to avoid injury. Ancillary staff, who include domestic staff and porters, as well as clinical staff may sustain injury. Healthcare workers who handle sharps should:

- Minimize the handling of sharps; avoid passing sharps from hand to hand (Pratt, 2003b)
- Avoid resheathing needles. They should never be cut or bent as this is when most accidents occur (Wormser et al., 1984)
- Never disconnect syringes from needles
- Consider themselves responsible for disposing of a sharp if they have used it: injuries may occur because the user has been careless of disposal. Protective devices are available to help to prevent needlestick injury. They are, however, expensive, and their effectiveness in the clinical situation still needs to be evaluated (Orenstein et al., 1995) (see below).

■ PRACTICE APPLICATION 12.3 ■

Safer Devices

In addition to safe practices when dealing with sharps, it is important that other strategies are considered in an effort to reduce the risk of sharps injuries. These strategies include the use of safer devices and eradicating the unnecessary use of needles (May and Brewer, 2001).

Activity

➤ Read the material covering Safer devices, including Box 5 (pp. 49–50), in May and Brewer (2001).

➤ Discuss the characteristics of safer sharps devices with your mentor or a member of the infection prevention and control team.

➤ Access the Safer Needles Network website below and investigate the devices available for injection. Identify safer devices that are in use in your placement/workplace.

Resources

Medicines and Healthcare products Regulatory Agency (MHRA) – www.mhra.gov.uk.

Safer Needles Network – www.needlestickforum.net/.

Disposal of sharps

Healthcare workers should adhere to the following examples of good practice:

- Sharps containers should comply with BSI regulations: they should be rigid and impermeable to leakage and puncture. No other type of containers should be used.

- Sharps should be placed in a designated container immediately after use. They should never be stored in open containers at the bedside, transported in pockets or carried in the hands.

- Sharps containers should be conveniently sited in all clinical areas. In critical care units, they should be placed at every bed space; in wards and units, they should be placed on the drugs trolley as well as in the treatment room.

- Sharps containers must be kept out of the reach of children, people who are confused, have dementia, or some other mental health problem, such as those who may self-harm.

- No attempt must ever be made to retrieve items from a sharps container or to empty it.

- Sharps containers of the appropriate size must be available. Accidents are more likely when large objects are forced into small containers.

- Where appropriate, patients, clients, carers and residents should be educated about safe disposal. For example, a person with diabetes responsible for administering their own insulin should be supplied with sharps containers at home, which are then collected by authorized handlers of clinical waste (see Chapter 5).

- Sharps containers should be discarded when no more than three-quarters full, and sealed and stored in a secure, dry place ready for collection. They must be incinerated.

Dealing with sharps injuries

The immediate priority following a sharps injury is to implement first aid measures. This may reduce the risk of infection with a BBV (May and Brewer, 2001). Documentation of the incident is vital. The incident is reported to the occupational health department (or the emergency department if it occurs out of hours), post-exposure prophylaxis (PEP) is implemented as appropriate, with counselling and follow-up testing. Following an analysis of the incident, it may be necessary for staff to have further training to ensure competence, and for procedures and equipment to be re-evaluated in order to reduce further occurrences.

First aid

The first aid following a sharps injury is to:

- Encourage the wound to bleed without sucking or squeezing
- Wash it thoroughly with warm running water and soap (May and Brewer, 2001)
- Apply a waterproof dressing.

Documentation and reporting

Complete the necessary documentation. This will involve filling in an incident/accident form and documenting the patient/client or resident's identity if known. Report the injury to the responsible manager as per local policy.

Input from occupational health department

In hospital, the staff member immediately reports to the occupational health department (OHD), or to the emergency department or a designated doctor when the OHD is closed. All other health and social care settings must have policies and arrangements in place that ensure that their staff have access to immediate expert advice, intervention as necessary and follow-up. The need to report all incidents should be emphasized.

Active and/or passive immunization against hepatitis B is used prophylactically (Pratt, 2003b). Staff exposed to HIV may be offered PEP with antiretroviral drugs (see below).

■ PRACTICE APPLICATION 12.4 ■

Post-exposure Prophylaxis

A decision to offer PEP following an exposure that could transmit HIV is based on an assessment of risk.

Activity

Using the resources below, find answers to the following questions:

➤   What factors will be considered in the risk assessment?

➤   How soon after exposure should drugs be commenced?

➤   Which antiretroviral drugs might be prescribed, and for how long?

➤   What side-effects are associated with antiretroviral drugs?

➤   Think about the support and counselling that victims will need.

➤   What follow-up testing will be planned?

Resources

British National Formulary – www.bnf.org.

Campbell S (2004) Management of HIV/AIDS transmission in health care. *Nursing Standard* 18(27): 33–5.

May D and Brewer S (2001) Sharps injury: prevention and management. *Nursing Standard* 15(32): 45–52.

Pratt R (2003b) Prevention and control of viral hepatitis. *Nursing Standard* 17(33): 43–52.

Contamination of the conjunctivae and mucous membranes

The following precautions are recommended when dealing with blood and body fluid contamination of the conjunctivae and mucous membranes:

- Irrigation of the area with water
- Recording and reporting the incident as above.

Spillage of blood and body fluids

Any spillage of blood and body fluids must be dealt with immediately by covering with sodium dichloroisocyanurate (NaDDC) powder, granules or hypochlorite solution. A plastic apron and gloves should be worn.

When using NaDDC:

- Leave the powder or granules in contact with the fluid for two minutes
- Scoop up the debris with disposable wipes
- Discard everything in a yellow plastic bag for incineration
- Clean the area with water and detergent
- Ensure that ventilation is optimal during this procedure, as NaDDC may release chlorine, which is toxic.

When using hypochlorite solution:

- Cover the spillage with paper towels to absorb the excess fluid
- Pour the hypochlorite solution over the towels. Use a 1 per cent solution containing 10,000 parts per million (ppm) of available chlorine
- Leave this for at least two minutes
- Scoop all the debris into a yellow plastic bag for incineration
- Clean the area with water and detergent
- In domiciliary settings, employ the same procedure, using a solution consisting of one part household bleach to 10 parts water.

Emergencies are unavoidable, and it is inevitable that accidental exposure to blood or body fluids will occasionally occur. Routine good practice enables staff to cope in these situations.

SELF-ASSESSMENT

1. Which of the following are classified as body fluids for the purposes of standard (universal) precautions?
   (a) semen
   (b) urine
   (c) wound discharge
   (d) synovial fluid

2. Which of the following are transmitted parenterally?
   (a) hepatitis B
   (b) hepatitis C
   (c) hepatitis D
   (d) hepatitis E

3. All people infected with the HBV become chronic carriers. True? or False?

4. An effective vaccine is available for hepatitis C. True? or False?

5. Which items of PPE are used to prevent exposure to BBVs?

6. Sharps bins should be sealed and discarded when they are no more than three-quarters full. True? or False?

7. Which first aid measures are required following a sharps injury?

REFERENCES

Bond WW, Favero MF, Peterson MJ et al. (1983) Inactivation of hepatitis B virus in intermediate to high level disinfectant chemicals. *Journal of Clinical Microbiology* **18**: 535–8.

Boxall EH (1993) Risks to surgeons and patients from HIV and hepatitis. *British Medical Journal* **306**: 652–3.

Briggs M and Thomas J (1994) Obstacles to hepatitis B vaccine uptake by health care staff. *Public Health* **108**: 137–48.

Campbell S (2004) Management of HIV/AIDS transmission in health care. *Nursing Standard* **18**(27): 33–5.

Castella A, Vallino A, Argentero P et al. (2003) Preventability of percutaneous injuries in healthcare workers: a year long study in Italy. *Journal of Hospital Infection* **55**: 290–4.

Centers for Disease Control and Prevention (CDC) (1993) Update: investigations of persons treated by HIV-infected health care workers. *Journal of the American Medical Association* **269**: 2622–3.

Chapman R, Collier J and Hayes P (2006) Liver and biliary tract disease. In N Boon, N Colledge and B Walker (eds) *Davidson's Principles and Practice of Medicine*, 20th edn. Churchill Livingstone, Edinburgh.

Dalgleish AG and Malkovsy M (1988) Surgical gloves as a mechanical barrier against human immunodeficiency viruses. *British Journal of Surgery* **75**: 171–2.

Department of Health (DH) (1998) *UK Health Departments Guidance for Clinical Health Care Workers: Protection Against Infection with Blood-borne Viruses.* DH, London.

Department of Health (DH) (2002) *Hepatitis C Strategy for England.* Available www.dh.gov.uk.

Department of Health (2006, modified 2007) *Immunisation against Infectious Diseases* (*The Green Book*), Chapter 18. TSO, Norwich. Available www.dh.gov.uk/en/Policyandguidance/Healthandsocialcaretopics/Greenbook/DH 4097254.

Drescher J, Wagner A, Haverich A et al. (1994) Nosocomial hepatitis B infections in cardiac transplant recipients transmitted during transvenous endomyocardial biopsy. *Journal of Hospital Infection* **26**: 81–2.

Duthie R, Morgan-Capner P, Wilson M et al. (1994) Problems in management of health care workers exposed to HBeAg positive body fluids. *Journal of Hospital Infection* **26**: 129–32.

Forseter G, Joline C and Wormser GP (1990) Blood contamination of tourniquets used in routine phlebotomy. *American Journal of Infection Control* **18**: 386–90.

Goldmann DA (1991) The role of barrier precautions in infection control. *Journal of Hospital Infection* **18** (Supplement A): 515–23.

Green SE and Grompertz RK (1992) Glove perforation during surgery. *Annals of the Royal College of Surgery* **74**: 306–8.

Hanson PJ, Gor D and Jeffries DJ (1989) Chemical inactivation of HIV on surfaces. *British Medical Journal* **298**: 862–4.

Havlichek DH, Greenman E and Plaisier K (1991) High prevalence of historical risk factors for blood-borne infections among in-patients in a community hospital. *American Journal of Infection Control* **19**: 67–72.

Health Protection Agency (HPA) (2006) *The Eye of the Needle: United Kingdom Surveillance of Significant Occupational Exposure to Bloodborne Viruses in Healthcare Workers*. Available www.hpa.org.uk/.

Henderson D, Fahey B, Willy M et al. (1990) Risk for occupational transmission of human immunodeficiency virus type 1 (HIV-1) associated with clinical exposures. *Annals of Internal Medicine* **113**: 740–6.

Heponstall J, Porter K and Gill ON (1993) Occupational transmission of HIV: summary of published reports. PHLS internal report, September.

Jagger J, Hunt EH and Pearson RD (1990) Sharp object injuries in hospital: causes and strategies for prevention. *Americal Journal of Hospital Infection* **18**(4): 227–31.

Jenner E (1990) Preaching safe practice. *Nursing Times* **86**(28): 68–9.

Korniewicz DM, Laughon BE, Butz A et al. (1989) Integrity of vinyl and latex procedure gloves. *Nursing Research* **38**: 144–6.

Korniewicz DM, Kirwin M, Cresci K et al. (1994) Barrier protection with examination gloves: double versus single. *American Journal of Infection Control* **22**: 12–15.

Leentvaar-Kuijpers G, Dekker MM, Cuutinho RA et al. (1990) Needlestick injuries, surgeons and HIV risks. *Lancet* **335**: 546–7.

Lifson AR (1988) Do alternative modes for transmission of human immunodeficiency exist? A review. *Journal of the American Medical Association* **259**: 1352–6.

Main J (1991) Therapy of chronic viral hepatitis. *Journal of Hospital Infection* **18** (Supplement A): 177–83.

May D and Brewer S (2001) Sharps injury: prevention and management. *Nursing Standard* **15**(32): 45–52.

Moore RM and Kaczmarek RM (1990) Occupational hazards to health care workers: diverse, ill-defined, and not fully appreciated. *Journal of the American Medical Association* **18**: 316–27.

Mulhall AB, King S and Wiggington E (1993) Maintenance of urinary drainage systems: are practitioners more aware of the dangers? *Journal of Clinical Nursing* **2**: 135–40.

Orenstein R, Reynolds L, Karabaic M et al. (1995) Do protective devices prevent needlestick injuries among health care workers? *American Journal of Infection Control* **23**: 344–51.

Peireira LJ, Lee GM and Wade FJ (1990) The effect of surgical handwashing routines on the microbial counts of operating room nurses. *American Journal of Infection* **18**: 354–64.

Poole CJ, Miller S and Fillingham G (1994) Immunity to hepatitis B among health care workers performing exposure prone procedures. *British Medical Journal* **309**: 94–5.

Pratt R (2003a) *HIV and AIDS: A Foundation for Nursing and Healthcare Practice*, 5th edn. Arnold, London.

Pratt R (2003b) Prevention and control of viral hepatitis. *Nursing Standard* **17**(33): 43–52.

Rennie-Meyer K (2007) Preventing the spread of infection. In C Brooker and A Waugh (eds) *Foundations of Nursing Practice: Fundamentals of Holistic Care*. Mosby, Edinburgh.

Rogers G and Campbell L (2003) Hepatitis C: its prevalence, implications and management. *Nursing Times* **99**(50): 31–2.

Shaw DJ and Bell DM (1993) Risk of occupational infection with blood-borne pathogens in operating and delivery room settings. *American Journal of Infection Control* **21**: 343–51.

Spence MR and Dash GP (1990) Hepatitis B: perceptions, knowledge, and vaccine acceptance among registered nurses in high risk occupations in a university hospital. *Infection Control and Hospital Epidemiology* **11**: 129–33.

Thomas JA, Fligelstone LJ, Jerwood TE et al. (1993) Theatre footwear: a health hazard? *British Journal of Theatre Nursing* **3**(7): 5–9.

Van Rijwisjk L (1992) Gloves and other rubber-based devices: benefits, problems and guidelines. *Wounds: A Compendium of Research and Practice* **4**: 65–73.

Watterson L (2004) Monitoring sharps injuries: EPINet™ surveillance results. *Nursing Standard* **29**(19): 33–8.

Wilson J and Breedon P (1990) Universal precautions. *Nursing Times* **86**(37): 67–9.

Wormser GP, Joline C and Duncanson F (1984) Needlestick injuries during the care of patients with AIDS. *New England Journal of Medicine* **310**: 1461–2.

World Health Organization (WHO) (2004) *Weekly Epidemiological Record No 28. Hepatitis B Vaccines*. WHO position paper **79:** 255–63. WHO, Geneva.

████████████ FURTHER READING AND INFORMATION SOURCES ████████

Advisory Committee on Dangerous Pathogens (1995) *Protection against Blood Borne Infections in the Workplace: HIV, Hepatitis*. HMSO, London.

British Liver Trust – www.britishlivertrust.org.uk.

Hainsworth T (2006) Key issues in diagnosing and treating hepatitis C infection. *Nursing Times* **102**(24): 23–4.

Health Protection Agency Centre for Infections (2005) Occupational transmission of HIV: summary of published reports. *CDR Weekly* **15**(10). Available www.hpa.org.uk/cdr/archives/archive05/News/news1005.htm.

National Audit Office (NAO) (2003) *A Safer Place to Work: Improving the Management of Health and Safety Risks to Staff in the NHS*. TSO, London.

Terence Higgins Trust – www.tht.org.uk.

UK Haemophilia Society – www.haemophilia.org.uk.

CHAPTER 13

Sexually transmitted infections

CHAPTER OUTCOMES

After reading this chapter, you should be able to:

➤ Explain why sexually transmitted infections are a significant health problem in the UK

➤ Outline public health measures taken to reduce the incidence of sexually transmitted infections

➤ Define the term 'sexual health'

➤ Describe the functions of sexual health clinics

➤ Discuss the common infections transmitted by the sexual route, name the organisms responsible and outline the methods used in diagnosis, prevention and treatment

Introduction

The sexually transmitted infections (STIs) discussed in this chapter are syphilis, gonorrhoea, *Chlamydia*, genital warts, herpes simplex, candidiasis (candidosis), trichomoniasis, bacterial vaginosis and human immunodeficiency virus (HIV).

In the UK, the diagnosis and treatment of STIs (also known as sexually acquired infections) are available in sexual health clinics (also known as genitourinary medicine clinics), from GPs, some family planning clinics and privately. STIs represent a significant health problem within the UK as many of the infections can lead to permanent problems such as infertility and, in pregnant women, can damage the fetus.

Incidence of sexually transmitted infections

There is a well-established system of recording the number of cases of STIs. Every sexual health clinic is required to submit quarterly returns to the Department of Health. These figures are vital for planning control measures, including health promotion campaigns, but the data underestimate the real incidence of infection: some infections are undiagnosed, and cases seen outside NHS sexual health clinics are excluded.

Over the past 15 years, there has been a substantial increase in high-risk sexual activity in the UK, resulting in a deterioration in sexual health (Ritchie, 2006). The incidence of STIs has increased overall and there have been increases associated with specific types of infection, notably syphilis, *Chlamydia* and gonorrhoea, especially among people under 20 (Brown et al., 2004). STIs are an important public health problem because they contribute to a range of poor health outcomes including cervical cancer, neonatal disorders and infertility coupled with psychological problems arising from sexual coercion and abuse (Department of Health, 2001). Health education aimed at young people is important in view of research findings which suggest that despite the well-established benefits of condoms in preventing STIs (Steiner and Cates, 2006), many young people engage in unprotected sexual activity yet fail to perceive themselves to be at risk (Fenton et al., 2001). In 2001, the Department of Health launched *Better Prevention, Better Services, Better Sexual Health: The National Strategy for Sexual Health and HIV* (see below). This has been followed by the introduction of a national screening programme for *Chlamydia* (Flannigan, 2006).

According to the Health Protection Agency report (2007) *Testing Times – HIV and other Sexually Transmitted Infections in the UK: 2007*, cases of syphilis are still high, genital herpes and warts have both increased, and these increases are linked to new HIV infections and STIs diagnosed in men who have sex with men (MSM).

PRACTICE APPLICATION 13.1

Improving Sexual Health

In *Better Prevention, Better Services, Better Sexual Health: The National Strategy for Sexual Health and HIV* (Department of Health, 2001, available www.dh.gov.uk/en/Publicationsandstatistics), the Department of Health sets out a strategy for improving sexual health in England.

Activity

Access the document and use it to answer the following questions:

➤ What are the adverse effects of poor sexual health (p. 7)?

➤ What percentage of 14–15-year-olds think that the contraceptive pill protects against infection (p. 8)?

➤ Which groups are most likely to suffer sexual ill-health (p. 9)?

Discuss the role of health and social care professionals in the prevention of HIV and STIs with your mentor.

Sexual health and the role of sexual health clinics

The control of STIs has been considered an important area of public health endeavour since the early part of the 20th century. The Public Health (Venereal Diseases) Regulations of 1916 required all local authorities to provide clinics where diagnosis and free treatment were available in strict confidence. Contact tracing became an essential feature of the service, contributing to its success. A second advance was made in 1924 with the establishment of the Venereal Disease Reference Laboratory: for the first time, it was possible to standardize methods of diagnosis and treatment and to collate statistics.

Nowadays, a broad view of sexual health is taken – it is seen as the integration of all aspects of sexual being including its physical, emotional, intellectual and social components. Sexual health is therefore an integral part of holistic health and involves much more than helping people to avoid infection. Health professionals working in this clinical setting provide information and advice, perform tests to diagnose infection and give treatment. Sexual health clinics play a central role in meeting government health targets through efforts to reduce the incidence of HIV and other STIs. Public health issues addressed include:

- The availability of a confidential self-referral service without a waiting list for anyone wishing to discuss sexual health matters
- Examination and testing for genital infections
- Health education and counselling
- Partner notification
- Free prescriptions.

Given the sensitive nature of visiting a sexual health clinic for advice, investigations and treatment for an STI, it is essential that people are made to feel comfortable and are assured that strict confidentiality will be maintained. It is important to ensure that they will complete a course of treatment, follow advice and return for further testing or treatment, as necessary (see below).

PRACTICE APPLICATION 13.2

Achieving Concordance in the Sexual Health Clinic

Concordance with treatment is increased through sexual health clinics because it is possible to process many specimens immediately. Diagnosis is swift and accurate, and treatment can begin at the same visit. With uncomplicated gonorrhoea, for example, it is often possible to give a single-dose treatment, thereby eliminating the need to follow a course of treatment. The person's reception in the clinic and the attitude of staff also play an important role in securing willingness to return for follow-up tests.

Activity

Discuss with your mentor or a health professional working in a sexual health clinic how the attitude of staff could influence a person's concordance with advice.

Sexually transmitted infections

It is important to remember that certain STIs are not exclusively sexually transmitted. For example, candidiasis (candidosis) is also associated with diabetes mellitus and some types of antibiotic use. Moreover, HIV is also transmitted by other means including exposure to infected blood or body fluids. Chapter 12 covers this aspect of HIV transmission, and also that of various hepatitis viruses, which are sexually transmitted.

People attending a sexual health clinic with a suspected STI are screened for other STIs as they may coexist, for example gonorrhoea and *Chlamydia*.

Syphilis

Syphilis is caused by the spirochaete *Treponema pallidum*, which is exclusively a human pathogen. Syphilis is a past example of a 'new' disease. It appeared suddenly in Europe in the late 15th century, engendering the same fear and speculation as HIV does today. There are two theories to explain its origins:

- **The Colomban theory** – syphilis endemic in the West Indies was brought to Europe by sailors returning with Columbus.
- **The unitarian theory** – syphilis is a form of yaws, a tropical treponemal infection caused by a spirochaete indistinguishable from *T. pallidum*. Yaws is a skin condition spread by direct skin contact. It was prevalent in the West Indies throughout the 15th century, reaching Europe as a result of slave trading. It has been suggested that in a colder climate where everyday skin contact was minimal, transmission gradually became dependent on sexual contact. Infection results in a wide range of symptoms; in the past, syphilis was called the 'great imitator'. Today, although still considered serious, the infection appears less virulent than when the first cases appeared in the 15th century.

According to Brown et al. (2004), there has been an eightfold increase in new cases of syphilis between 1997 and 2002. During the period 2002–06, the incidence of syphilis in MSM increased by 117 per cent (Health Protection Agency, 2007).

Stages of acquired syphilis

In adults, syphilis is transmitted mainly by sexual intercourse. The incubation period is 9–90 days. Traditionally, its progress has been described in four stages – primary, secondary, latent and tertiary. Increasingly, it is divided into two main stages – early and late.

Early stage syphilis

- **Primary syphilis** – A chancre (ulcer) appears at the site of infection on the genitalia, rectum, mouth or rarely finger. The early signs of infection are easily overlooked, as chancres are painless and often difficult to see. In the absence of treatment, the chancre heals within 2–6 weeks. Spirochaetes spread rapidly to other parts of the body, probably within a few hours.
- **Secondary syphilis** – About two months after infection, the person may experience a vague, flu-like illness with malaise, fever, aching joints and lymph node enlargement.

Symptoms may be mild and dismissed because they are so nonspecific. Some people develop a rash. People are highly infectious because the surfaces of the lesions team with treponemes. The other manifestations of secondary syphilis include elongated ulcerated lesions ('snail-track' ulcers) and flattened warty growths (condylomata lata). Again, these are easily overlooked, or their significance may not be appreciated.

- **Early latent stage** – The untreated person has no clinical signs of syphilis, but they remain sexually infectious within the first two years following infection (Scott, 2006). Diagnosis is by positive serological tests, or testing cerebrospinal fluid for abnormalities.

Late stage syphilis

- **Late latent stage** – This stage may persist for years. The person appears well but shows serological evidence of infection if tested. They are no longer sexually infectious.

- **Tertiary syphilis** – This arises years later. There are different forms – the formation of gummata, cardiovascular or neurosyphilis:

  - Chronic ulcers called 'gummata' can develop anywhere on the skin, in the tissues, or form visceral lesions. Gummata cause particular damage if they involve bone, cardiovascular or nervous tissue.

  - Syphilis affecting the cardiovascular system causes aortitis (inflammation of the lining of the aorta), which can lead to the formation of an aortic aneurysm (swelling in the wall of an artery), damage to the aortic valve, or angina.

  - Neurosyphilis leads to tabes dorsalis (locomotor ataxia – a lack of coordination with disturbed sensation in the legs) and dementia (general paralysis of the insane). The mechanism by which *T. pallidum* evokes damage remains obscure: it does not produce toxins, and it evokes only a weak immune response.

Congenital syphilis

Congenital (prenatal) syphilis is transmitted vertically from mother to fetus via the placenta. It causes spontaneous miscarriage, stillbirth or the delivery of an infant with the signs and symptoms of syphilis (see below). The earlier the maternal infection occurs during pregnancy, the more grave the prognosis for the infant. Congenital syphilis is extremely rare in the UK, having been eliminated by routinely testing all pregnant women as part of their antenatal screening programme.

INFORMATION BOX 13.1

The hallmarks of congenital syphilis

Early – appearing within two weeks of delivery

  ➤ Skin lesions – a weeping, crusted rash principally affecting the peripheries, followed by a maculopapular rash and condylomata lata reminiscent of adult secondary syphilis. Scarring may result in areas subject to friction, such as the mouth

➤ Mucous membranes – discharging lesions develop in the nose, mouth, throat, larynx and pharynx, interfering with feeding. Fissures around the mouth, nose and anus

➤ Lymphadenopathy (any disease of the lymph nodes, but in this case an enlargement of the lymph nodes)

➤ Rhinitis, discharge from the nose ('snuffles')

➤ Viscera – hepatosplenomegaly (enlargement of the liver and spleen), with altered plasma protein levels

➤ Neurological – meningitis

➤ Choroiditis (inflammation of the choroid layer of the eye)

➤ Bone lesions – osteochondritis (inflammation of bone cartilage) and periostitis (inflammation of the periosteum – the membrane covering bones)

Late effects and stigmata – these result from maldevelopment of the tissues through the damage caused by treponemes at or soon after birth. They include:

➤ A perforated nasal septum

➤ Saddle nose

➤ Maldeveloped, notched, peg-shaped teeth (Hutchinson's incisors)

➤ Scarring (rhagades) from the early rashes around the nose, mouth and anus

➤ Keratitis leading to corneal scarring

➤ Effusion of the joints (Clutton's joints)

➤ Bony deformities, especially of the palate, maxilla and long bones (for example the tibia). Bossing of the parietal and frontal cranial bones

➤ Eighth cranial nerve (the auditory or vestibulocochlear nerve) deafness

Any of the conditions arising during the adult form of tertiary syphilis may also develop

Diagnosis

Diagnosis at the primary stage involves scraping exudate from the surface of the chancre for microscopy. Treponemes are too small and too difficult to visualize even under the high power of the light microscope so a special technique called dark ground microscopy is used (Chapter 3). Treponemes are also identified using more advanced techniques, such as fluorescent antibody tests. Most people with syphilis are, however, detected because they have been alerted to the risk through contact tracing or during routine testing for other STIs. The diagnosis is then made by serological testing (see below).

INFORMATION BOX 13.2

Serological tests for syphilis

Serological tests may be nonspecific (non-treponemal) or specific treponemal anti-body tests.

Nonspecific tests

➤ Venereal Disease Research Laboratory (VDRL) test – a rapid precipitation test

➤ Rapid plasma reagin (RPR) test

Specific antibody tests

➤ Treponemal antigen-based enzyme immunoassay (EIA) – measures immunoglobulins IgG and IgM. Used for screening

➤ Fluorescent treponemal antibody-absorbed test (FTA-ABS) – sometimes used in early diagnosis as it yields a result at an earlier stage in the course of disease than most other tests. Too expensive for routine screening

➤ *Treponema pallidum* haemagglutination assay (TPHA) – a highly specific agglutination test for treponemal antigens that can be used in routine screening

➤ *Treponema pallidum* particle agglutination assay (TPPA)

NB The Wasserman reaction (WR), a complement fixation test, has been superseded by modern tests that are more accurate.

Treatment

Treatment involves the intramuscular administration of high doses of procaine benzylpenicillin given for 10–14 days; the exact regimens depend on the stage of disease and also vary between clinics. There have been no recorded cases of treponemal resistance to penicillin. People allergic to penicillin are usually given doxycycline, a tetracycline, or erythromycin. The injections are painful, and daily attendance can disrupt usual activities. Thus, as well as giving medication, the nurse has an important role in maintaining concordance, especially with clients who feel well or for whom the diagnosis was unexpected. People are asked to refrain from sexual activity until the course of treatment has finished and must return to the clinic to ensure that it has been successful. They may need to undergo neurological investigations. They must also be warned about the possibility of experiencing the Jarisch–Herxheimer reaction: fever, headache, nausea, chills, myalgia (muscle aches), tachycardia (increased heart rate) and dizziness (caused by hypotension – low blood pressure) within 6–12 hours of receiving antibiotics. The cause of the reaction is unknown, but it is thought to be due to the release of endotoxins from the treponemes as they are destroyed. The Jarisch–Herxheimer reaction is usually short-lived and is not harmful. People are advised to rest in bed and take fluids and antipyretics (drugs that reduce temperature). Once the course of treatment has been completed, the infection is eradicated, but previous exposure does not produce immunity: it is thus possible to develop syphilis more than once. Asymptomatic contacts of the infected person are also treated with doxycycline.

Gonorrhoea

Gonorrhoea is caused by a Gram-negative diplococcus, *Neisseria gonorrhoeae* (also known as the gonococcus or GC). It attaches to the urethral and cervical mucosae by pili, laboratory strains without pili being non-pathogenic. The bacteria survive in neutrophils (a type of polymorphonuclear leucocyte or white blood cell) (Figure 13.1). The adult vaginal wall is not invaded, probably because its tough squamous epithelium is inhospitable to the delicate bacteria. *N. gonorrhoeae* rapidly succumbs to cold and drying. It is unable to survive long outside the host, explaining why transmission is primarily via the sexual route. The eyes of infants become infected during passage down the birth canal in the presence of cervical secretions containing gonococci. This causes ophthalmia neonatorum (pus discharging from the eyes of an infant that starts within 21 days of birth).

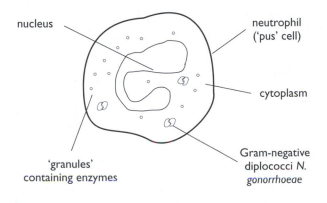

Figure 13.1 Neutrophil containing *Neisseria gonorrhoeae*

In both sexes, acute infection presents as urethritis (inflammation of the urethra), with discharge and pain on micturition. The incubation period is between 2 and 10 days. Approximately a third of infected women remain asymptomatic. The consequences are serious both from the perspective of the individual and in public health terms. Gonococci migrate from the cervix to the uterus and uterine tubes, where they cause severe scarring that may result in occlusion, thus impairing fertility. Escape from the fimbriated ends of the uterine tubes may lead to peritonitis (inflammation of the peritoneum), but this is less common. More often, female carriers experience symptoms of vague, debilitating chronic ill-health and are highly infectious. Gonococcal vulvovaginitis (inflammation of the vulva and vagina) in young girls may be a sign of sexual abuse. In men, untreated infection causes scarring, urethral stricture, epididymitis and prostatitis (inflammation of the epididymis of the testes and prostate gland respectively).

The involvement of the joints, with the development of gonococcal arthritis, is another late occasional complication of infection in either sex.

Diagnosis

Diagnosis is by the examination of wet films of material collected using swabs. The survival of *N. gonorrhoeae* outside the host is so poor that microscopy must be performed in the clinic as soon as the swabs have been obtained.

Treatment

Treatment choices depend on whether the infection is uncomplicated or not and the site involved. Treatment is usually successful using oral amoxicillin with probenecid to delay its renal clearance. Penicillin-resistant strains were first reported in the 1970s. These release beta-lactamase enzymes, which destroy the beta-lactam part of the penicillin molecule (see Chapter 4), rendering it ineffective. A variety of antibacterial drugs are used to treat gonorrhoea (see below). Advice is given to avoid sexual activity until the success of treatment is confirmed. People carrying resistant strains must be given another antibiotic, such as spectinomycin. Infection does not result in immunity so it is possible to develop gonorrhoea more than once. Contacts are also traced and contacted.

■ PRACTICE APPLICATION 13.3 ■

Drugs for Treating Gonorrhoea

Antibacterial drugs used to treat uncomplicated gonorrhoea are usually administered as a single dose; this is usually orally, but may be by intramuscular injection.

Activity

Use the resource below to find out about the drugs used to treat uncomplicated gonorrhoea:

➤ Find examples of a single-dose penicillin, cephalosporin, other beta-lactams and a quinolone antibacterial drug.

➤ Note the doses, route of administration and the side-effects.

Resource

British National Formulary – www.bnf.org.

Chlamydia

Chlamydia trachomatis is an intracellular pathogen (Flannigan, 2006). It is the most commonly diagnosed STI worldwide. Its incidence in the UK is increasing (Clutterbuck, 2004), especially among the under twenties, with the highest increase in young men (Flannigan, 2006).

It infects the urethra and in men is responsible for most cases of nonspecific urethritis (nongonococcal urethritis). Complications include prostatitis and epididymitis. In women, its behaviour is similar to that of *N. gonorrhoeae* and it may be carried asymptomatically. The cervix is a common site of infection. It ascends the genital tract, causing salpingitis (inflammation of the uterine tubes), pelvic inflammatory disease and impaired fertility. Infection with *Chlamydia* is serious and highly damaging, meriting early detection and treatment. The need for a national screening programme for *Chlamydia* was recognized in *The National Strategy for Sexual Health and HIV* (Department of Health, 2001). Initial uptake was promising (Flannigan, 2006) and from 2007 all Primary Care Trusts have been required to have a screening programme in place. Opportunistic screening outside clinical areas (for example the workplace) is possible because new technology (nucleic acid amplification testing) requires the person to supply only a urine sample without an uncomfortable clinical examination. Because the infection can remain asymptomatic for so long, a diagnosis does not suggest that infidelity has taken place. It is important for people to receive this information because it helps to encourage the uptake of screening.

Treatment

The antibacterial drugs azithromycin (single dose), doxycycline (7-day course) or erythromycin (14-day course) are used to treat *Chlamydia*.

Genital warts

Genital warts are caused by the human papilloma virus (HPV). Of all newly diagnosed STIs, 22 per cent were genital warts; they were the most common sexually transmitted virus infections diagnosed in sexual health clinics during 2006 (Health Protection Agency, 2007). The incubation period is 2–3 months, but the virus can remain latent for years so contact tracing is not practical. The mode of transmission is poorly understood. Entry is thought to occur via minor abrasions in the mucous membranes developing through trauma during sexual intercourse. Warts are unsightly, catch on clothing and contribute to the development of malignancy, and are a source of anxiety for patients (Chandler, 1996). HPV types 16 and 18 appear to have the greatest oncogenic (cancer-causing) potential and are important causative agents of cervical cancer, both in women who have warts and in those whose partners are affected. Annual cervical smears are recommended for those at risk, and some authorities now recommend tests for HPV to complement cytology (examination of cells using a microscope).

A vaccine against HPV types 6, 11, 16 and 18 has recently been licensed for females aged 9–26 years. The vaccine has been added to the NHS immunization programme and will be introduced in the autumn of 2008 for girls aged 12–13 years, with a later catch-up programme for girls aged up to 18 years (Department of Health, 2007). The vaccine protects against the virus types that cause around 70 per cent of cervical cancers. Cervical screening will still be important because of this and because many women will not have been vaccinated.

Treatment

The treatment options include:

- Application of topical creams or solutions containing either podophyllin (cyto-toxic agent) or its extract podophyllotoxin, or imiquimod (immune response modifier) (see below)
- Cryotherapy (use of low temperature)

- Electrofulguration (use of electrical current to destroy the warts)
- Surgical removal.

PRACTICE APPLICATION 13.4

Topical Treatments for Genital Warts

The topical preparations used for treating genital warts are:

➤ Imiquimod cream (5 per cent)

➤ Podophyllin solution (0.5 per cent)

➤ Podophyllotoxin cream (0.15 per cent)

Activity

Use the resource below to find out the following:

➤ How often each preparation should be applied and the duration of treatment.

➤ The advice given to patients.

➤ The cautions involved with each preparation.

➤ Potential side-effects.

➤ The circumstances in which a health professional should apply the preparations.

Resource

British National Formulary – www.bnf.org.

In the past people, were obliged to attend clinics for all their treatment, but providing the lesions meet certain criteria and are sited in an area where they may be visualized (with a mirror if necessary), self-treatment is now possible, although it should still occur under the supervision of a health professional.

Herpes simplex

Herpes simplex virus (HSV) is a DNA virus responsible for cold sores (involving the oral mucosae) and genital ulceration. By the age of five years, over 60 per cent of the population have become infected. There are two types, distinguished on the basis of biochemical and antigenic properties:

- HSV-1, primarily isolated from oral lesions
- HSV-2, primarily isolated from genital lesions, and less common.

There is an increasing tendency for HSV-1 to be isolated from genital lesions. People already infected with HVS-1 can become infected with HVS-2 and vice versa.

Primary oral herpes infection

Primary oral herpes infection usually occurs early from contact with an asymptomatic salivary carrier or someone who has an actively discharging lesion. Characteristic vesicles appear around the mouth or eyes, sometimes associated with febrile illness. Encephalitis is a rare complication that may be fatal. Infection, however, is more often mild and overlooked.

Recurrent oral herpes infection

Recurrent oral herpes infection occurs throughout adult life. After primary infection, the virus migrates up the sensory nerves to their associated ganglia where it lies dormant, occasionally becoming active through some challenge to the immune system (a cold, influenza or sometimes even exposure to sunshine or during menstruation). Virus particles travel back down the nerves, and as these supply a localized area on the face, crops of vesicles develop at the same site, usually around the nostrils or lips.

Primary genital herpes

Primary genital herpes infection is acquired sexually, probably through small breaks in the mucosae. The main viral reservoirs are the cervix and the male genital tract. Painful ulceration develops on the glans and shaft of the penis or the vulva, where it may interfere with micturition. Health professionals are well placed to offer general advice and support to people with genital herpes (see below). Individuals feel most unwell during the prodrome (time between the onset of symptoms and the appearance of a rash or other lesions) before the lesions have fully developed. Treatment of first-episode HSV is with oral antiviral agents, for example aciclovir, valaciclovir or famciclovir. Antiviral drugs, for example aciclovir, are used with caution during pregnancy. Aciclovir should only be used in situations where the potential benefits are greater than any risk to the fetus or woman.

INFORMATION BOX 13.3

General advice and support for people with genital herpes

A diagnosis of genital herpes will affect all aspects of the person's life and health – there will be psychological and social implications and not just the physical effects of the infection. Individuals may feel unclean, that their sex life is at an end and stigmatized by misinformed opinion on the nature of herpes. It is easy to see why those affected may experience low mood, especially when one considers the recurring nature of herpes.

The following will be very helpful:

➤ Provide information about all aspects of genital herpes – treatments, recurrence, risk to sexual partners and pregnancy.

➤ Teaching that allows people to recognize when they have genital herpes.

➤ Teaching that allows people to recognize the 'early warning' signs of a recurrent episode of herpes.

> ➤ Provide written, audio or electronic back-up information about genital herpes, including treatment, complementary therapies and self-help groups.

> ➤ Provide a relaxed and non-judgemental environment in which people have the opportunity to talk through their feelings about having genital herpes with a well-informed health professional.

> ➤ Provide advice about simple symptomatic remedies, for example paracetamol, for the systemic illness that occurs with the primary infection; advice to rest and to take extra fluids.

> ➤ Provide information about keeping the lesions clean and dry.

> ➤ Provide advice about when to stop having sexual intercourse; during the primary infection, for example, this would be until the lesions have healed and all other symptoms of genital herpes have passed.

> ➤ Stress the importance of women telling health professionals about a pregnancy or a plan to conceive in the future.

> ➤ Encourage people to return for follow-up consultations and make sure that tests for other STIs are completed.

> ➤ If necessary, encourage sexual partners to visit the clinic.

> ➤ Ensure that the individual is involved in decisions about his or her management.

Recurrent genital herpes

Recurrent genital herpes infection occurs throughout life. The same antiviral drugs aciclovir, valaciclovir or famciclovir are used during recurrence if necessary. Some of those affected may, however, prefer to use complementary therapies, for example tea tree oil. Delivery during primary infection acquired late in pregnancy may result in the baby developing fatal encephalitis (brain inflammation) unless an elective caesarean section is performed.

Candidiasis (candidosis)

Candidiasis is caused by *Candida*, a yeast-like, spore-forming fungus. It causes a white, highly irritant vaginal discharge, often most troublesome just before menstruation. The infection is also known as 'thrush' (a lay term). There are numerous species, the most common being *Candida albicans*. Spores are visible when wet films are Gram stained and examined under the microscope. Hyphae are difficult to visualize.

Candida occasionally causes balanitis (inflammation of the glans penis) in men. It is not always sexually transmitted but is most common in sexually active women, especially during the childbearing years. Infection is said to be more common in women taking oral contraceptives, but there is little supporting evidence for this (Odds, 1988). Some women suffer from repeated attacks, which may be the result of reinfection. Boiling or disinfecting clothing is, however, not effective as a treatment, even though it is recommended in 'self-help' material for patients (Rashid et al., 1991).

The incidence is higher among diabetics than members of the general population and may be a sign of undetected diabetes mellitus. It has been suggested that an elevated blood glucose level alters vaginal pH by interfering with lactic acid production. The situation may be similar in pregnancy, when *Candida* infection is also common. Increased oestrogen levels stimulate the formation of glycogen from glucose, again resulting in the excess production of lactic acid. Vaginal candidiasis is also associated with the use of antibiotic drugs.

The personal, social and economic consequences of vulval/vaginal *Candida* infection tend to be overlooked. Many women suffer recurrent inconvenience, embarrassment and discomfort. The irritation is often most intense at night, interfering with sleep and the following day's activities. Micturition becomes painful. Time is lost from school or work, and underperformance may result (Odds, 1988). Contact tracing is not routinely performed, many cases being self-treated as topical fungicide creams, vaginal creams and pessaries are available without prescription.

Candida has been responsible for healthcare-associated outbreaks, mainly among the critically ill (Lee et al., 1991). Infection often develops in the mouth or large bowel in response to antibiotic therapy and can be transmitted via the hands of health professionals (Findik et al., 1996). It is a common complication of immunosuppression, including HIV disease.

Treatment

Treatment is usually possible with vaginal creams or pessaries containing, for example, clotrimazole, econazole, miconazole or nystatin, with a vulval cream to control itching. Many over-the-counter products are conveniently single dose. Women should be warned that many of the preparations might damage latex contraceptive diaphragms or condoms. If self-treatment is unsuccessful, women may be given fluconazole or itraconazole orally. Contraception is vital during treatment with fluconazole, as it is teratogenic (capable of causing embryonic or fetal malformation) and high dose long-term use has been associated with multiple fetal abnormalities. Recurrent vaginal candidiasis may require longer term treatment and sexual partners who are symptomatic should be treated.

Trichomoniasis

Trichomoniasis is caused by *Trichomonas vaginalis*, a highly motile, flagellated protozoon that may be carried asymptomatically or cause an offensive, frothy, yellow-green vaginal discharge. Speculum examination reveals an inflamed cervix and vaginal walls. In severe cases, the vulva, perineum and insides of the thighs may become sore. The distress and inconvenience experienced by patients are frequently overlooked. The organisms are easily visualized in wet microscope preparations made from vaginal swabs and examined under low power, but they are difficult to isolate from men even though they may be present in prostatic fluid or cause mild urethral discharge. *Trichomonas vaginalis* forms cysts under adverse environmental conditions.

Sexual transmission is thought to be the most usual mechanism of dispersal because partners often show evidence of infection if examined thoroughly and it is sometimes possible to identify chains of infection when there have been multiple partners (Krieger et al., 1993). Non-sexual transfer has been suggested but never demonstrated.

Treatment

Treatment is administered orally with metronidazole (either as a large single dose or a 7-day course), or tinidazole (large single dose). Both partners should be treated. This may be difficult to organize because routine contact tracing is not performed.

Bacterial vaginosis

Bacterial vaginosis is not always sexually transmitted, although it is often diagnosed in conjunction with other STIs. It is a distressing condition most commonly diagnosed among women during the fertile years, especially if they have had several partners or a recent change of partner (Temple, 1994). It also occurs in women who are not sexually active. It has attracted more attention since it was established that affected women are more likely to experience late miscarriage or preterm delivery (Hay et al., 1994).

The most commonly reported symptom is an unpleasant, fishy odour from the genital area, not linked to poor hygiene. Some women also complain of a frothy, non-irritant grey discharge. According to Dapaah and Dapaah (2003), approximately 50 per cent of women are asymptomatic. Bacteriological examination of the vagina reveals an abnormally high number of anaerobic bacteria coupled with a reduction in the *Lactobacillus* count, suggesting a disturbance in the usual ecology of the vaginal flora and perhaps general ill-health. *Gardnerella vaginalis* is one of the bacteria most frequently isolated. An association was initially made between this organism and the presence of vaginal irritation in 1955 (Gardner and Dukes, 1955). However, it may also be present in healthy women. Diagnosis involves placing a piece of pH indicator paper inside the vagina to test the pH. A value greater than 4.5 indicates infection but is not specific. Swabs from the vaginal wall and cervix are cultured to demonstrate the presence of anaerobes and a reduction in lactobacilli.

Treatment

Treatment is with metronidazole 0.75 per cent vaginal gel (5-day course), clindamycin 2 per cent vaginal cream (3–7-day course), or a single oral dose of tinidazole. Women should be warned that clindamycin might damage latex contraceptive diaphragms or condoms.

Human immunodeficiency virus

Human immunodeficiency viruses (HIV-1 and HIV-2) are RNA retroviruses. The virus multiplies aggressively, damaging the host by progressively destroying the immune system, especially the CD4 (T helper) lymphocytes (Chapter 2). These play a key role in activating the immune response, especially cell-mediated immunity. New CD4 lymphocytes are produced to replace those lost, but the immune system cannot sustain this effect indefinitely (Cooper and Mergigan, 1996). The result is profound immunosuppression, with the appearance of characteristic opportunistic infections (Table 13.1) and tumours (for example Kaposi's sarcoma and lymphomas). Many of the opportunistic infections and tumours are considered to be AIDS-defining by the US Centers for Disease Control and Prevention (Atlanta) and the World Health Organization.

Reverse transcriptase, an enzyme released by HIV, manufactures DNA blueprints of viral RNA. This reversal of the usual mechanism of nucleic acid synthesis permits HIV to take control of normal cellular function. Several new copies of the virus are made but lie dormant until some event or environmental insult triggers their release, the host cell being destroyed in the process. The total number of CD4 lymphocytes can be taken as a reflection of the extent of HIV infection. As the number of CD4 lymphocytes falls, the risk of opportunistic infection increases dramatically.

A discussion of HIV as a parenterally transmitted infection can be found in Chapter 12.

Table 13.1 Opportunistic infections associated with HIV disease

Microorganism	Presentation
Bacteria	
Mycobacterium (*M. tuberculosis, M. avium intercellulare, M. kansasii*)	Pulmonary or disseminated infection
Shigella	Diarrhoea
Salmonella	Diarrhoea
Viruses	
Herpes simplex	Mucocutaneous lesions of the gastrointestinal tract
Herpes zoster	Shingles
Cytomegalovirus	Central nervous system (CNS), gastrointestinal and pulmonary lesions
Fungi	
Candida	Oesophageal and pulmonary lesions
Cryptococcus	Pulmonary, CNS and disseminated infection
Aspergillus	CNS and disseminated infection
*Coccidioides immitis**	Disseminated infection
*Histoplasma capsulatum**	Disseminated infection
Protozoa	
Pneumocystis jiroveci (previously *carinii*)	Pneumonia
Cryptosporidium	Diarrhoea
Toxoplasma	Pneumonia, CNS and disseminated infection
*Leishmania**	Lesions in the spleen, liver and bone marrow. Anaemia

*When patients have travelled to areas where the microorganism is endemic

Transmission of HIV

Transmission occurs sexually, through exposure to infected blood and body fluids, and perinatally. Situations in which exposure is possible (Pratt, 2003) include:

- Iatrogenic transmission to healthcare professionals, or to people with haemophilia who have received blood products that have not undergone heat treatment (Chapter 12)
- Injecting drug users (Chapter 12)
- Sexual transmission
- Vertical transmission from infected mothers to infants (see above).

In Europe (including Eastern Europe), North America and Australia, the transmission of HIV is mainly associated with intravenous drug use and/or sex between men; this is also the usual transmission for a viral subtype in Thailand (Wilkins, 2006). In Africa, India and Thailand, however, the transmission of HIV is mainly associated with heterosexual sexual activity (Wilkins, 2006).

Historical aspects of HIV infection

HIV was first reported in the USA in 1979. As the number of affected individuals increased, it became apparent that the characteristic opportunistic infections and Kaposi's sarcoma occurred in young, previously healthy MSM. In the UK, the first cases were reported in gay men who had had sexual contact with people from the USA. By 1983, a syndrome had been recognized. Towards the end of that year, HIV was identified as the causative agent, an antibody test being developed in 1984. This is a test for antibodies produced in response to HIV. HIV infection is now an established health problem worldwide.

A prevalence study of HIV infection undertaken in 1998 indicated that the number of individuals living with HIV in the UK had grown considerably over the previous three years, the estimated figure being 30,000 (Department of Health, 1999). By 2002, this estimate had increased to 49,500 adults over 15 years of age living with HIV in the UK (Brown et al., 2004) (see below). A recent report estimates that the prevalence of HIV has increased in the UK and that 73,000 people are now infected with HIV, with a third of them undiagnosed (Health Protection Agency, 2007).

PRACTICE APPLICATION 13.5

Trends in HIV Infection

Regular estimates of the number of people in the UK living with HIV are important for targeting health promotion for groups at the greatest risk and planning services.

Activity

Using Brown et al. (2004) or Dougan et al. (2007), find answers to the following questions:

> New HIV cases diagnosed in the UK doubled in the five years to 2002 (Brown et al., 2004). What was the main cause of this?

> In 2002, which group accounted for 80 per cent of newly diagnosed HIV acquired in the UK?

> ➤ In 2004, how many MSM were estimated to be living with HIV in the UK and what percentage of these was undiagnosed?

Using the report *Testing Times – HIV and other Sexually Transmitted Infections in the UK: 2007* (Health Protection Agency, 2007), find answers to the following questions:

> ➤ What was the estimate of new diagnoses of HIV in the UK during 2006?

> ➤ Looking at particular groups or parts of the UK, were there differences in the new HIV diagnoses?

Consider your findings and discuss the trends with your mentor or a health professional working in a sexual health clinic.

Resources

Brown AE, Sadler KE, Tompkins SE et al. (2003) Recent trends in HIV and other STIs in the United Kingdom. *Sexually Transmitted Infections* **80**: 159–66.

Dougan S, Evans BG, Macdonald N et al. (2007) HIV in gay and bisexual men in the United Kingdom: 25 years of public health surveillance. *Epidemiology and Infection* 136: 145–56. Published online, doi:10.1017/S0950268807009120.

Worldwide, it is estimated that there are 39.5 million people living with HIV (UNAIDS/WHO, 2006). Of the 4.3 million new cases in 2006, most of these occurred in sub-Saharan Africa, with increases in Central Asia and Eastern Europe (UNAIDS/WHO, 2006).

Manifestations and stages of HIV infection

In adults, HIV infection is possible via the sexual route in both sexes. For MSM, the risk of this is especially high for the receptive partner during anal intercourse. The rectal mucosa is much more delicate than the vaginal mucosa, and the virus probably gains access via tears and abrasions. Although sexual transmission of HIV between lesbians is extremely rare, safe sexual practices are still important (see www.avert.org).

Antibodies appear about three months after exposure. Antibodies are produced during the earliest stage of the disease; this is known as the primary infection stage. The progress of HIV infection is usually described in four stages (see also below):

- **Primary infection stage** – according to Wilkins (2006), most people will experience some symptoms 2–6 weeks following exposure to HIV. These include a transient, nonspecific illness: fever, general malaise, myalgia, pharyngitis, lymphadenopathy and a rash

- **Asymptomatic infection stage** – people usually feel well during this stage, but in some cases there may be persistent generalized lymphadenopathy (PGL)

- **Symptomatic infection stage** – there is damage to the immune system, which worsens over time, thus allowing the development of opportunistic infections and early changes that lead to AIDS-defining malignancies. This stage has similarities with AIDS-related complex (ARC), a term previously used to describe the appearance of the first signs and symptoms of opportunistic infection

■ **Acquired immune deficiency syndrome (AIDS)** – involves the full manifestation of the disease, with weight loss, fever and diarrhoea. Kaposi's sarcoma does not develop in all cases but it can affect the skin, mucous membranes or internal organs.

■ PRACTICE APPLICATION 13.6 ■

Stages of HIV Infection

Both the World Health Organization and the Centers for Disease Control and Prevention in the US publish definitions of the stages of HIV infection.

Activity

Using the resources below:

➤ Find out the detailed criteria used to define each stage of HIV infection.

➤ Why are there differences between the criteria used in poorer countries and those used in more affluent developed countries?

Resources

AVERT, an international HIV/AIDS charity providing comprehensive information about the stages of HIV infection – www.avert.org/hivstages.htm.

Centers for Disease Control and Prevention – www.cdc.gov/hiv/.

WHO HIV/AIDS Programme (2006) *WHO Case Definitions of HIV for Surveillance and Revised Clinical Staging and Immunological Classification of HIV-related Disease in Adults and Children.* Available www.who.org.

Other problems associated with AIDS

People with HIV infection may present with diverse physical problems and mental health problems (for example dementia). These include diseases affecting the gastrointestinal tract, the liver, respiratory tract, mucosae and skin (mucocutaneous), the eyes and nervous system. There is an increased risk of some malignant conditions, such as invasive cervical cancer, penile cancer, lymphomas and Kaposi's sarcoma.

Three areas are outlined below (information about opportunistic infections is included in Table 13.1 above):

■ Gastrointestinal involvement becomes increasingly common as the disease progresses because the gut is host to many potentially pathogenic agents able to cause opportunistic infection as the immune system fails. Lymphoid tissue in the gastrointestinal mucosa may be invaded by the virus and operate as a reservoir (Winson, 1994). Over 80 per cent of those with progressive HIV infection eventually develop diarrhoea, vomiting, malnutrition and wasting, which contribute to mortality. Quality of life is severely affected by *Candida* infections in the mouth and oesophagus, leading to anorexia and dysphagia (difficulty swallowing), and by ulceration through cytomegalovirus and other opportunistic infections.

- Cerebral involvement occurs late, indicated by memory loss, poor concentration and AIDS-associated dementia. In rare cases, encephalopathy develops before the appearance of opportunistic infection.

- Healthcare-associated infection is a major risk for hospital patients with HIV disease, staphylococcal infection being a particular problem (Goetz et al., 1994).

A full coverage of presenting problems is beyond the scope of this book and readers are directed to Wilkins (2006).

Treatment of HIV infection and AIDS

Treatment should begin as early and as intensively as possible and should be targeted against the virus itself (Gallo, 1996). Before 1995, antiviral drugs were given to slow down viral replication. This prolonged the period before the immune system collapsed and delayed the development of opportunistic infections but did not lead to a cure. A number of new drugs have, however, now become available, the aim of therapeutic intervention being to prevent the replication of HIV. If these drugs are successful, it may be possible to halt the disease itself.

Zidovudine (azidothymidine or AZT) was the first nucleoside shown to improve survival and decrease the incidence of symptoms arising from opportun-istic infection (Abouker and Swart, 1993). Zidovudine inhibits the action of reverse transcriptase so that the virus cannot reproduce. Used alone, however, it is only of short-term benefit as HIV rapidly develops resistance to it. Fortunately, other nucleosides became available in 1994, and there is a new group of drugs called 'protease inhibitors' that are able to disrupt other metabolic reactions vital for the multiplication and survival of HIV. Triple therapy with two nucleosides and an HIV protease inhibitor seems to be the most effective treatment currently available (Collier et al., 1996). This is because a combination of agents can be used to destroy HIV at different stages in its life cycle, and the use of more than one antiviral drug reduces the risk of resistance (Lipsky, 1996). Concurrent therapy with appropriate antimicrobial agents is used to reduce the incidence of opportunistic infection.

Public health measures

See Chapter 12.

Women and HIV infection

An estimated 17.7 million women are infected worldwide (UNAIDS/WHO, 2006). Women with HIV infection are found mainly in Africa (Quintanilla, 1996), the vast majority being of childbearing age. This is significant in public health terms as it increases the risk of vertical transmission. Vertical transmission is possible during:

- **Pregnancy** – HIV crosses the placenta. It is a significant route for transmission.

- **Delivery** – HIV present in cervical secretions or blood contaminates the infant. This appears to be a frequent mechanism as most infection occurs at or near delivery.

- **Breastfeeding**, via the milk.

It is difficult to determine the most important route of transmission because all infants born to infected mothers have maternal antibodies at birth (passive immunity), which do not clear until the child is 18 months old.

An opportunity to consider the advice about breastfeeding given to women with HIV is provided below.

■ PRACTICE APPLICATION 13.7 ■

Breastfeeding by Women with HIV

The advice given to women depends on the circumstances. Advice given to women living in affluent developed countries, such as the UK, is very different to that given to women in poorer or developing countries. Breastfeeding is recommended by the World Health Organization in countries where safe water supplies cannot be guaranteed because the risk of gastroenteritis outweighs the risk of transmitting HIV via breast milk (Cutting, 1992).

Activity

Using the resources below, find out:

➤   The advice regarding breastfeeding given to HIV-positive women in the UK.

➤   The reasons, apart from lack of safe water, why the World Health Organization may endorse breastfeeding in poorer or developing countries.

Resources

Cutting W (1992) Breastfeeding and HIV infection: advice depends on the circumstances. *British Medical Journal* **305**: 788–9.

Department of Health (DH) (2004) *HIV and Infant Feeding: Guidance from the UK Chief Medical Officers' Expert Advisory Group on AIDS.* Available www.dh.gov.uk/en/Publicationsandstatistics.

World Health Organization – www.who.org/.

HIV during childhood

The first case of HIV during childhood was reported to the US Centers for Disease Control and Prevention in Atlanta in 1982, but the number has since escalated. Childhood HIV has received comparatively little publicity but the problem is considerable – an estimated 2.3 million children under the age of 15 years are infected (UNAIDS/WHO, 2006). HIV infection progresses more rapidly in children because their immune system is immature. Most succumb to bacterial infections through depleted B lymphocyte activity, and a high proportion develop AIDS within their first year (Newell, 1994). In some centres, there is a policy to prescribe co-trimoxazole routinely to all children of HIV-positive women as protection against opportunistic infection, especially *Pneumocystis jiroveci* (previously *carinii*), which is that most commonly encountered.

SELF-ASSESSMENT

1. Sexual health is primarily concerned with avoiding STIs. True? or False?

2. The primary lesions of syphilis are:

   (a) gummata
   (b) chancres
   (c) condylomata lata
   (d) snail-track ulcers

3. In the UK, primary prescriptions for syphilis are subject to the standard prescription charge. True? or False?

4. Gonorrhoea is caused by *Neisseria meningitidis*. True? or False?

5. *Chlamydia* may be carried asymptomatically. True? or False?

6. The lesions caused by human papilloma virus are treated with:

   (a) penicillin
   (b) aciclovir
   (c) trimethoprim
   (d) imiquimod

7. Herpes simplex virus type 2 is isolated only from oral lesions. True? or False?

8. The organism causing trichomoniasis is:

   (a) fungal
   (b) protozoal
   (c) helminthic
   (d) viral

9. Name six opportunistic infections associated with HIV disease.

10. The 2006 estimate for the number of people worldwide living with HIV is:

    (a) 50 million
    (b) 17.7 million
    (c) 39.5 million
    (d) 4.3 million

REFERENCES

Abouker JP and Swart AM (1993) Preliminary analysis of the Concorde Trial. *Lancet* **341**: 889–90.

Brown AE, Sadler KE, Tompkins SE et al. (2004) Recent trends in HIV and other STIs in the United Kingdom. *Sexually Transmitted Infections* **80**: 159–66.

Chandler MG (1996) Genital warts: a study of patient anxiety and information needs. *British Journal of Nursing* **5**(3): 174–9.

Clutterbuck D (2004) *Sexually Transmitted Infections and HIV.* Mosby, Edinburgh.

Collier A, Coombes R, Schoenfield D et al. (1996) Treatment of human immunodeficiency virus infection with saquinavir, zidovudine and zalcitabine. *New England Journal of Medicine* **334**: 1011–17.

Cooper DA and Mergigan TC (1996) Clinical treatment. *AIDS* **10** (Supplement A): S133–4.

Dapaah S and Dapaah V (2003) Sexually transmissible and reproductive tract infections in pregnancy. In DM Fraser and MA Cooper (eds) *Myles Textbook for Midwives*, 14th edn. Churchill Livingstone, Edinburgh.

Department of Health (DH) (1999) *Unlinked Anonymous Prevalence Monitoring Programme in the United Kingdom.* DH, London.

Department of Health (DH) (2001) *Better Prevention, Better Services, Better Sexual Health: The National Strategy for Sexual Health and HIV.* Available www.dh.gov.uk/en/Publicationsandstatistics.

Department of Health (DH) (2007) *HPA Vaccine Recommended for NHS Immunisation Programme.* Available www.gnn.gov.uk/.

Fenton KA, Korovessis C, Johnson AM et al. (2001) Sexual behaviour in Britain: reported sexually transmitted infections and prevalent genital *Chalmydia trachomatis* infection. *Lancet* **358**: 1851–4.

Findik D, Ural O and Baysal B (1996) Bacterial colonisation and yeast carriage on the hands of nurses. *Journal of Hospital Infection* **34**: 234–5.

Flannigan J (2006) Chlamydia: the nurse's role in diagnosis, treatment and health promotion. *Nursing Standard* **20**(41): 59–64.

Gallo RC (1996) AIDS as a clinically curable disease: the growing optimism. *AIDS, Patient Care and STDs* **10**(1): 7–9.

Gardner JL and Dukes CD (1955) *Haemophilus vaginalis* vaginitis: a newly defined specific infection previously classified 'non-specific vaginitis'. *American Journal of Obstetrics and Gynecology* **69**: 962–76.

Goetz AM, Squier C, Wagener MM et al. (1994) Nosocomial infections in the human immunodeficiency virus-infected patient: a two year survey. *American Journal of Infection Control* **23**: 334–9.

Hay PE, Taylor-Robinson D, Lamont RF et al. (1994) Abnormal bacterial colonisation of the genital tract and subsequent pre-term delivery and late miscarriage. *British Medical Journal* **308**: 295–8.

Health Protection Agency (HPA) (2007) *Testing Times – HIV and other Sexually Transmitted Infections in the UK: 2007.* Available www.hpa.org.uk/.

Krieger JN, Verdon M, Siegal N et al. (1993) Natural history of urogenital trichomoniasis. *Journal of Urology* **149**: 1455–8.

Lee W, Burnie UP, Matthews RC et al. (1991) Hospital outbreaks with yeasts. *Journal of Hospital Infection* **18** (Supplement A): 237–40.

Lipsky JJ (1996) Antiretroviral drugs for AIDS. *Lancet* **348**: 800–3.

Newell ML (1994) Mother to child transmission of HIV-1: The AIDS letter. *Royal Society of Medicine Services* 41. Royal Society of Medicine.

Odds FC (1988) *Candida and Candidosis*. Baillière Tindall, London.

Pratt RJ (2003) *HIV and AIDS: A Foundation for Nursing and Healthcare Practice*, 5th edn. Arnold, London.

Quintanilla K (1996) Can HIV be transmitted through breastmilk? *Nursing Times* **92**(31): 35–7.

Rashid S, Collins M and Kennedy RJ (1991) A study of candidosis: the role of fomites. *Genitourinary Medicine* **67**: 137–42.

Ritchie G A (2006) Strategies to promote sexual health. *Nursing Standard* **20**(48): 35–40.

Scott GR (2006) Sexually transmitted infections. In NA Boon, NR Colledge and BR Walker (eds) *Davidson's Principles and Practice of Medicine*, 20th edn. Churchill Livingstone, Edinburgh.

Steiner MJ and Cates W (2006) Condoms and sexually transmitted infections. *New England Journal of Medicine* **354**: 2642–3.

Temple CA (1994) Diagnosis and treatment of bacterial vaginosis. *Nursing Times* 14(90): 43–4.

UNAIDS/WHO (2006) *AIDS Epidemic Update*. Available www.unaids.org/en/.

Wilkins E (2006) Human immunodeficiency virus infection and the human acquired immunodeficiency syndrome. In NA Boon, NR Colledge and BR Walker (eds) *Davidson's Principles and Practice of Medicine*, 20th edn. Churchill Livingstone, Edinburgh.

Winson G (1994) Gastrointestinal problems in patients with AIDS. *Nursing Times* **90**(25): 36–9.

FURTHER READING AND INFORMATION SOURCES

Adler MW (2003) Sexual health of the nation. *Sexually Transmitted Infections* **79**: 85–7.

AVERT, an international HIV/AIDS charity providing comprehensive information about the stages of HIV infection – www.avert.org/hivstages.htm.

Mahilum-Tapay L, Laitila V, Wawrzyniak J et al. (2007) New point of care *Chlamydia* Rapid Test – bridging the gap between diagnosis and treatment: performance evaluation study. *British Medical Journal* **335**: 1190–4.

Peate I (2007) Syphilis: clinical presentation, diagnosis and treatment. *Nursing Standard* **22**(10): 48–55.

Phillips AN, Gazzard BG, Clumeck N et al. (2007) When should antiretroviral therapy for HIV be started? *British Medical Journal* **334**: 76–8.

Pratt RJ (2003) *HIV and AIDS: A Foundation for Nursing and Healthcare Practice*, 5th edn. Arnold, London.

Royal College of Nursing (RCN) (2001) *Sexual Health Strategy: Guidance for Nursing Staff*. RCN, London.

CHAPTER 14

Epidemiology: changing trends of communicable diseases

CHAPTER OUTCOMES

After reading this chapter, you should be able to:

➤ Define the common epidemiological terms – 'endemic', 'epidemic', 'incidence', 'pandemic' and 'prevalence'

➤ Interpret the classic epidemiological curve and its derivations

➤ Describe the points to look for when critically interpreting epidemiological data

➤ Describe the organism(s) responsible for cholera, Creutzfeldt–Jakob disease, enteric fevers, Legionnaires' disease, malaria, meningococcal meningitis, rabies, severe acute respiratory syndrome, toxoplasmosis, tuberculosis and the viral haemorrhagic fevers

➤ Describe the main features including transmission, prevention, diagnosis and treatment of the communicable diseases listed above

Introduction

This chapter provides an outline of epidemiological principles and the basic terms of epidemiology. There is a discussion about the control of communicable diseases and infections that are notifiable by law.

A selection of communicable diseases are covered in more detail; some are rare in the UK, such as rabies, whereas others, including tuberculosis, are increasingly common in the UK.

Introduction to epidemiology

Epidemiology is the study of diseases and the ways in which they are distributed within the population. This traditionally meant contagious disease, but today the scope of epidemiology has expanded to include all diseases whether transmissible or not. Contagious diseases may occur in epidemics or pandemics, or they may be endemic within a community.

- **Epidemics** – In hospital, epidemics are recognized when the same organism infects two or more people. In the community, a sudden increase in the number of infections of the same kind in a specific area (for example a school or hotel) is defined as an epidemic.

- **Pandemics** – A pandemic is the simultaneous occurrence of a large number of the same infection. The Black Death (bubonic plague) that swept across Europe in the 14th century is an example of a pandemic. In more modern times, the influenza pandemic of 1918 killed 20 million people worldwide.

- **Endemic disease** – This is disease always present in a population. The number of cases varies depending on factors allowing the organisms to multiply and the susceptibility of potential hosts. Malaria is endemic in several regions of the world, including parts of Africa.

Epidemiological patterns: the distribution of contagious disease

The classical epidemiological curve and its three derivations – single point, secondary spread with longer incubation period and the cyclical curve – are discussed.

Classical epidemiological curve

The classical epidemiological curve is drawn when the number of new cases of an infection is plotted against time (Figure 14.1). On the left-hand side of the graph, the number of people infected rises gradually, reaching a peak at the midpoint. On the right-hand side, recovery proceeds faster than the emergence of new infections until the epidemic wanes.

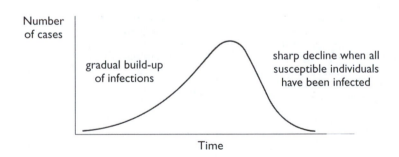

Figure 14.1 Classical epidemiological curve

Much of our knowledge about the behaviour of contagious disease has come from studying the pattern of infection in geographically isolated regions. Spitzbergen, an island on the edge of the Arctic Circle, was once used to study the distribution of respiratory infections. Until the 1930s, it received no visitors throughout the winter. In spring, respiratory disease was absent from the population, the first colds appearing with the arrival of the earliest trade ship, being brought by the crew. The epidemic curve rose to its peak as an increasing number of the islanders caught colds from one another. As the year progressed, the number of new cases declined.

Single-point epidemiological curve

Other epidemiological curves include the single-point curve. In an outbreak of food-borne disease (see Chapter 11) with a short incubation period, many people will be affected simultaneously if the food is eaten at the same time. Their simultaneous recovery results in a single-point curve (Figure 14.2).

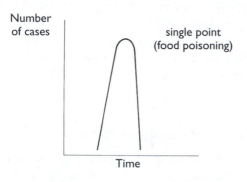

Figure 14.2 Single-point epidemiological curve

Secondary spread and longer incubation period

When the incubation period is longer (weeks or months), with the possibility of secondary spread, the curve develops a second peak (Figure 14.3). This is typical of an outbreak of *Salmonella* in a household where person-to-person transmission has occurred.

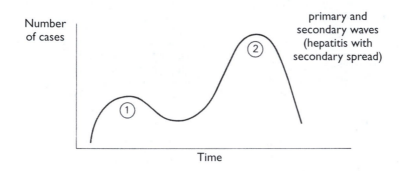

Figure 14.3 Epidemiological curve illustrating secondary spread

Cyclical epidemiological curve

Many infectious diseases appear cyclically every few years (Figure 14.4). Before the availability of vaccine, measles and whooping cough followed this pattern. Outbreaks resulted when a cohort of children lacking immunity had developed and waned once all were infected. Between outbreaks, cases occurred sporadically.

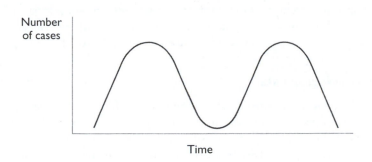

Figure 14.4 Epidemiological curve with cyclical infection

Factors affecting the incidence of infectious disease

Infectious agents depend on a supply of new victims. Thus, transmission is more likely when a large number of susceptible people are gathered together. Poor standards of hygiene, overcrowding and poverty increase the risk of spread. Early man probably escaped relatively unscathed because the total population was small and mobile, moving from one locality to another in search of food. Then, with better health resulting through improved hygiene, nutrition, living conditions and the introduction of public health measures such as vaccination, contagious diseases again caused less morbidity and mortality. The discovery of antibiotics led to an expectation that they would be eliminated altogether. This has not, however, been possible because of the emergence of antibiotic-resistant strains of bacteria. More-over, many people still live in poor conditions, and this has contributed to the resurgence of infectious diseases. Several outbreaks have occurred in recent years, notably the Stanley Royd Hospital incident in which 19 frail patients died as a result of *Salmonella* food poisoning (Department of Health, 1986a) and an outbreak of Legionnaires' disease in Stafford (Department of Health, 1986b). These provided stimulus for the Acheson Report (Department of Health, 1988), which proposed better strategies for the control of communicable disease. An outbreak of *Escherichia coli* 0157 (Chapter 11) in central Scotland in 1996, which caused 20 deaths, led to further recommendations being made (Pennington Group, 1997). Many further outbreaks of *E. coli* have occurred in the UK since Professor Pennington's report; at the time of writing, an outbreak linked to bought cold meat products in Scotland has affected at least 9 people, including the death of an older woman.

It is clear that infections remain a major health problem. In developing countries, millions of people die from tuberculosis and malaria every year. The speed of air travel means that many apparently well people incubating these conditions develop symptoms after their arrival in other countries, importing infectious diseases to the Western world. There are, however, other problems of infection in Western coun-tries. Recent years have witnessed the emergence of 'new' diseases caused by trans-missible agents made possible by advances in technology and more accurate methods of surveillance. Both the acquired immune deficiency syndrome (AIDS) and bovine spongiform encephalopathy (BSE) are caused by transmissible agents, and some cancers have been linked to infection. For example, there is an established association between the papilloma wart virus and cervical cancer, the Epstein–Barr virus and Burkitt's lymphoma and some hepatitis viruses and liver cancer (Campbell, 2006).

Interpreting epidemiological data

Epidemiological studies provide information about the ways in which microorganisms are spread and the types of people most likely to be infected, and suggest risk factors. They also reveal genuine changes in the pattern of infection occurring over time, for example as a result of the emergence of antibiotic resistance. Information about epidemiological data, such as prevalence and incidence of disease, is provided below.

INFORMATION BOX 14.1

Epidemiological data

To evaluate the results of epidemiological investigations, it is essential to have key knowledge about the way in which the information was collected. The results of different studies are often compared, but this is not meaningful unless the data were collected from similar groups of patients in the same type of clinical setting. Data collected prospectively, when the event occurred, are likely to be more accurate than data collected retrospectively (after the event) (Kreger et al., 1989). Now that surveillance data are routinely stored on computer, prospective studies are easier to conduct and more accurate (Gransden, 1991). Data may be collected as part of a prevalence or incidence study, the proposed use affecting the interpretation of findings.

Prevalence

The prevalence is the number of the existing cases of a condition in a population at a single point in time (Brooker, 2008). Prevalence studies give little explanation of risk factors so they are not useful as a means of suggesting control measures. The extent of a problem may be underestimated because each case is counted only once. Infected patients who have successfully completed their antibiotic treatment or have died at the time of data collection are excluded. Prevalence studies may, however, reveal problems that merit more detailed investigations.

Incidence

Incidence studies report the number of new cases of a condition arising within a population over a period of time. They are more expensive and more time-consuming but suggest possible risk factors contributing to the development of infection. From this approach, it has become apparent that critically ill patients are most susceptible to healthcare-associated infection (HCAI) (Evans et al., 1992). In the most sophisticated experimental incidence studies, different treatment regimens are tested. Patients are assigned to an experimental group to receive treatment (antibiotics or immunization, for example), and the number of infections developing is compared with that seen in a control group that has not received treatment. Donowitz (1986) used this approach to show that the incidence of infection declined in a group of critically ill children when hand hygiene was scrupulously performed, cotton gowns making no difference.

International recommendations

The World Health Organization holds overall responsibility for the administration of international health programmes to control disease, including infectious conditions such as malaria, HIV, tuberculosis and so on. The latest *International Health Regulations* (IHR) came into force in June 2007 (World Health Organization, 2005a).

An example of successful collaboration between member nations is shown by the eradication of smallpox in 1970. A more recent example is the World Health Organization (2005b) recommendations for preventing pandemic avian influenza. Other areas dealt with under the IHR include:

- Control of the spread of serious infectious conditions such as cholera, yellow fever and plague
- The disinfection of aircraft
- The control of vermin in ships.

The World Health Organization provides advice about controlling infection by:

- Assisting individual nations to collect and analyse data, which it then disseminates to other countries.
- Acting as a resource for health workers by collecting, consolidating and publishing epidemiological data from different countries.
- Providing technical advice and training to encourage countries to standardize the methods they use to collect and present epidemiological data so that comparison is possible between them all. This is necessary because of the enormous difference between the methods used to notify, investigate, diagnose and report diseases. Interpretation is straightforward if a universal method is employed.
- Offering blueprints for the role of public health laboratories in the surveillance and control of infectious disease so that information concerning new technology is shared.

Control of communicable disease in the UK

The Health Protection Agency plays a key role in the control of infectious conditions. It comprises a network of laboratories in England and Wales and a central infections unit in London. The Health Protection Agency, which was formed in 2003, incorporated the existing Public Health Laboratory Service (formed in 1946) along with other agencies involved in protecting the public against risks that include chemical hazards and radiation. Health Protection Scotland, a body formed in 2004, provides the same services in Scotland.

The Health Protection Agency provides infection control services to hospitals, public health microbiology such as testing water, food and milk, and specialist microbiology and epidemiological surveillance at national, regional and local levels. It also contributes to the control of communicable diseases by surveillance, investigating outbreaks and formulating policies for their control. A sudden increase in the number of infections caused by a specific organism in England or Wales is reported to the agency, which can then monitor the outbreak and help control it. Staff assemble, analyse and disseminate data relating to all communicable diseases. The early recognition of a problem and prompt action by the Health Protection Agency can contain an emerging outbreak.

Notifiable infections

Notifiable infectious conditions are reported to the Health Protection Agency to help to trace contacts who may have been exposed to infection so that they can be monitored and treated as necessary. In the case of food or waterborne infection, it is important to determine and eliminate the source. The data generated at local and national level help to monitor fluctuations in the incidence of infection and identify potential outbreaks, allowing preventive action or the recognition of a particular need for health promotion. Responsibility for notification falls to local authorities, which have a statutory responsibility to control infectious conditions within their boundaries. They can add to the statutory list of notifiable infectious conditions (for England and Wales) shown below. For example, HIV disease is not notifiable, but there is a confidential voluntary referral scheme. Similarly, sexually transmitted infections do not appear in the list because they are reported anonymously to the Department of Health.

INFORMATION BOX 14.2

Notifiable diseases (England and Wales)

Public Health (Control of Disease) Act 1984

Cholera	Plague	Smallpox
Food poisoning	Relapsing fever	Typhus

Public Health (Infectious Diseases) Regulations 1988

Acute encephalitis	Ophthalmia neonatorum
Acute poliomyelitis	Paratyphoid fever
Anthrax	Rabies
Diphtheria	Rubella
Dysentery (bacillary and amoebic)	Scarlet fever
Leprosy	Tetanus
Leptospirosis	Tuberculosis
Malaria	Typhoid
Measles	Viral haemorrhagic fever
Meningitis	Viral hepatitis
Meningococcal septicaemia	Whooping cough
Mumps	Yellow fever

Changing trends of communicable diseases

A selection of communicable diseases – their transmission, prevention, diagnosis and treatment – are now discussed in more detail. The diseases discussed are:

- Malaria
- Meningitis
- Toxoplasmosis
- Creutzfeld–Jakob disease (CJD)
- Enteric fevers
- Cholera
- Legionnaires' disease
- Tuberculosis (TB)
- Severe acute respiratory syndrome (SARS)
- Viral haemorrhagic fevers
- Rabies

Malaria

Malaria is caused by protozoal parasites belonging to the genus *Plasmodium* (Table 14.1). The vector is the female *Anopheles* mosquito. Infection causes intermittent fever with haemolytic anaemia (anaemia caused by the destruction of red blood cells – erythrocytes).

Table 14.1 Malarial parasites

Genus	Distribution	Severity	Fever
Plasmodium falciparum (malignant malaria)	Tropics	+++	Every 2 days
Plasmodium vivax	Temperate zones	++	Every 2 days
Plasmodium malariae	Subtropics	++	Every 3 days
Plasmodium ovale	Variable and patchy	++	Every 2 days

The life cycle of *Plasmodium* is complex (Figure 14.5). The protozoa are injected into the human host by the mosquito, and then pass through a stage of division called the 'exoerythrocytic' (occurring outside the erythrocytes – red blood cells) stage. Some plasmodia enter the erythrocytes (erythrocytic stage), where they undergo asexual division. Their increasing number causes the cell to rupture, the escaping plasmodia being free to enter and destroy more erythrocytes in turn, thus giving rise to the haemolytic anaemia. Bouts of fever recur when the plasmodia enter the bloodstream. Their frequency depends on the length of time taken to complete the asexual stages of reproduction and to escape.

Malaria is a huge global health problem. According to the World Health Organization (2007a), malaria causes in excess of a million deaths each year, with most of these occurring in Africa; those most at risk being infants, small children and pregnant women. Malaria is responsible for enormous suffering and economic loss. This is especially true of *P. falciparum*, which causes the most severe form of the disease.

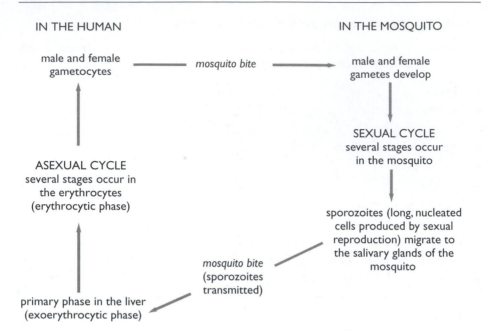

IN THE HUMAN

IN THE MOSQUITO

male and female gametocytes ——— *mosquito bite* ———→ male and female gametes develop

SEXUAL CYCLE
several stages occur
in the mosquito

ASEXUAL CYCLE
several stages occur in
the erythrocytes
(erythrocytic phase)

sporozoites (long, nucleated
cells produced by sexual
reproduction) migrate to
the salivary glands of the
mosquito

mosquito bite
(sporozoites
transmitted)

primary phase in the liver
(exoerythrocytic phase)

Figure 14.5 Simplified description of the life cycle of *Plasmodium*

Most cases of malaria occurring in the UK are contracted abroad, although travellers incubating the disease may not exhibit symptoms until after their arrival (Chiodini, 2006). Unfortunately, travellers do not always take appropriate preventive measures (Hill, 2006). There have been a number of cases of 'airport malaria' caused when mosquitoes have been transported to the UK in aircraft and then escaped (Conlon, 1990). It is interesting to note that malaria was once endemic in the UK, the disease occurring in marshy areas of southeast England, only being eradicated as recently as the early part of the last century.

Transmission

Person-to-person infection does not occur, and isolation is unnecessary unless a patient arriving from overseas with pyrexia and a presumptive diagnosis of malaria is considered to be at risk of harbouring another tropical fever.

Prevention

Draining the stagnant water used by *Anopheles* as a breeding ground controls malaria. Small areas (puddles, ponds, wells and water butts) may be covered by a thin film of oil, and the introduction of fish preying on the larvae is a helpful measure. Vital personal prevention involves:

■ Measures to avoid mosquito bites – mosquito nets sprayed with long-acting insecticide are effective, mosquito-proof clothing when mosquitoes are particularly active after dusk and screens are recommended inside the home.

- Insecticide sprays and so on to kill adult *Anopheles* within homes, and repellents for topical application. Insect repellents, for example permethrin, can be used to treat mosquito nets and added to rinsing water after washing clothes.

- Chemoprophylaxis, for example chloroquine with proguanil, doxycycline, mefloquine, proguanil with atovaquone (Malarone®) (see below).

PRACTICE APPLICATION 14.1

Malaria chemoprophylaxis

Numerous drugs are used in malarial chemoprophylaxis, but resistance is widely reported so travellers should be advised to seek the latest information from travel centres. It may be necessary to take several drugs in combination to reduce the possibility of the plasmodia developing resistance. Drug regimens differ between regions according to the levels of risk and existing drug resistance.

Activity

Using the resources below, find out about the drugs used for malaria prophylaxis including:

➤ The factors taken into account when a drug is selected.

➤ The differences between regions.

➤ The duration of treatment.

➤ Common side-effects.

Resources

British National Formulary provides information for UK residents travelling to regions where malaria is endemic – www.bnf.org.

Health Protection Scotland – www.hps.scot.nhs.uk.

National Travel Health Network and Centre (NaTHNaC) – www.nathnac.org/.

The interiors of aircraft should be treated with insecticide to reduce the risk of importing malaria. It has been suggested that public awareness of the dangers of malaria in relation to travel should be increased, especially as prophylaxis is highly cost-effective (Behrens and Roberts, 1994). A campaign by the World Health Organization to eradicate malaria failed because of the problem of drug resistance and a lack of cooperation on the part of some member states. Prevention would be more of a reality if an effective vaccine could be developed. Research aimed at producing an effective vaccine against malaria is ongoing (see www.malaria-vaccines.org.uk/).

Diagnosis

Diagnosis is confirmed by the microscopic examination of stained blood films, which reveal the malarial parasites.

Treatment

Chloroquine has traditionally been the mainstay of treatment and prophylaxis for *P. falciparum* malaria, but increasing resistance means that it is no longer used for treatment. A number of other drugs are available, including:

- quinine in conjunction with, or followed by, doxycycline or clindamycin
- proguanil with atovaquone (Malarone®)
- artemether with lumefantrine (Riamet®).

Malaria caused by other plasmodia (*P. malariae*, *P. ovale*, *P. vivax*) is still treated with chloroquine, although resistance has been reported. Primaquine is used after the course of chloroquine for malaria caused by *P. vivax* and *P. ovale* in order to kill all the parasites, thus preventing relapses.

Meningitis

Meningitis is an inflammation of the meninges (three membranes covering the brain and spinal cord) and infective meningitis is caused by a range of microorganisms (Table 14.2).

Table 14.2 Some microorganisms causing meningitis

Bacterial	Viral	Fungal	Protozoal
Streptococcus pneumoniae	Echovirus	*Candida*	Amoeba
Haemophilus influenzae type b	Coxsackie virus	*Cryptococcus neoformans*	*Toxoplasma*
Neisseria meningitidis	Mumps virus	*Histoplasma*	
Escherichia coli	Epstein–Barr virus	*Coccidioides*	
Group B streptococci	HIV		
Listeria monocytogenes	Influenza		
Mycobacterium tuberculosis	Herpes simplex		
(usually insidious onset)	Varicella zoster		

An in-depth discussion of all types of meningitis is beyond the scope of this book. The discussion concentrates on bacterial meningitis, especially meningococcal meningitis caused by *N. meningitidis* (meningococcus). Viral meningitis is milder than bacterial infections, and most people recover spontaneously. Bacterial meningitis has a mortality rate of 3–6 per cent, tends to be severe and can have an extremely rapid rate of onset (Kornelisse et al., 1995). An individual with meningococcal disease, especially infants and children, can deteriorate and die within hours of feeling unwell. It is thus hardly surprising that considerable fear and anxiety surrounds meningitis.

The typical symptoms and signs of bacterial meningitis are listed below.

Until recently, *Haemophilus influenzae* caused 40 per cent of all cases of meningitis in early infancy and early childhood, but since the introduction of a vaccination in 1992 in the UK, the incidence of this organism has declined sharply.

INFORMATION BOX 14.3

Signs and symptoms of meningitis

➤ Early on – vague flu-like symptoms

➤ Fever, but the extremities may be cold

➤ Increased respiratory rate

➤ Headache

➤ Nausea and vomiting

➤ Confusion

➤ Increasing drowsiness

➤ Altered consciousness

➤ Neck stiffness

➤ Abdominal pain

➤ Painful joints and muscles

➤ Photophobia (intolerance of bright light) and phonophobia (intolerance to noise)

➤ Seizures

NB A characteristic rash will be present in meningococcal septicaemia – a dark red/purple petechial rash that does not disappear with pressure.

In infants and babies, there may be signs and symptoms in addition to the fever, vomiting, drowsiness and seizures listed above. These may include:

➤ Irritability and not wanting to be handled

➤ Poor feeding or rejecting feeds

➤ Abnormal cry – whimpering or high-pitched

➤ Poor muscle tone – floppy

➤ Bulging fontanelle ('soft spot') as pressure increases in the skull

➤ Reduced responses

➤ Pallor or skin mottling

➤ Retraction of the neck with an arched back

Meningococcal meningitis is caused by *N. meningitidis*, a Gram-negative, aerobic coccus that affects primarily children and young adults, although people of any age can become infected. There are three serological groups: A, B and C. In 1994, sero-type B caused 70 per cent of all cases of meningococcal meningitis in the UK. The path resulting in clinical infection occurs in three stages:

1. Growth of the organism in the nasopharynx. This causes local inflammation but in most cases does not progress, and the individual becomes a carrier.

2. Invasion of the bacteria into the blood, with the appearance of a petechial rash comprising small red/purple haemorrhagic spots and life-threatening meningo-coccal septicaemia.

3. Invasion of the meninges and infection of the cerebrospinal fluid (CSF). Acute symptoms and fatality can develop within 12 hours.

Transmission

N. meningitidis is carried asymptomatically in the nasopharynx of 5–10 per cent of healthy people, transmission being via droplets. The rate of carriage rises dramatically with overcrowding, which in the past has been associated with a higher incidence of infection. Spread also occurs by contact: saliva and nasal secretions easily contaminate bedding, and when they are shaken, the bacteria are liberated into the surrounding air, settling as dust that is inhaled. *N. meningitidis* dies rapidly in the environment.

Preventing the spread of meningococcal meningitis

Prevention is as follows:

- **Isolating the patient** for the first 24–48 hours of antibiotic therapy may be recommended. A single room is usually appreciated for longer because the symptoms of meningitis include intolerance of light and noise.
- **Chemoprophylaxis** for close contacts and staff who have performed mouth-to-mouth resuscitation. Susceptible carriers identified by throat swabbing are given rifampicin, ciprofloxacin or ceftriaxone.
- The **vaccination** of named people at risk. The effects of vaccination are short-lived, and it is protective only against serotypes A and C. During 1999, a long-acting vaccine against group C meningococcal infection was introduced in the UK (Chapter 2). Further research continues in the development of a vaccine effective against serotype B.

Diagnosis

Diagnosis is made by clinical examination and is confirmed by culturing CSF obtained by lumbar puncture.

Treatment of meningococcal meningitis

Treatment is with benzylpenicillin or a cephalosporin, for example cefotaxime. Patients allergic to penicillin and cephalosporins are given chloramphenicol. The prompt administration of parenteral benzylpenicillin before transfer to hospital to suspected cases increases the chances of survival (Cartwright et al., 1992). If meningitis is suspected from the history and examination, treatment is commenced at once, that is, before confirmation is obtained from culturing the CSF.

Toxoplasmosis

Toxoplasmosis is caused by the protozoan *Toxoplasma gondii*, which is carried asymptomatically by many wild and domestic animals. Its life cycle is complex (Figure 14.6).

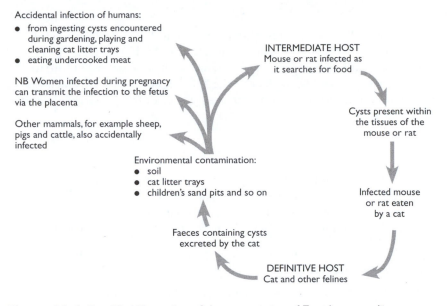

Accidental infection of humans:
- from ingesting cysts encountered during gardening, playing and cleaning cat litter trays
- eating undercooked meat

NB Women infected during pregnancy can transmit the infection to the fetus via the placenta

Other mammals, for example sheep, pigs and cattle, also accidentally infected

INTERMEDIATE HOST
Mouse or rat infected as it searches for food

Cysts present within the tissues of the mouse or rat

Environmental contamination:
- soil
- cat litter trays
- children's sand pits and so on

Infected mouse or rat eaten by a cat

Faeces containing cysts excreted by the cat

DEFINITIVE HOST
Cat and other felines

Figure 14.6 Simplified illustration of the transmission of *Toxoplasma gondii*

Transmission

Human infection occurs when infected meat is consumed, or during contact with infected pets or livestock. Cats frequently harbour *Toxoplasma gondii*, having consumed infected prey. Human infection is possible through handling cat faeces (for example litter trays or gardening in earth soiled by cats). It is usually asymptomatic, or the symptoms of malaise, myalgia and fatigue are mild so that diagnosis is never established. Sometimes people develop choroidoretinitis (inflammation of the choroid and retina layers of the eye), which requires treatment. For some people, however, toxoplasmosis is serious:

- **The immunocompromised** – especially people with HIV disease. Reactivation of latent infection occurs, giving rise to severe disseminated toxoplasmosis or encephalitis (inflammation of the brain).

- **Organ transplant recipients** – infection acquired from the donated organ becomes active with immunosuppressive therapy.

- **Pregnant women** – vertical transmission occurs via the placenta from mother to fetus when primary infection occurs during pregnancy. Fetal infection can result in stillbirth, low birth weight and an infant with hepatosplenomegaly (enlarged liver and spleen), central nervous system defects, eye problems, jaundice and haemolytic defects including anaemia. Some infants are asymptomatic at birth, but may develop later-onset cirrhosis, encephalitis and eye damage, becoming blind after a latent period lasting many years.

Diagnosis

A rapid, safe, accurate screening test that became available in 1994 may lead to a more comprehensive screening programme in the UK (Hohlfeld et al., 1994). The test was developed in France, where the awareness of the risk associated with maternal toxoplasmosis is much higher than in the UK because there is a much higher incidence of infection, associated with eating rare meat. In France, screening during pregnancy is mandatory.

Treatment

The treatment of toxoplasmosis depends on the circumstances and an expert should be consulted. The drugs used include pyrimethamine with sulfadiazine, or pyrimethamine with another antimicrobial, such as clindamycin. Spiromycin (supplied on a named-patient basis from the manufacturer) may be used during pregnancy.

Creutzfeldt–Jakob disease

Creutzfeldt–Jakob disease (CJD) is one of a range of diseases known collectively as the 'transmissible spongiform encephalopathies' (TSEs). They are characterized by slow progression during which the brain develops minute perforations, eventually assuming a spongy appearance. The TSEs also include bovine spongiform encephalopathy (BSE), known colloquially as 'mad cow disease', and scrapie, which infects sheep. All have long incubation periods but eventually progress rapidly and are inevitably fatal.

CJD is one of a rare group of fatal diseases, which destroy neural tissue through the accumulation of abnormal prion proteins (Turner, 2004). Prions are self-replicating proteins that do not contain nucleic acid. They are insoluble and very resistant to degradation, so they accumulate in nerve cells, disrupting function. Eventually cell death occurs. CJD is a degenerative condition. It is characterized by progressive brain damage. The incubation period ranges from 4 to 30 years. In the past, most cases of CJD affected people aged 40–60, but cases are now seen in teenagers, possibly representing a new strain (new variant CJD or vCJD).

Transmission

Transmission probably occurs via contaminated blood and body fluids. Most reported cases follow the transfusion of blood or blood products. Other potential routes of transmission include:

- Tissue grafts of corneas or dura mater (the outer meningeal membrane)
- Injections of contaminated human growth hormone obtained from cadaver pituitary glands, although this has been replaced by growth hormone derived from recombinant DNA
- Surgical procedures using contaminated instruments.

Prevention

Decontamination of equipment, such as surgical instruments, is difficult because the prion responsible for CJD is highly resistant to the physical and chemical methods normally used (Chapter 5). For example, exposure of contaminated materials to steam heat at 134 °C may not inactivate it completely. Disposable surgical instruments may be used in certain types of surgery in order to reduce the risk of transmission to another person. Standard (universal) precautions are required in hospital but there is no evidence at present that CJD poses a health risk to families in the domiciliary setting (Department of Health, 2004, modified 2007).

Diagnosis

Diagnosis is on clinical grounds. CJD is differentiated from other forms of presenile dementia by its rapid onset and progression. Death usually occurs within a year of diagnosis. The typical spongiform changes in the cerebral cortex are seen at postmortem. No treatment is currently available.

Enteric fevers

Enteric fevers are caused by *Salmonella enterica* serovar Typhi and *Salmonella enterica* serovar Paratyphi (causing typhoid and paratyphoid fevers respectively). The incubation period is approximately 14 days. In the case of typhoid fever, infection is usually severe, producing malaise, fever and aching muscles (see below). Fever may continue for weeks, and septicaemia develops about 10 days after the onset of infection, with bacteria appearing in the blood, urine and stools. Bacteria may be carried for months, sometimes years. The usual seat of infection is the gallbladder, but other organs, including the liver, may be involved. Paratyphoid fever is generally milder and of shorter duration. The enteric fevers mainly affect those living in poorer parts of the world where sanitation and clean water are lacking (Xavier, 2006). In the UK, they are usually associated with people neglecting to take proper precautions when travelling abroad or contact with somebody who has been overseas.

INFORMATION BOX 14.4

Signs, symptoms and complications of typhoid fever

Onset of disease

➤ Fever – the temperature rises in a typical 'stepladder' fashion

➤ Slow pulse relative to the increase in body temperature

➤ Malaise

➤ Headache

➤ Muscle aches

➤ Constipation

End of first week/second week

➤ Appearance of rose-coloured rash ('rose spots') on the abdomen and back

> Profuse 'pea soup' diarrhoea, which may be blood-stained

> Abdominal distension

> Enlarged spleen

> Cough

> Apathy

> Temperature remains elevated

End of second week/third week

> Delirium

> Drowsiness (progressing to altered consciousness and death in untreated cases)

> Temperature remains elevated

> Complications (see below)

Potential complications

> Myocarditis (inflammation of the myocardium), pneumonia, cholecystitis (inflammation of the gallbladder) and so on, caused by toxaemia

> Intestinal haemorrhage

> Perforation of the bowel

Transmission

Transmission is by the faecal-oral route. Both bacteria are virulent, only a low infective dose being needed to cause disease.

Diagnosis

A diagnosis is made by stool or blood culture and an agglutination test for antibodies (the Widal reaction).

Prevention

Prevention is achieved by eliminating the source of infection, including carriers, and public health measures focusing on the provision of safe water supplies, food preparation and the pasteurization of milk. Travellers to regions where typhoid is endemic may receive active immunization, but this is not highly effective (World Health Organization, 2000).

Treatment

Treatment depends on severity, the region of origin and bacterial resistance to drugs. The antibacterials used include chloramphenicol, ciprofloxacin, cefotaxime and azithromycin. In addition, appropriate supportive measures, such as the correction of fluid and electrolyte imbalance, may be required.

Cholera

Cholera is caused by *Vibrio cholerae*, an aerobic, Gram-negative bacterium. Cholera is an acute intestinal infection, which occurs in regions without clean water or proper sanitation. It no longer occurs in the UK (see below), but is endemic throughout Asia, Africa and Central and South America.

INFORMATION BOX 14.5

Epidemiological research and cholera in London

During the 19th century, Britain was seriously affected by four cholera pandemics, 14,000 people dying of it in 1866. During the 1854 epidemic, Dr John Snow carried out a piece of epidemiological research plotting the cases of cholera on a map of London. He identified a concentration of cases in Soho (a district in London) around the public water pump in Broad Street. At Snow's instigation, the pump handle was removed, and the epidemic, which was already abating, soon came to an end.

The incubation period ranges from a few hours to five days. Many infections are mild, but severe, life-threatening illness occurs in 5–10 per cent of cases. The bacteria release an enterotoxin that alters the metabolism of the cells in the gastrointestinal mucosa so that they secrete a large quantity of fluid faster than it can be reabsorbed, resulting in copious diarrhoea and vomiting. Adults can lose up to a litre of fluid in one hour. Stools and vomitus are watery and specked with small white flocculi (fragments of the intestinal epithelium – 'rice water stools'). This is followed by massive dehydration, circulatory collapse and renal failure unless treated. Mortality, without proper medical intervention to replace fluid and electrolytes, is high.

Transmission

Transmission is by the faecal-oral route usually in parts of the world where cholera is endemic. Infections sometimes occur in travellers (Hainsworth, 2004). The infective dose is high, many vibrios being required to cause symptoms. Thus, person-to-person transmission is rare. Contaminated water is usually responsible for sudden outbreaks affecting large numbers of people. Chronic carriage is unusual, although the contacts of acutely infected patients may carry vibrios asymptomatically for a few days.

Prevention

Oral vaccination is available but this does not reduce the importance of public health measures. Prevention depends on good-quality water supplies without contamination from human sewage, food safety and scrupulous personal hygiene precautions.

Diagnosis

Diagnosis is made by microscopy confirmed by faecal culture.

Treatment

Tetracyclines, such as doxycycline, reduce diarrhoea and the duration of vibrio excretion, but the mainstay of treatment is fluid and electrolyte replacement with oral rehydration solution or intravenous rehydration. Vibrios are developing resistance to tetracycline so trimethoprim may be given instead.

Legionnaires' disease

Legionnaires' disease is caused by *Legionella pneumophila*, a tiny, motile, Gram-negative bacillus found in soil and water that grows between 20 °C and 40 °C. Legionnaires' disease is not uncommon, but patients are slow to seroconvert, and the bacteria are difficult to detect and isolate. The first recorded outbreak occurred in 1976 among delegates attending a convention of the American Legion in Philadelphia (Fraser et al., 1977). Epidemics have since occurred in several countries, mainly in hotels and hospitals. The largest outbreak in the UK occurred in Stafford District General Hospital in 1985. The design of the ventilation system was faulty, leading to contamination of the water supply (Department of Health, 1986b); there were 28 deaths. Approximately 300 cases are reported annually in the UK every year, often associated with travel, but there is occasional reporting of outbreaks in the UK (Makin, 2005).

Transmission

Epidemiological links between *Legionella* infection and contaminated hospital water are now well documented, with air conditioning, ventilation systems and water from cooling towers presenting a potential risk (Vincent-Houdek et al., 1993). *Legionella* has been isolated from shower units, nebulizers, humidifiers, cold- and hot-water circuits, water tanks and calorifiers (Liu et al., 1993). Contamination occurs between different parts of the system, calorifiers operating as an important source (Bartlett et al., 1983). However, the source of infection may sometimes originate outside the hospital premises, so this, too, must be included in any epidemiological investigation (Vincent-Houdek et al., 1993).

Simulation experiments suggest that the mode of transmission is via contaminated aerosols from humidifiers and respiratory equipment but not from showers (Woo et al., 1986). If contaminated water becomes airborne in aerosols less than 5 μm in diameter, the bacteria can be inhaled. This leads either to subclinical (without any signs or symptoms) infection, mild infection not involving the lungs (Pontiac fever) or fulminant pneumonia, which can be fatal. Person-to-person spread has never been reported so patients need not be isolated.

Prevention

The immunocompromised are especially vulnerable so prevention, especially in hospital, is important (Vincent-Houdek et al., 1993). Control measures involve maintaining the hot-water temperature at 60 °C and chlorinating incoming water. It is also vital to maintain the system in good working order, closing down redundant parts of the circuit that cannot be maintained at an adequate temperature and monitoring the speed of flow. Water containers and humidifiers should be cleaned and descaled at regular intervals and kept dry if the system is closed down (Health and Safety Commission, 1991). The value of bacteriological sampling in routine prevention is debated (Liu et al., 1993).

Treatment

In the UK, the antimicrobial treatment of choice is erythromycin with the addition of rifampicin for severe infection. Other antimicrobial drugs used include those of the quinolone group and doxycycline.

Tuberculosis

According to the World Health Organization (2007b), around 1.6 million people die each year from tuberculosis (TB), which is a curable infection. However, it is estimated that 2 million lives are lost to the disease. TB is a chronic infection involving the lungs and sometimes other parts of the body that is caused by *Mycobacterium tuberculosis*, the acid-fast bacillus. An association with overcrowding and poverty was first made in the 1870s, when infection was rife in the UK. Gradual improvements in housing, nutrition and hygiene helped to reduce the incidence, and with the availability of antibiotics, infection became less common. Throughout the 1980s, it was generally considered that the incidence of TB was declining, but during the 1990s, there was resurgence in the UK, the US and many other countries, leading the World Health Organization to declare a global health emergency in 1993. It is now considered a serious global problem and a major cause of morbidity and mortality (Dye et al., 2005). The first reversal in the previous trend was recorded in the US, where resurgence was attributed to an increase in the incidence of HIV and to a relaxation of infection control programmes.

In the UK, the increase is confined to particular groups. Most of the increase in cases has occurred in London and other inner city areas. The Health Protection Agency (2007) states that 8,497 cases of TB were reported in the UK (including Scotland) during 2006; most cases affected people aged 15–44 years, and 40 per cent of reported cases (3,362) were in London.

In most parts of the country, incidence remains low, but health workers should not dismiss the possibility of TB in cases of ongoing ill-health (Williams, 2006). Groups at particular risk include:

- **The socially deprived**, especially if they are malnourished, the homeless being particularly at risk (Watson, 1993). Most cases are caused by the reactivation of old lesions when health is compromised.
- **Those with debilitating illnesses** depressing cell-mediated immunity (Wilkins, 2006), including people with HIV (Charatan, 1991, 1994). This is because damage to the immune system allows dormant infections to reactivate.
- **Travellers**. In many parts of the world (for example Africa and Asia), the inci-

dence of tuberculosis is high and travellers may already be infected on their arrival in the UK (Davies and Williams, 1993). Notifications of tuberculosis support this view, as cases are most common in London and the West Midlands, both of which are areas that attract a high proportion of immigrants to the UK. The Health Protection Agency (2007) reports that 72 per cent of cases of TB occur in people born outside the UK.

■ **Healthcare professionals** who have been in contact with infectious patients (Uttley and Pozniak, 1993).

Transmission

Transmission occurs by inhaling infectious airborne particles released in aerosols. The length of contact between the source and the potential new case increases the risk of transmission because the longer the period of exposure, the greater the risk of inhalation. Mycobacteria have tough, waxy walls, and the host response is primarily cell mediated rather than humoral. The bacilli multiply slowly and when phagocytosis (Chapter 2) occurs, they are able to resist destruction by lysosomal enzymes. Instead, they continue to grow within macrophages and escape when the macrophages die, leading to their growth in the extracellular environment. Tuberculosis (primary) infection is possible with and without the full manifestation of the disease (post-primary or secondary infection).

Tuberculosis (primary) infection

Inhaled bacteria set up a single focus of infection in the lung, with involvement of the hilar and mediastinal lymph nodes (the primary complex). There is a local inflammatory reaction followed by healing to leave a calcified lesion visible on a chest X-ray. There are usually few symptoms, and recovery is often spontaneous. The individual is not infectious to others and reacts negatively to bacteriological tests, although he or she usually has a positive tuberculin skin test. However, at the time of primary infection, bacteria are carried to the regional lymph nodes within the macrophages, gain access to the bloodstream and are carried to extrapulmonary (outside the lungs) sites. Extrapulmonary manifestations are severe – acute tuberculous bronchopneumonia, miliary tuberculosis, tuberculous meningitis and involvement of the bones, joints or kidneys. Even in the patient who apparently resists primary infection, the bacilli remain dormant for years, any condition compromising cell-mediated immunity reactivating them.

Post-primary (secondary) infection

Post-primary (secondary) infection, the form mainly seen nowadays, occurs either through reactivation of the bacilli within old primary lesions or through reinfection. Pulmonary infection results in the development of one or more lesions near the apex of the lung. These do not usually involve the hilar lymph nodes. The infection is chronic and destructive, resulting in fibrosis, tissue loss and cavity formation. Spontaneous recovery is not a feature of post-primary tuberculosis, and people may be infectious to others before treatment becomes effective.

Diagnosis

The confirmation of a diagnosis of active tuberculous infection is made by isolation and culture of the bacteria from sputum or gastric (stomach) washings. Obtaining sputum may require the help of a physiotherapist. In addition, people have a positive tuberculin skin test and may exhibit clinical signs and symptoms of disease (cough, weight loss, night sweats, low grade pyrexia and malaise), although these may be too nonspecific to allow a firm diagnosis.

Prevention

Prevention involves:

- **Immunization** – Guidelines from the National Institute of Health and Clinical Excellence (2006) do not recommend routine bacille Calmette–Guérin (BCG) vaccination for children aged 10–14, while routine Mantoux skin testing before vaccination is not required for children under the age of 6 unless they were born in or have recently visited a country with a high incidence of tuberculosis.

  According to the *British National Formulary* (British Medical Association/Royal Pharmaceutical Society of Great Britain, 2007), skin testing is not required for children under the age of six as long as they have not spent longer than one month in a country where the incidence of TB is more than 40 per 100,000, and have not been in contact with a person who has TB.

  BCG vaccination should be offered to new entrants to the UK, who have no evidence of vaccination, if they meet certain criteria, for example are from a country in which there is a high incidence of TB (National Institute of Health and Clinical Excellence, 2006).

  Since discontinuing routine Mantoux skin testing and BCG vaccination for all children at secondary school, the Department of Health has concentrated on vaccinating groups identified as being at high risk for TB infection (see below).

- **Radiography** – This is used in conjunction with the segregation and treatment of known cases, with a follow-up of contacts.

- **Specialist healthcare practitioners** – Specialist tuberculosis nurses, other members of the TB team and specialist community public health nurses undertake testing and contact follow-up and so on.

- **Pasteurization of milk** – In the UK, pasteurization has eradicated the risk of contracting TB from drinking milk from cows with bovine tuberculosis. However, bovine tuberculosis infection within cattle herds is viewed very seriously. The Department for Environment, Food and Rural Affairs has a programme in place for surveillance, testing cattle for TB and the slaughter of any suspect cattle.

■ PRACTICE APPLICATION 14.2 ■

BCG Vaccination for High-risk Groups in the UK

In 2005 (and reiterated in 2007), advice from the Joint Committee on Vaccination and Immunisation led the Department of Health to change the BCG programme, whereby the existing routine BCG vaccination programme for children at secondary school was replaced by a programme that targeted vaccination for those individuals at the greatest risk of TB.

Activity

➤ What reasons were given by the Department of Health in 2005 to support the change?

➤ Which groups are targeted in the current BCG programme?

➤ Which additional groups does the *British National Formulary* recommend should have BCG vaccination?

Resources

British National Formulary – www.bnf.org

Department of Health (DH) (2005) *Tuberculosis: Improvements to BCG Immunisation Programme.* Available www.dh.gov.uk/en/Publicationsandstatistics.

Joint Committee on Vaccination and Immunisation (JCVI) (2007) *BCG Statement.* Available www.advisorybodies.doh.gov.uk/jcvi/index.htm.

Treatment

See Chapter 4.

Multidrug resistant-tuberculosis and extensively drug-resistant tuberculosis

Multidrug resistant-tuberculosis (MDR-TB) is a dangerous development that complicates treatment. MDR-TB is defined as TB caused by organisms that are resistant to at least rifampicin and isoniazid (World Health Organization, 2007c).

The more recent identification of bacterial strains that cause extensively drug-resistant tuberculosis (XDR-TB) is extremely worrying, as treatment options are very limited. XDR-TB is a global issue with cases in many counties on most continents. In the UK, a recent case of XDR-TB was diagnosed in Glasgow during March 2008. In 2006, a new definition for XDR-TB was agreed – it is characterized by the drug resistance pattern of MDR-TB with additional resistance to any fluoroquinolone antibacterial drugs, and at least one of three second-line anti-TB drugs – amikacin, capreomycin or kanamycin – given by intramuscular injection (World Health Organization, 2007c). Both MDR-TB and XDR-TB are major threats in countries where there are high levels of HIV disease.

Severe acute respiratory syndrome

Severe acute respiratory syndrome (SARS) is caused by a coronavirus (other coronaviruses cause 'colds' and gastrointestinal infections; see Chapter 9). It is an important emerging infectious disease. Following the identification of a patient in Hong Kong in February 2003, outbreaks have been reported from Asia, North America and Europe. SARS is very serious infection and is highly contagious. The mortality rate is high and risk of death appears to be associated with increasing age. The route of transmission is via droplet spread through close personal contact. Outbreaks have occurred in hospital as well as the community and health workers are particularly at risk. So far Hong Kong has been the worst city affected and the experience of staff implementing the most stringent infection control protocols with strict patient isolation carries important messages for infection control teams in other countries (Leung et al., 2004).

Viral haemorrhagic fevers

The viral haemorrhagic fevers are caused by RNA viruses – Lassa fever by an arenavirus and Ebola fever and Marburg fever by filoviruses. They are endemic in Africa, especially the countries in central and western regions (Winter, 2005). Rodents and monkeys in parts of tropical Africa carry these viruses, which are extremely virulent. In 1967, seven animal handlers in the German town of Marburg died after contact with infected laboratory monkeys imported from Uganda, these being the first cases of viral haemorrhagic fever reported in Europe. Occasional cases are reported in people who have been in the bush and in health professionals working abroad. In recent years, a number of outbreaks have been reported. The mortality rate can be 80 per cent or higher. In a large outbreak of Marburg fever in the Democratic Republic of the Congo in 1998–2000, the mortality was over 83 per cent, and in an outbreak that started in Angola in 2004, the mortality was over 90 per cent (World Health Organization, 2005c). More recent outbreaks in 2007 include cases of Marburg fever in Uganda and Ebola fever in the Democratic Republic of the Congo (World Health Organization, 2007d, 2007e).

Early symptoms are nonspecific, and many people familiar with the onset of malaria attribute vague feelings of malaise to this infection. However, the disease progresses rapidly, with a decline in blood count, haemorrhage into the internal organs, and the appearance of a bleeding rash, seizures and death. Blood splashing is common, and the spillage of infectious secretions can be difficult to contain in primitive field hospitals. Even with intensive supportive treatment, the mortality rate is very high, death typically occurring within 10 days of infection.

Transmission

Transmission is by blood and body fluids. The viral haemorrhagic fevers are highly infectious. The long incubation period of 21 days means that travellers can arrive in the UK apparently healthy, developing symptoms after their arrival. The occasional cases of viral haemorrhagic fever seen in the UK tend to be reported in cities with good links to major airports.

Prevention

Prevention is achieved by avoiding exposure to potentially infected wildlife. The most stringent form of isolation in a specialist unit is used when caring for infected patients (see Chapter 5). Greater care is now being taken during contact with mammals imported from tropical Africa. There are currently no vaccines against the viral haemorrhagic fevers.

Diagnosis

The diagnosis is made by testing for viruses in the blood.

Treatment

There is no specific treatment currently available. Some victims have recovered with intensive supportive measures.

Rabies

Rabies causes infection of the brain and spinal cord. It is caused by a rhabodovirus able to infect all warm-blooded animals. Cases have been recorded for more than 2,000 years, and the disease has always been much feared because of its dramatic manifestations and because, in untreated cases, it is invariably fatal. The victim develops seizures and hydrophobia (intense fear of water), falls into a coma and perishes. In some cases involving the brainstem, the infection follows a less dramatic course but nevertheless ultimately results in paralysis and death. The incubation period varies from one to eight weeks.

Transmission

Transmission is via saliva in a bite from an infected animal, or saliva having contact with mucous membrane. Viruses travel from the site of infection along the peripheral nerves to the brain. Transmission has also been recorded through corneal grafts from infected donors and from handling the tissues of infected animals.

Prevention

Prevention was previously achieved by enforcing quarantine on all imported livestock. Rabies was well established in the British Isles throughout the Middle Ages, and despite legislative measures, cases were reported until 1903. In Europe, however, rabies is endemic in wildlife so there is the potential for its transmission to domestic animals and humans. There have been fears that it might return to the UK because of a relaxation in the quarantine laws or via the Channel Tunnel, but these fears must be kept in perspective. In 1996, a woman developed rabies having been bitten by an infected bat that was not believed to have arrived via the transport system.

Vaccination is available for people at risk, for example those travelling to areas where rabies is present in wild and domestic animals, or who have occupations that include contact with animal species that are susceptible to rabies (see below). Many countries in Europe and other parts of the world operate a mandatory system of vaccination and microchip registration, with documentation for pet animals. Pet animals with the relevant up-to-date documentation (a 'pet pass-port'), including evidence of effective vaccination, are allowed to travel between counties without the need for quarantine (which is expensive and distressing for both pet and owner). In the UK, a Pet Travel Scheme (PETS) operates to allow eligible pet animals that have a microchip and have been vaccinated to travel outside the UK and return, if the necessary criteria are met (see Further Reading). Animals that do not qualify for the scheme are still required to spend six months in quarantine when they first enter or return to the UK. A vital precaution, because in early 2008 a dog in UK quarantine died from rabies.

Diagnosis

Diagnosis is made by clinical examination and a history of contact with an infected animal.

Treatment

A suspect wound should be thoroughly cleansed with soap and running water for some minutes as soon as possible. Post-exposure prophylaxis is achieved by infiltrat-ing rabies immunoglobulin directly into and around the wound if possible, and administering a course of vaccine (see below). Dual treatment is given because the immunoglobulin provides rapid, albeit short-acting immunity to cover the delay associated with active immunity from the vaccine.

PRACTICE APPLICATION 14.3

Rabies: Pre- and Post-exposure Prophylaxis

It is important that people at risk of contact with animals with rabies have the appro-priate course of vaccinations. Post-exposure prophylaxis involves wound first aid and possibly immunoglobulin and a course of vaccination.

Activity

Using the resources below, answer the following questions:

➤ Which specific groups of people should be offered pre-exposure vaccination?

➤ How many doses of vaccine are required for pre-exposure prophylaxis?

➤ What wound care advice is given after the wound has been washed?

➤ What factors are used to decide whether a person needs post-exposure prophylaxis?

➤ How many doses of vaccine are given for post-exposure prophylaxis?

Resources

British National Formulary – www.bnf.org.

Health Protection Scotland – www.hps.scot.nhs.uk.

National Travel Health Network and Centre (NaTHNaC) – www. nathnac.org/.

SELF-ASSESSMENT

1. An epidemic is a substantial increase in the number of cases of a condition simultaneously affecting several people. True? or False?

2. Explain the difference between the incidence and the prevalence of a disease.

3. The more severe type of malaria is caused by:

   (a) *Plasmodium ovale*
   (b) *P. falciparum*
   (c) *P. vivax*
   (d) *P. malariae*

4. According to the World Health Organization, where do most cases of malaria occur and which groups are most at risk?

5. A young adult with meningitis caused by *Neisseria meningitidis* will usually have:

   (a) early flu-like symptoms
   (b) headache
   (c) fever with cold extremities
   (d) nausea and vomiting

6. What type of transmissible agent causes Creutzfeldt–Jakob disease?

7. Contaminated water is usually responsible for sudden large outbreaks of cholera. True? or False?

8. What antibacterial drugs are usually used to treat Legionnaires' disease?

9. How is pulmonary tuberculosis diagnosed?

10. What are MDR-TB and XDR-TB?

REFERENCES

Bartlett CL, Kurtz JB, Hutchinson JG et al. (1983) Legionella in hospital and hotel water supplies. *Lancet* **2**: 1315.

Behrens RH and Roberts JA (1994) Is travel prophylaxis worthwhile? Economic appraisal of prophylaxis measures against malaria, hepatitis A and typhoid in travellers. *British Medical Journal* **309**: 918–22.

British Medical Association (BMA)/Royal Pharmaceutical Society of Great Britain (2007) *British National Formulary No 53.* BMJ Publishing, London.

Brooker C (ed.) (2008) *Churchill Livingstone's Medical Dictionary*, 16th edn. Churchill Livingstone, Edinburgh.

Campbell K (2006) Understanding how viruses can cause malignant disease. *Nursing Times* **102**(36): 30–1.

Cartwright K, Reilly S, White D et al. (1992) Early treatment with parenteral penicillin in meningococcal disease. *British Medical Journal* **305**: 143–7.

Charatan F (1991) Tuberculosis soars in New York. *British Medical Journal* **303**: 209–10.

Charatan F (1994) New York makes progress in fight against tuberculosis. *British Medical Journal* **308**: 807–8.

Chiodini J (2006) Malaria in UK travellers: assessment, prevention and treatment. *Nursing Standard* **20**(34): 49–58.

Conlon C (1990) Imported malaria. *Practitioner* **243**: 841–3.

Davies PD and Williams CS (1993) Tuberculosis is increasing in England and Wales. *Tubercle and Lung Disease* **74**: 350–1.

Department of Health (DH) (1986a) *Report of the Committee of Inquiry into the Outbreak of Salmonella Food Poisoning at Stanley Royd Hospital.* HMSO, London.

Department of Health (DH) (1986b) *Report of the Committee of Inquiry into the Outbreak of Legionnaires' Disease in Stafford in 1985* (Badenoch Report). HMSO, London.

Department of Health (DH) (1988) *Report of the Committee of Inquiry into Future Development of the Public Health Function* (Acheson Report). HMSO, London.

Department of Health (DH) (2004, modified Feb 2007) *Transmissible Spongiform Encephalopathy Agents: Safe Working and the Prevention of Infection.* Guidance from the Advisory Committee on Dangerous Pathogens and the Spongiform Encephalopathy Advisory Committee. DH, London. Available www.dh.gov.uk/en/policyandguidance.

Donowitz LG (1986) Failure of the overgown to prevent nosocomial infection in a paediatric intensive care unit. *Paediatrics* **77**: 35–8.

Dye C, Watt C J, Bleed DM et al. (2005) Evolution of tuberculosis control and prospects for reducing tuberculosis incidence, prevalence and deaths globally. *Journal of the American Medical Association* **293**: 2767–75.

Evans R, Burke JP, Classen D et al. (1992) Computerised identification of patients at high risk for hospital-acquired infection. *American Journal of Infection Control* **20**: 4–10.

Fraser DW, Tsai T and Orenstein W (1977) Legionnaires' disease: description of an epidemic and of pneumonia. *New England Journal of Medicine* **297**: 1183–97.

Gransden WR (1991) Predictors for bacteraemia. *Journal of Hospital Infection* **18** (Supplement A): 308–16.

Hainsworth T (2004) The value of cholera vaccination in promoting travel health. *Nursing Times* **100**(22): 30–1.

Health Protection Agency (HPA) (2007) *Tuberculosis in the UK: Annual Report on Tuberculosis Surveillance and Control in the UK 2007.* Available www.hpa.org.uk/.

Health and Safety Commission (HSC) (1991) *The Prevention and Control of Legionellosis Including Legionnaires' Disease: Approved Code of Practice.* HMSO, London.

Hill DR (2006) The burden of illness in international travel. *New England Journal of Medicine* **354**: 115–17.

Hohlfeld P, Daffos F and Costa JM (1994) Pre-natal diagnosis of congenital toxoplasmosis with a polymerase chain reaction test on amniotic fluid. *New England Journal of Medicine* **331**: 695–9.

Kornelisse FR, de Groot R and Neijens HJ (1995) Bacterial meningitis: mechanisms of disease and therapy. *European Journal of Paediatrics* **154**: 85–96.

Kreger BE, Craven DE and Carling PC (1989) Gram-negative bacteraemia: reassessment of aetiology, epidemiology and ecology in 612 patients. *American Journal of Medicine* **68**: 332–3.

Leung TF, Ng PC, Cheng FW et al. (2004) Infection control for SARS in a tertiary paediatric centre in Hong Kong. *Journal of Hospital Infection* 56: 215–22.

Liu WK, Healing DE, Yeomans JT et al. (1993) Monitoring of hospital water supplies for Legionella. *Journal of Hospital Infection* **24**: 1–9.

Makin T (2005) Legionella bacteria and water systems in health care premises. *Nursing Times* **101**(39): 48–51.

National Institute for Health and Clinical Excellence (NICE) (2006) *Tuberculosis: Clinical Diagnosis and Management of Tuberculosis, and Measures for its Prevention and Control.* Clinical guideline 33 (developed by The National Collaborating Centre for Chronic Conditions). Available www.nice.org.uk.

Pennington Group (1997) *Report on the Circumstances Leading to the 1996 Outbreak of Infection with E. coli O157 in Central Scotland: the Implications for Food Safety and the Lessons To Be Learnt.* TSO, Edinburgh.

Turner G (2004) Emerging concerns related to CJD. *Nursing Times* **100**(34): 28–30.

Uttley AHC and Pozniak A (1993) Resurgence of tuberculosis. *Journal of Hospital Infection* **23**: 249–53.

Vincent-Houdek M, Muytjens HL, Bongaerts GPA et al. (1993) Legionella monitoring: continuing story of nosocomial prevention. *Journal of Hospital Infection* **25**: 117–24.

Watson JM (1993) Tuberculosis in Britain today. *British Medical Journal* **306**: 221–2.

Wilkins E (2006) Human immunodeficiency virus infection and the human acquired immunodeficiency syndrome. In N Boon, N Colledge and B Walker (eds) *Davidson's Principles and Practice of Medicine*, 20th edn. Churchill Livingstone, Edinburgh.

Williams V (2006) Tuberculosis: clinical features, diagnosis and management. *Nursing Standard* **20**(22): 49–53.

Winter G (2005) Global virus alert. *Nursing Standard* **19**(44): 24–6.

Woo AH, Yu AH and Goetz A (1986) Potential in-hospital modes of transmission of *Legionella pneumophila*. Demonstration experiments for dissemination by showers, humidifiers and rinsing of ventilation bag apparatus. *American Journal of Medicine* **80**: 567–73.

World Health Organization (WHO) (2000) *Typhoid Vaccines: WHO Positional Paper.* WHO, Geneva.

World Health Organization (WHO) (2005a) *International Health Regulations.* Available www.who.org.

World Health Organization (WHO) (2005b) *Responding to the Avian Influenza Pandemic Threat: Recommended Strategic Actions.* WHO, Geneva.

World Health Organization (WHO) (2005c) *Marburg Haemorrhagic Fever.* Fact sheet. Available www.who.int.

World Health Organization (WHO) (2007a) *Malaria.* Fact sheet 94. Available www.who.int.

World Health Organization (WHO) (2007b) *Tuberculosis.* Fact sheet 104. Available www. who.int.

World Health Organization (WHO) (2007c) *XDR-TB Extensively Drug-resistant Tuberculosis. What, Where, How and Action Steps.* Available www.who.int.

World Health Organization (WHO) (2007d) *Marburg Haemorrhagic Fever in Uganda – Update.* Available www.who.int.

World Health Organization (WHO) (2007e) *Ebola Haemorrhagic Fever in the Democratic Republic of the Congo – update 3.* Available www.who.int.

Xavier G (2006) Management of typhoid and paratyphoid fevers. *Nursing Times* **102**(17): 49–52.

FURTHER READING AND INFORMATION SOURCES

Boyne L (2005) Providing a travel health service in primary care. *Practice Nurse* **30**(8): 25–8.

Burnet M and White DO (1972) *The Natural History of Infectious Disease.* Cambridge University Press, Cambridge.

Department for Environment, Food and Rural Affairs (DEFRA) (2007) *Pet Travel Scheme.* Available www.defra.gov.uk/animalh/quarantine/pets/index.htm.

Department of Health (DH) (2006, modified 2007) *Immunisation against Infectious Diseases (The Green Book).* TSO, Norwich. Available www.dh.gov.uk/en/Policyandguidance/ Healthandsocialcaretopics/Greenbook/DH_4097254.

Goodyear L (2004) *Travel Medicine for Health Professionals.* Pharmaceutical Press, London.

Health Protection Agency (2003, updated 2007) *Travel Health.* Available www.hpa.org.uk/ infections/topics_az/travel/default.htm.

Health and Safety Commission (HSC) (2000) *Approved Code of Practice and Guidance. Legionnaires' Disease: the Control of Legionella Bacteria in Water Systems.* HSC, London.

Jefferson T, Foxlee R, Del Mar C et al. (2008) Physical interventions to interrupt or reduce the spread of respiratory viruses: systematic review. *British Medical Journal* **336**: 77–80.

Kimball A (2006) *Risky Trade: Infectious Disease in the Era of Global Trade.* Ashgate, London.

Lee G and Leese J (eds) (2001) *Health Information for Overseas Travel.* TSO, London.

MVT: Malaria Vaccine Trials – www.malaria-vaccines.org.uk.

Meningitis Research Fund – www.meningitis.org.uk.

Royal College of Nursing (RCN) (2005) *Delivering Travel Health Services: RCN Guidance for Nursing Staff.* RCN. London

Stop TB Partnership – www.stoptb.org.

Webber R (1996) *Communicable Disease Epidemiology and Control.* CAB International, London.

World Health Organization (WHO) (2007) *The World Health Report 2007 – A Safer Future: Global Public Health Security in the 21st Century.* Available www.who.org/.

World Health Organization (WHO) (2007) *International Travel and Health.* Available www.who.org/.

Answers to self-assessment questions

Chapter 1

1. False
2. (b)
3. False
4. (a)
5. The ability of a pathogen to cause disease
6. True
7. False
8. True
9. True
10. See Practice Application 1.4

Chapter 2

1. False
2. Redness, heat, swelling, pain, loss of function
3. Ability of some leucocytes (e.g. neutrophils) to engulf foreign material
4. True
5. See Practice Application 2.1
6. Antigen specificity, clonal selection, clonal expansion, clonal suppression and the formation of memory cells, and antibodies (immunoglobulins)
7. True
8. False
9. (d)
10. (c)

Chapter 3

1. False
2. Gram stain, wet film, dark ground illumination
3. All bacteria in a colony are derived from the same original cell and are therefore identical
4. True

5. See Practice Application 3.3

Chapter 4

1. True
2. See Information box 4.1
3. True
4. (b) and (d)
5. (b) and (c)
6. (c)
7. When the body's normal commensal flora is suppressed by antibiotics and replaced by drug-resistant organisms
8. See p. 92

Chapter 5

1. True
2. See p. 103
3. False
4. (a) and (d)
5. All of these
6. True
7. True
8. See p. 124

Chapter 6

1. False
2. True
3. Difficult to eradicate, many people become carriers, some strains are more readily disseminated than others, antibiotic resistance
4. False
5. Exposure to a wide range of different antibiotics promotes the survival of antibiotic-resistant strains
6. True
7. See p. 143

317

Chapter 7

1. True
2. A collection of microorganisms and their extracellular products bound to a solid surface
3. (d)
4. True
5. See Figure 7.1
6. 40 cm men and 25 cm women

Chapter 8

1. True
2. Inflammatory response, collagen synthesis, angiogenesis, epithelialization
3. See p. 167
4. See p. 185
5. See Information box 8.3
6. False

Chapter 9

1. (d)
2. True
3. True
4. See pp. 192–4
5. See pp. 194–6
6. (b) and (d)
7. False
8. See p. 203

Chapter 10

1. See Figure 10.1
2. False
3. See p. 211
4. True
5. 2 per cent chlorhexidine in 70 per cent alcohol

Chapter 11

1. See pp. 223–4
2. All of these

3. True
4. All of these
5. See p. 234
6. True
7. False
8. See pp. 237–9

Chapter 12

1. All of these
2. (a), (b) and (c)
3. False
4. False
5. See pp. 253–4
6. True
7. See p. 256

Chapter 13

1. False
2. (b)
3. False
4. False
5. True
6. (d)
7. False
8. (b)
9. See Table 13.1
10. (c)

Chapter 14

1. True
2. See Information box 14.1
3. (b)
4. See p. 293
5. All of these
6. Abnormal prion proteins
7. True
8. See p. 305
9. See p. 307
10. See p. 308

Glossary

Abscess A localized collection of purulent material contained within a fibrin membrane.

Acquired immunity Immunity (usually long-lasting) that is stimulated by exposure to a microbial antigen. It results from having the disease or receiving a vaccine containing antigenic substances, which leads to the production of antibodies or specific T cells.

Acute bronchitis Inflammation of the bronchi. *See* Bronchitis.

Aerobe A microorganism able to grow in oxygen. Strict (obligate) aerobes must have oxygen for their growth and survival.

Agar Inert polysaccharide (complex carbo-hydrate) derived from seaweed, solid at room temperature; it is used to solidify culture media.

Agglutination The aggregation or clumping together of cells or particles.

Agranulocyte A white blood cell without granules in its cytoplasm.

Allergic reaction Hypersensitivity to a specific allergen (an antigen that produces allergy), for example pollen, dust, drugs or food. An abnormal immune response occurs that results in the release of chemical mediators such as histamine, prostaglandins and 5-hydroxytryptamine (5-HT), inflammation and an anaphylactic reaction. There are usually local effects such as bronchospasm, rashes and diarrhoea, or, rarely, a widespread systemic reaction – anaphylactic shock.

Amoeba A microscopic unicellular protozoon. Some species have evolved as human parasites.

Anaerobe A microorganism that can grow and flourish without the presence of oxygen. Strict (obligate) anaerobes cannot grow in the presence of oxygen, whereas some facultative microbes can grow with or without oxygen.

Anaphylactic shock A severe hypersensitivity reaction to a foreign protein mediated by mast cells and basophils.

Angiogenesis The formation of new blood capillaries, such as during wound healing.

Antibiotic-associated diarrhoea Also known as 'pseudomembranous colitis'. A serious condition linked to superinfection with *Clostridium difficile* in patients who have received broad-spectrum antibiotics, which suppress the normal intestinal flora. Large areas of the intestinal epithelium undergo necrosis causing profuse watery diarrhoea. Antibiotic-associated colitis causes intestinal ulceration that can lead to potentially life-threatening perforation and peritonitis.

Antibiotics Strictly speaking, they are chemicals produced by living organisms, which are able to inhibit the growth of other organisms. In common usage, the term refers to antibacterial drugs whatever their source.

Antibodies (immunoglobulins) Proteins secreted by B lymphocytes that are able to bind to antigens during the immune response. They appear in the blood and tissue fluids of the host in the presence of specific antigens.

Antigenicity The ability of microorganisms and their products to induce antibody production, a property that is utilized during immunization.

Antigens Foreign cells or molecules that stimulate the immune system of the host and bind to antibodies or lymphocytes.

Antimicrobial agent Any substance that destroys microorganisms or inhibits their growth.

Aseptic technique Procedures that exclude pathogenic microorganisms from a particular environment, for example the use of sterile equipment and non-touch technique.

Atelectasis Collapse of the alveoli.

Attenuation The process by which vaccines are produced that retain microbial antigenicity without pathogenicity; that is, they induce antibody production without causing the disease.

Autoclaving The application of moist heat (steam under pressure) to achieve sterilization.

Autolysis The self-destruction of an organism through the release of its own enzymes.

Bacillus A genus of Gram-positive microorganisms. Also a general name for any rod-shaped bacterium.

Bacteraemia The presence of bacteria in the blood (bloodstream infection).

Bacteria Unicellular microorganisms, widely distributed within a variety of environments. Some may be pathogenic (disease-producing), whereas others perform useful functions, for example producing an environment that is hostile to harmful pathogens in the body.

Bactericidal agent A substance able to kill bacteria.

Bacteriological growth curve A typical sequence of events through which a newly inoculated culture of bacterial cells passes. It encompasses an initial lag phase (without multiplication, as the cells adapt to their new surroundings), a logarithmic phase (of optimal growth), a stationary phase (the total number of cells present remaining static as the rate of multiplication equals the number of cells dying through lack of nutrients) and a final decline phase (the number of cells decreasing as the nutrient supply is expended).

Bacteriophage (phage) A virus that parasitizes bacteria.

Bacteriostatic agent A substance able to prevent bacterial replication but unable to kill bacteria.

Bacteriuria The presence of bacteria in the urine – 100,000 or more pathogens per ml of freshly voided urine representing an infection.

Barrier nursing *See* Isolation.

Basophil A phagocytic granulocyte present in the blood, which contains heparin and histamine.

B cells B lymphocytes. Part of the humoral immune response, these become plasma cells, which produce antibodies (immunoglobulins).

Binary fission A method of microbial reproduction in which the microorganism divides into two genetically identical 'daughter' cells.

Biofilm A collection of microorganisms and their extracellular products, for example proteins, bound to a solid surface.

Blood–brain barrier The arrangement of capillary endothelial cells and specialized cells (astrocytes) surrounding the brain and spinal cord that allows the passage of some but not all chemical substances. This selective chemical permeability is commonly referred to as the blood–brain barrier.

Body fluids These include blood, all blood products (for example plasma, plasma-depleted blood and white cell infusions), cerebrospinal fluid, amniotic fluid, pleural fluid, peritoneal fluid, pericardial fluid, synovial fluid, semen, vaginal fluid, saliva, unfixed tissues and organs, urine and faeces.

Bradykinin A chemical (peptide) mediator of the inflammatory response. It causes vaso-dilation, contraction of involuntary muscle, increased blood vessel permeability and pain.

Bronchitis Inflammation of the bronchial mucosa. Acute bronchitis is caused by a variety of viruses and bacteria. Chronic bronchitis, which is classified as a chronic obstructive pulmonary disease (COPD), is characterized by inflammation, excess mucus production, reduced mucociliary clearance and the eventual impair-ment of gaseous exchange. The chronic condition is made worse by repeated respiratory infections.

Capsule A mucus layer surrounding the cell wall of some types of bacterium. Helps to prevent desiccation when adverse environmental conditions are encountered.

Carrier An individual harbouring micro-organisms and able to transmit them without manifesting the signs and symptoms of infection.

Cell-mediated immunity Part of the immune response involving the action of T lymphocytes, which release regulatory chemicals and destroy foreign or abnormal cells.

Cellulitis The diffuse inflammation of connective tissue.

Cellulose A polysaccharide (complex carbohydrate) found as a component of plant cell walls.

Cell wall The outer layer that surrounds the cell membrane of certain cell types: some bacteria and all plant cells.

Chancre The primary lesion of syphilis; a hard, painless, highly infectious ulcer.

Chemoprophylaxis The prevention of infection by administering antibacterial drugs before signs and symptoms appear.

Chemotaxis The movement – attraction (positive) or repulsion (negative) – of cells in response to chemicals, for example leucocytes (white blood cells) are attracted to areas of infection by the release of bacterial substances.

Chemotherapy The use of chemical substances to treat disease in palliation and cure. Covers antimicrobial drugs and drugs used to treat malignancy. In common usage, chemotherapy has come to mean the cytotoxic drugs used in cancer treatment.

Cilia Microscopic 'hair-like' processes found on the surface of some cells, for example respiratory mucosa and uterine tubes. Their ability to beat in a rhythmic way enables mucus to be cleared from the lungs, the process of mucociliary clearance.

Cleaning A procedure to remove vegetative microorganisms in order to maintain the appearance, structure and effective functioning of the clinical environment and its contents.

Clinical infection Pathogenic invasion eliciting a response from the host (pyrexia and inflammation).

Clinical waste Waste generated by healthcare facilities (both human and animal). Disposal by incineration reduces the risk associated with hazardous waste, be it toxic or infectious.

Coagulase A bacterial enzyme capable of clotting plasma. It is produced by some staphylococci.

Coccus A general name for any spheroidally shaped bacterium, for example *Streptococcus* and *Staphylococcus.*

Cohort A group of individuals sharing a particular characteristic. Infection control in healthcare facilities is assisted by 'cohorting' similarly infected individuals together during outbreaks of infection.

Collagen Strong fibres giving strength to connective tissues such as skin, bone and tendons.

Colonization The establishment of pathogenic microorganisms at a particular body site with little or no host response to the pathogen. Colonization can lead to a large number of microorganisms, which form a reservoir for infection and cross-infection.

Colony A collection of bacteria growing on a solid culture medium that is large enough to be seen by the naked eye.

Commensals Microorganisms that live in close association with their host. In their correct location, they do no harm and may even have a beneficial effect.

Communicable An infectious disease, one that is transmitted directly or indirectly from one person or animal to another.

Complement proteins A group of proteins that are activated on exposure to components in bacterial cell walls and parasites. They enhance phagocytosis and some complement proteins perform additional functions important in the overall immune response.

Condylomata lata Flattened, wart-like lesions appearing during the secondary stage of syphilis at anatomical sites that are usually moist.

Conjugation A method by which bacteria exchange genetic material via sex pili. It is of particular importance in Gram-negative bacilli.

Contagious *See* Communicable.

Creutzfeldt-Jakob disease (CJD) One of a range of diseases, known collectively as the 'transmissible spongiform encephalopathies' (TSEs). It is caused by abnormal prion proteins.

Cross-infection An infection acquired from outside the individual. *See* Exogenous infection.

Croup Laryngeal spasm associated with a viral infection involving the larynx and trachea.

Cystitis Inflammation of the urinary bladder, usually caused by bacteria such as *Escherichia coli.*

Cytokines A generic term used to describe cellular signalling molecules, such as the interferons and interleukins, involved in the modulation of body defences. Cytokines produced by lymphocytes are sometimes called lymphokines.

Cytotoxic Describes the ability to kill or destroy cells.

Decontamination Encompasses cleaning, disinfection and sterilization.

Dermatophyte Superficial fungal infection of the skin involving the hair and nails.

Diploid Describes a cell containing a full set of paired chromosomes.

Disinfection Process causing the destruction of vegetative microorganisms but not their spores.

Ectoparasite A parasite that lives upon the surface of the host, for example the flea. *Compare* Endoparasite.

Electron microscopy Using a beam of electrons rather than light to produce images of extremely small particles such as virus particles.

ELISA (enzyme-linked immunosorbent assay) A method that utilizes enzyme-labelled antibodies to detect and measure other antibodies and antigens.

Encrustation The deposition of crystalline solids, mainly calcium and magnesium salts, on the surface of a urinary catheter and drainage apparatus.

Endemic disease A disease always present in a given population.

Endocarditis Inflammation of the endocardium (the lining of the heart) and heart valves. Bacterial endocarditis is commonly caused by staphylococci and streptococci.

Endogenous infection Self-infection, the organisms responsible originating from the same individual. *Compare* Exogenous infection.

Endoparasite A parasite that lives within the host, for example a tapeworm. *Compare* Ectoparasite.

Endotoxin An intracellular toxin contained in the cell wall of some Gram-negative bacteria, the toxin being released only when the bacterial cell is destroyed. The effects may include fever, malaise and inflammation. *Compare* Exotoxin.

Eosinophil A weakly phagocytic granulocyte playing a role in the allergic response and protecting the body against parasites.

Epidemic The same condition simultaneously affecting several people.

Epidemic infection A substantial increase in the number of people becoming carriers or infected with a particular organism.

Epithelialization The growth of epithelium over the surface of a wound.

Epithelium The tissue that covers the external body surfaces, forms glands and lines the body cavities. It is one of the four basic tissues.

Eukaryotic Desribes a cell with a true nucleus. The genetic material is enclosed within a nuclear membrane. *Compare* Prokaryotic.

Exogenous infection (cross-infection) Caused by organisms originating from an external source – other patients, staff or the environment. *Compare* Endogenous infection.

Exotoxin A toxin released through the bacterial cell wall into the extracellular fluid. These are secreted by Gram-positive bacteria and can have widespread effects. For example, the toxin of *Clostridium botulinum* inhibits the transmission of nerve impulses to cause paralysis. *Compare* Endotoxin.

Extensively drug-resistant tuberculosis (XDR-TB) Tuberculosis caused by bacterial strains that exhibit the drug resistance pattern of MDR-TB with additional resistance to any fluoroquinolone antibacterial drugs, and at least one of three second-line anti-TB drugs amikacin, capreomycin or kanamycin given by intramuscular injection (WHO, 2007).

Facultative Describes a microorganism that can adapt and survive in different environmental conditions. *See* Anaerobe.

Fibroblast A connective tissue cell producing collagen.

Flagellum A microscopic projection from the surface of some cells, such as spermatozoa, and some microorganisms. It is concerned with cell movement.

Fluorescent antibody technique A method of detecting antibodies by the use of fluorescent dyes. The antibody, when attached to the dye, can be seen by using ultraviolet light with a special fluorescent microscope.

Fomite Any item that has been in contact with an infectious source and is in turn able to transfer infection.

Food-borne infection (invasive intestinal gastroenteritis) An infective condition caused by the activity of bacteria multiplying within the gastrointestinal tract.

Food intoxication Food-borne disease caused by bacterial toxins present in food.

Fungus A diverse group of simple plants that includes mushrooms, moulds and yeasts. Some are human pathogens, but many others are used in the food and pharmaceutical industries.

Gangrene Massive tissue death (necrosis) resulting from loss of blood supply. Infection may be present in some types.

General paralysis of the insane A manifestation of tertiary syphilis involving the nervous system (neurosyphilis), characterized by memory loss, incontinence and disintegration of the personality, with a sudden or insidious onset.

Genus A biological subdivision of a family of plants or animals. A genus may contain several related species.

Gram staining A staining method used to identify and classify some bacteria. Gram-positive microorganisms stain violet and Gram-negative ones pink.

Granulation tissue The new moist, red/pink tissue that forms in the wound bed.

Granulocyte A leucocyte (white blood cell) containing granules of enzymes within its cytoplasm. Includes basophils, neutrophils and eosinophils.

Gummata The lesions of tertiary syphilis. Obstruction to the blood supply results in necrosis and the formation of chronic ulcers that are probably not infectious.

Haemolysin A chemical produced by many bacteria that causes disruption of the red blood cell membrane.

Healthcare-associated infection (HCAI) An infection not present or incubating at the time of admission or healthcare intervention (Bennett and Brachman, 1979).

Hepatitis Inflammation of the liver often caused by viruses, for example hepatitis B virus.

Histamine A powerful chemical mediator released by many tissues and blood cells. Released during inflammation, it causes vasodilation, increased blood flow and increased blood vessel permeability. It is also implicated in the signs and symptoms of some allergic conditions, for example hay fever.

Hospital-acquired infection (HAI) Infection arising from hospital stay or treatment. Also known as nosocomial infection. *See* Healthcare-associated infection.

Humoral immunity Part of the immune response involving B lymphocytes, plasma cells and the production of antibodies.

Hypersensitivity reaction Abnormal sensitivity to an allergen.

Immunity A state of resistance to an infectious agent, either intrinsic or acquired.

Immunization The administration of antigens to induce a state of immunity.

Immunocompromised person An individual whose immune system is prevented from responding to pathogens in the normal way, through poor health or the action of drugs, or because he or she is undergoing an invasive procedure.

Immunodeficiency An impairment of humoral or cell-mediated immunity, which may be congenital or acquired. Causes include a failure to produce antibodies, HIV/AIDS and chemotherapy.

Immunoglobulins *See* Antibodies.

Immunosuppression The condition in which the activity of the immune system is depressed through treatment (radiotherapy or drugs) or disease.

Incidence The number of new cases of a disease occurring in a population over a specific period of time.

Incubation period The time from contact with an infectious disease until the signs and symptoms appear.

Infection The successful invasion, establishment and growth of microorganisms within the tissues of a host.

Infectious *See* Communicable.

Inflammation The response of the tissues to trauma (physical, chemical, extremes of temperature, or pathogenic invasion). The classic hallmarks of inflammation are erythema (redness), heat, swelling, pain and possible loss of function (depending on the site and extent of the injury).

Inoculum The material, such as urine or sputum, containing microorganisms that is used to inoculate culture medium in the laboratory.

Interferons (IFNs) Antiviral proteins produced by T lymphocytes and other cells. They act as cellular signalling chemicals to modulate the immune response by stimulating other immune cells; macrophages, for example, are activated to become killer cells. *See* Cytokines.

Interleukins (ILs) A group of cellular signalling chemicals. They are produced by a variety of cells involved in immune processes, for example macrophages. Interleukins also act as growth factors needed for the production of blood cells. *See* Cytokines.

Invasive device/procedure One that bypasses the body's natural defences against infection, for example urinary catheterization, intravenous cannulation, intubation or incision.

Isolation Various measures used to contain an infectious disease or protect vulnerable individuals. *See* Protective isolation.

Kaposi's sarcoma A malignant neoplasm in which there is growth of new blood vessels first appearing as brown, red or purple lesions on the skin. Spread occurs to other areas with metastasis to the lymph nodes and viscera. Often occurs in immunocompromised individuals, such as those with HIV disease.

Latent infection An infection in which the individual is infected by the microorganism without the signs of disease being obvious.

Leucocytes Generic name for all white blood cells: neutrophils, eosinophils, basophils, monocytes and lymphocytes.

Leucopoiesis The formation of leucocytes.

Live attenuated vaccine A vaccine produced from living microorganisms, for example that for MMR (measles, mumps and rubella). The microorganisms are changed to remove their ability to cause disease while still being able to stimulate antibody production. *See* Attenuation.

Lymphocytes Agranulocytic leucocytes (white blood cells), types include T and B cells.

Lymphokines Chemicals released by T cells. They control all the cells of the immune system by activating or suppressing other cells involved in the immune response.

Lysozyme A bactericidal enzyme found in many body fluids, for example tears, saliva and nasal secretions.

Macrophages Large phagocytic cells derived from monocytes. They play an important nonspecific scavenging role in the inflammatory response, and are also involved in many specific immune responses.

Malaise A general (nonspecific) feeling of illness or discomfort.

Mast cell A tissue cell with granules containing histamine and other chemicals. Mast cells have similarities with basophils and both are involved in the initiation of inflammation by the release of histamine.

Memory cells Cells derived from B and T lymphocytes, which persist in the body. They 'remember' a specific antigen and are able to respond quickly if that antigen is encountered again.

Meningitis Inflammation of the meninges (the three membranes covering the brain and spinal cord). Meningitis may be bacterial or viral.

Meticillin-resistant *Staphylococcus aureus* (MRSA) A strain of *Staphylococcus aureus* that is resistant to most antimicrobial agents, including meticillin (not used clinically) and flucloxacillin.

Microbe *See* Microorganism.

Microorganism An organism, usually too small to be seen without a microscope, for example bacteria, viruses, fungi and protozoa.

Monocyte A type of phagocytic leucocyte (white blood cell). Some are able to move into the tissues from the blood to become macrophages.

Multidrug resistant-tuberculosis (MDR-TB) Tuberculosis caused by organisms that are resistant to at least rifampicin and isoniazid (WHO, 2007).

Multiple organ dysfunction syndrome (MODS) A syndrome affecting critically ill people. Organ function is impaired and there may be kidney failure, abnormal blood coagulation (disseminated intravascular coagulation – DIC), acute respiratory distress syndrome (ARDS) and gastrointestinal failure. *See* Systemic inflammatory response syndrome.

Mycelium Filaments produced by moulds (a type of fungus). It is these filaments that can be seen on mouldy food.

Myocarditis Inflammation of the myocardium, the muscle layer of the heart.

Natural killer (NK) cell A type of lymphocyte able to destroy virus infected cells and those showing malignant change.

Necrosis The localized death of tissue in response to injury, poor blood supply or disease.

Neutrophil A phagocytic granulocyte playing a key role in the inflammatory response.

Nonspecific urethritis Nongonococcal urethritis. Urethritis associated with infection with *Chlamydia trachomatis*.

Normal flora The microorganisms that normally colonize the body.

Nosocomial infection *See* Hospital-acquired infection, Healthcare-associated infection.

Obligate Of a microorganism, requiring specific environmental conditions for its survival. *See* Aerobe and Anaerobe.

Opportunistic infection Infection caused by organisms that do not usually exhibit pathogenic properties but which become pathogenic in patients who are seriously ill, immuno-compromised, or undergoing invasive treatment.

Opsonin An antibody or complement protein that recognizes a foreign molecule (antigen). It attaches to the foreign molecule and labels it to enhance phagocytosis.

Opsonization The process by which bacteria are marked as foreign cells, rendering them more susceptible to phagocytosis.

Otitis media Acute otitis media is inflammation of the middle ear.

Pandemic The simultaneous occurrence of a large number of infections of the same kind.

Parasite An organism that lives in or on another living organism (the host). It confers no benefit upon the host, which it exploits for its physical needs.

Parenteral Literally meaning 'outside the alimentary tract'. Applies to therapy such as fluids, nutrients or drugs given via a route other than the alimentary tract, for example by injection.

Parenteral transmission Literally, the delivery of a substance by any route other than via the alimentary tract. Usually now taken to mean transmission via blood.

Pathogen An agent able to cause disease.

Pathogenicity The capacity of microorganisms to cause disease.

Pericarditis Inflammation of the pericardium (the double serous membranous sac enveloping the heart). This can be caused by bacteria or viruses.

Peritonitis Inflammation of the peritoneum (the two-layer serous membrane lining the abdominal cavity and covering some of the organs). It may be caused by bacterial infection or chemical irritation.

Petri dish A plastic dish that, when filled with agar, is used to grow bacteria in the laboratory.

pH The hydrogen ion concentration. A method of expressing acidity (hydrogen ions) or alkalinity (hydroxyl ions). It utilizes a logarithmic scale with a range from 0 to 14 (pH 0 representing the greatest concentration of hydrogen ions, pH 7 neutrality, the number of hydrogen and hydroxyl ions being equal,

and pH 14 the greatest concentration of hydroxyl ions).

Phage *See* Bacteriophage.

Phagocytes Cells that are capable of phagocytosis, for example the white blood cells (neutrophils and monocytes) and the macrophages in the tissues.

Phagocytosis The cellular engulfment of bacteria and particulate matter.

Phlebitis Inflammation of the vein. Usually caused by chemical or mechanical irritation but may become complicated by infection.

Plasma cells Transient immune cells derived from B lymphocytes. They produce specific antibodies.

Plasmid Extrachromosomal DNA present in the cytoplasm of some bacteria.

Pleomorphism A state in which the size and shape of bacterial cells becomes highly variable, sometimes ceasing to display the typical morphological characteristics of the species and thus making identification difficult.

Pneumonia Inflammation of the lung. In bronchopneumonia, the affected tissue is distributed widely around the bronchi. In lobar pneumonia, the area of consolidation is localized. Nosocomial pneumonia is a hospital-acquired infection of the lower respiratory tract developing at least 72 hours after admission.

Polymorphonuclear leucocyte A leucocyte (white blood cell) containing a many-lobed nucleus. This can be a neutrophil, an eosinophil or a basophil.

Prevalence The total number of cases of a disease present in a population at a single point in time.

Primary intention The type of healing that occurs in clean surgical wounds where the skin edges are in apposition.

Primary response The immune response that results from the first contact with an antigen. There is an initial lag phase of 2–3 weeks before antibody production reaches a protective level.

Prion An infectious agent that consists of protein but no nucleic acids. Prions are responsible for the transmission of the transmissible spongiform encephalopathies, such as Creutzfeldt–Jakob disease, bovine spongiform encephalopathy and scrapie in sheep.

Prokaryotic Describes a cell that lacks a true nucleus and nuclear membrane, the genetic material lying within the cytoplasm. *See* Eukaryotic.

Prophylaxis Measures taken to prevent disease, for example immunization and perioperative antimicrobial drug therapy. *See* Chemoprophylaxis.

Protective isolation Special measures taken to protect immunocompromised individuals from infection.

Protozoa Microscopic unicellular animals. Many are harmless, but others are responsible for human diseases including malaria, toxoplasmosis and cryptosporidiosis, which affect immunocompromised individuals.

Pseudomembranous colitis *See* Antibiotic-associated diarrhoea.

Puerperal sepsis A local infection, which results from childbirth, arising in the genital tract leading to septicaemia.

Pus Matter resulting from infection. It consists of bacterial cells, leucocytes, cell debris and tissue fluid.

Pyelonephritis (acute) Ascending urinary tract infection spreading outwards from the pelvis of the kidney to its cortex. In some cases, the source of infection is the blood rather than the lower urinary tract.

Reservoir of infection A source of microorganisms, for example a human carrier of the microorganism *Salmonella enterica* serovar Typhi that causes typhoid fever.

Reverse transcriptase A viral enzyme that catalyses the synthesis of nucleic acids.

Rickettsia A group of microorganisms that have the characteristics of both bacteria and viruses. They cause diseases such as typhus and Rocky Mountain spotted fever.

Risk assessment A method of identifying and assessing a particular risk or hazard. Subsequent management seeks to minimize the potential risk by the use of specific precautions, for example handwashing protocols.

Saprophyte A free-living microorganism obtaining nourishment from decaying animals and plant tissue.

Screening A preventive measure employed to identify potential or incipient disease.

Secondary intention The type of healing that occurs in a wound where there is tissue loss, for example a pressure ulcer. Here, the wound heals from the base.

Secondary response The immune response occurring when B lymphocytes encounter an antigen on a second or subsequent occasion. The memory cells produce antibodies very quickly (without a lag phase).

Septicaemia Multiplication of bacteria in blood. Septicaemia is a very serious condition, which can lead to overwhelming sepsis and systemic inflammatory response syndrome (SIRS).

Seroconversion The secretion of specific antibodies following exposure to an antigen.

Serology The study of blood sera with particular emphasis on the reactions concerned with immunological function and diagnosis.

Serotyping A method of classifying microbial strains based on their antigenic characteristics. The surface antigens are identified in the laboratory by using the specific antibodies.

Serum The plasma component of coagulated blood with all the cellular elements removed.

Severe acute respiratory syndrome (SARS) A highly infectious viral pneumonia caused by a coronavirus. It is an important emerging infectious disease first identified in Hong Kong in 2003. The mortality rate is high and outbreaks have been reported from Asia, North America and Europe.

Sharp Any item – needles, razors, lancets, scalpel blades, microscope slides, ampoules, wires and stitch-cutters – able to cut or penetrate skin or mucous membranes.

Slough Necrotic tissue that detaches from healthy tissue following infection.

Source of infection The site from which a microorganism responsible for an infection has emanated.

Species Smaller subdivisions within a genus.

Spirochaetes An order of slender, spiral-shaped bacteria. Genera included in the order are *Treponema*, *Leptospira* and *Borrelia*.

Spore A bacterial adaptation to unfavourable environmental conditions. Cells survive as their metabolism slows, and they become surrounded by a thick capsule. When favourable conditions return, the spore is able to germinate.

Standard (universal) precautions/ principles The measures taken to prevent and/ or control infection – environmental cleaning, personal protective equipment, fundamental hygiene, including handwashing and decontamination, and proper handling and disposal of sharps. Also the procedures to be followed in the case of accidents, especially needlestick injury and exposure to blood and body fluids.

Sterilization The destruction of all microorganisms and their spores.

Stevens–Johnson syndrome An adverse, potentially fatal reaction to co-trimoxazole characterized by a bullous rash, fever and ulceration of the mouth.

Strain Microorganisms of the same species that have different physical and chemical features.

Subclinical infection The presence of infection without any obvious signs or symptoms of the disease.

Superinfection A situation that occurs when the body's normal commensal flora is suppressed by antibiotics and replaced by drug-resistant microorganisms. *See* Antibiotic-associated diarrhoea.

Surveillance The process of monitoring the occurrence of diseases, for example notifiable infectious diseases, within a population.

Systemic inflammatory response syndrome (SIRS) A life-threatening condition, which can be triggered by overwhelming sepsis, major trauma, severe haemorrhage, acute pancreatitis and conditions that result in poor tissue perfusion and so on (Adams, 2003). The release of inflammatory mediators into the blood lead to an abnormal response with widespread effects and organ damage. *See* Multiple organ dysfunction syndrome (MODS).

Tabes dorsalis A manifestation of tertiary syphilis affecting the nervous system (neurosyphilis). It involves the posterior columns of the spinal cord and the associated sensory nerve roots, resulting in disordered gait and a loss of sense of position in the legs (locomotor ataxia).

T cells T lymphocytes that facilitate cell-mediated immunity. They differentiate into active T cells that destroy foreign cells carrying specific antigens and regulate the immune response.

Titre The measurement of antibody concentration, for example in the blood.

Toxin A poisonous substance, usually of microbial origin.

Toxoid A microbial toxin that has been modified to retain antigenicity without pathogenicity. It is used to produce immunity against specific diseases, for example tetanus. *See* Attenuation.

Transduction The transfer of genetic material from one bacterium to another by a bacteriophage.

Transformation The transfer of genetic material from one bacterium to another through the cell wall into the cytoplasm.

Universal precautions *See* Standard (universal) precautions/principles.

Vaccine An extract prepared from inactivated or weakened microorganisms that is used to induce a state of immunity to the pathogen in the recipient.

Vibrio A genus of comma-shaped bacteria. *Vibrio cholerae* causes cholera.

Virulence The ability of a microorganism to cause infection.

Virus A microorganism containing either DNA or RNA. Can only replicate inside a living host cell. Visualization is only possible using electron microscopy.

White blood cell *See* Leucocytes.

Yeast A simple, single-celled fungus, for example *Candida albicans*.

Ziehl–Neelsen stain A staining technique used in the identification of acid-fast bacilli such as *Mycobacterium tuberculosis*.

Zoonoses Diseases transmitted from animals to humans, for example anthrax and rabies.

References

Adams S. (2003) Shock, systemic inflammatory response and multiple organ dysfunction. In C Brooker and M Nicol (eds) *Nursing Adults: The Practice of Caring*. Mosby, Edinburgh, pp. 157–9, 167–9.

Bennett JV and Brachman PS (1979) *Hospital Infections*. Little, Brown, Boston.

World Health Organization (WHO) (2007) *XDR-TB Extensively Drug-resistant Tuberculosis: What, Where, How and Action Steps*. Available www.who.int.

Index

Page numbers printed in *italic* refer to tables or boxed material; those in **bold** to figures. Page numbers preceded by an asterisk (*) denote a glossary item